RETINAL DETACHMENT
DIAGNOSIS AND MANAGEMENT

THIRD EDITION

RETINAL DETACHMENT
DIAGNOSIS AND MANAGEMENT

THIRD EDITION

Carl D. Regillo, M.D., F.A.C.S.
Associate Professor of Ophthalmology
Wills Eye Hospital
Thomas Jefferson University School of Medicine
Philadelphia, Pennsylvania
Formerly, Co-Director, Retina Service
Naval Medical Center
San Diego, California

William E. Benson, M.D., F.A.C.S.
Director, Retina Service and Attending Surgeon
Wills Eye Hospital
Professor of Ophthalmology
Thomas Jefferson University School of Medicine
Philadelphia, Pennsylvania

Illustrated by
Laurel Cook-Lhowe

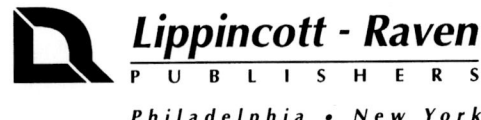

Philadelphia • New York

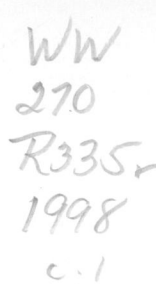

Manufacturing Manager: Dennis Teston
Production Manager: Jodi Borgenicht
Cover Designer: Karen K. Quigley
Indexer: Pamela Edwards
Compositor: Lippincott–Raven Desktop Division

© 1998 by Lippincott–Raven Publishers. All rights reserved. This book is protected by copyright. No part of it may be reproduced, stored in a retrieval system, or transmitted, in any form or by any means—electronic, mechanical, photocopy, recording, or otherwise—without the prior written consent of the publisher, except for brief quotations embodied in critical articles and reviews. For information write **Lippincott–Raven Publishers, 227 East Washington Square, Philadelphia, PA 19106-3780.**

Materials appearing in this book prepared by individuals as part of their official duties as U.S. Government employees are not covered by the above-mentioned copyright.

Printed and bound in China

9 8 7 6 5 4 3 2 1

Library of Congress Cataloging-in-Publication Data

Regillo, Carl D.
  Retinal detachment : diagnosis and management — 3rd ed. / Carl D. Regillo, William E. Benson; illustrator, Laurel C. Lhowe.
    p. cm.
  Includes bibliographical references and index.
  ISBN 0-7817-1646-2
  1. Retinal detachment. 2. Retinal detachment—Surgery.
I. Benson, William Edmunds. II. Benson, William Edmunds Retinal detachment.
  [DNLM: 1. Retinal Detachment—diagnosis. 2. Retinal Detachment—surgery. WW 270 R335r 1998]
RE603.B46 1998
DNLM/DLC
For Library of Congress   98-12131
                                                                           CIP

Care has been taken to confirm the accuracy of the information presented and to describe generally accepted practices. However, the authors and publisher are not responsible for errors or omissions or for any consequences from application of the information in this book and make no warranty, express or implied, with respect to the contents of the publication.

The authors and publisher have exerted every effort to ensure that drug selection and dosage set forth in this text are in accordance with current recommendations and practice at the time of publication. However, in view of ongoing research, changes in government regulations, and the constant flow of information relating to drug therapy and drug reactions, the reader is urged to check the package insert for each drug for any change in indications and dosage and for added warnings and precautions. This is particularly important when the recommended agent is a new or infrequently employed drug.

Some drugs and medical devices presented in this publication have Food and Drug Administration (FDA) clearance for limited use in restricted research settings. It is the responsibility of the health care provider to ascertain the FDA status of each drug or device planned for use in their clinical practice.

To "The Penguin," Teresa, Audrey, and Grant

Contents

Foreword by William Tasman		ix
Preface		x
1.	Primary Retinal Detachment	1
2.	Pathophysiology	14
3.	Predisposing Conditions	29
4.	History	45
5.	Differential Diagnosis	60
6.	Fundus Examination and Preoperative Management	75
7.	Scleral Buckling Procedure	100
8.	Pneumatic Retinopexy	135
9.	Alternative Techniques for the Treatment of Retinal Detachment	149
10.	Surgery of Complicated Cases	159
11.	Postoperative Complications of Primary Retinal Detachment Repair	175
12.	Prophylactic Therapy	194
Appendix		206
Subject Index		215

Foreword

When the First Edition of *Retinal Detachment: Diagnosis and Management* was published in 1980, pars plana vitrectomy had just been added to the arsenal of treatments for retinal detachment. Previously, treatment of retinal detachment had consisted largely of scleral buckling. The Second Edition, published in 1988, included pneumatic retinopexy and other innovative treatments of the 1980s.

Now, with the Third Edition, pneumatic retinopexy enjoys more widespread acceptance than it had a decade ago, and agents and techniques such as perfluorocarbon liquids, retinotomy, and silicone oil allow us to successfully restore vision in cases that were previously considered hopeless.

When the late Dr. Edward W. D. Norton wrote his foreword to the First Edition of *Retinal Detachment: Diagnosis and Management*, he commented on the superb qualifications of the author, Dr. William Benson. I echoed this opinion in the foreword to the Second Edition and still share this opinion today.

In the Third Edition, Dr. Carl Regillo joins Dr. Benson as coauthor. Dr. Regillo, a superb vitreoretinal surgeon and teacher, has contributed significantly to the literature in a relatively short period of time. Drs. Benson and Regillo have compiled an excellent volume that maintains the best of the previous editions—a clear, well-organized structure, and a handy size with an easy-to-read style. The illustrator, Laurel Cook-Lhowe, has created line drawings that are uniform in appearance and complementary to the text.

This volume represents the latest information related to retinal detachment. As the millennium approaches, I am tempted to speculate what new and exciting treatments will be in use when the Fourth Edition is published.

William Tasman, M.D.
Wills Eye Hospital
Jefferson Medical College
Philadelphia, Pennsylvania

Preface

This book is intended to provide residents, fellows, and practitioners of ophthalmology with a concise, up-to-date guide to the diagnosis and management of retinal detachment. As with the first two Editions, basic principles are stressed to give the reader the knowledge necessary to cope with individual cases or clinical situations not specifically discussed.

Much has changed in the field over the past 10 years since the last Edition of the book published in 1988. Our understanding of the interrelationship and the type of risk factors for retinal tears and detachment has continued to evolve over this time period. Even more of a change has been the growing popularity of alternative techniques to treat primary rhegmatogenous retinal detachment such as pneumatic retinopexy, balloon buckling, and vitrectomy. In an effort to adequately reflect such changes in treatment approach, the chapters on surgical technique have undergone the most significant revisions.

The overall organization of the book, however, is similar to the previous Editions. The first chapters address the basic mechanism and pathophysiology of retinal tears and detachments along with the conditions that predispose to them. A general history of the repair techniques follows. This is followed by the principles of fundus examination and preoperative evaluation and then the details of the various surgical techniques and complications themselves. Although individual chapters can stand alone, the reader will have a better perspective of the condition, particularly with regard to management, if the book is read from beginning to end. Concepts are then reinforced, as before, with an appendix that covers specific retinal detachment scenarios.

The approach to retinal tears and detachments reflect, in part, our training at Washington University in St. Louis and at Bascom Palmer Eye Institute in Miami (WEB) and Wills Eye Hospital in Philadelphia (CDR). However, we have changed with the times and also recognize that both within the United States and abroad, significant differences currently exist, particularly with regards to the specific technique preferred for managing a given retinal detachment presentation. To the best of our ability, we have tried to be impartial and present both sides of controversial issues.

Many individuals have helped make both the earlier versions and this Edition possible. First, our teachers and mentors deserve much credit. We are indebted to the numerous attendings at the above institutions present at the time of our respective training. We wish to recognize and thank the staff, residents, and fellows of Wills Eye Hospital and Naval Medical Center, San Diego for all the technical assistance and intellectual stimulation needed to prepare the Third Edition. We also wish to recognize the efforts and expertise of Mr. Jack Scully, Robert Curtin, and Roger Barone in the Audiovisual Department along with Ms. Judy Schaffer-Young and Gloria Lewis in the Library of Wills Eye Hospital. We were also fortunate to have the artistic talents of Ms. Laurel Cook-Lhowe once again to create and revise the illustrations. Finally, we wish to extend special thanks to our wives, Linda and Teresa, for their ongoing support and encouragement to rewrite the book as it never would have materialized without them.

RETINAL DETACHMENT
DIAGNOSIS AND MANAGEMENT

THIRD EDITION

1

Primary Retinal Detachment

A retinal detachment is a separation of the sensory retina from the retinal pigment epithelium (RPE) by an accumulation of fluid in the potential subretinal space. In a rhegmatogenous (Greek *rhegma*, rent) retinal detachment, the fluid gains access to this space through a break in the retina. A primary, or spontaneous, retinal detachment is a rhegmatogenous retinal detachment (RRD) in which the retinal break has not been caused by an antecedent event, such as trauma, or a condition, such as proliferative retinopathy. Primary detachments are often, but not always, preceded by posterior vitreous detachment (PVD).

POSTERIOR VITREOUS DETACHMENT

Mechanism

A meshwork of collagen fibers occupies the vitreous cavity. Hyaluronic acid molecules are interspersed between the fibers, supporting them. The fibers are most firmly attached to the retina and to the pars plana at the vitreous base, which extends for a few millimeters to each side of the ora serrata. Here, the collagen fibers insert into the basement membrane of the Müller cells of the retina and of the nonpigmented epithelium of the pars plana (Fig. 1-1). Less firm adhesions are found at the optic disc, at the macula, at areas of chorioretinal scarring, and along retinal blood vessels (57). A still weaker adhesion, probably mediated by extracellular matrix molecules (55), exists between the vitreous and the internal limiting membrane of the retina.

As one ages, changes occur within the hyaluronic molecule that appear to cause destabilization and aggregation of the collagen fibers (36,54). Initially, small cavities of liquefied vitreous form in the central vitreous. With time, they coalesce. Eventually, a hole presumably forms in the thinned posterior vitreous cortex that allows the liquid vitreous access to the retrohyaloid space and separates the posterior vitreous from the internal limiting membrane of the retina. The collagen meshwork collapses and moves forward; this phenomenon is PVD. In about one-half of patients, however, the separation is incomplete, and some remnants of cortical vitreous remain attached to the retina (32).

Autopsy studies have found PVD to be rare in persons under 30 years of age, but the prevalence increases from 10% in persons between 30 and 59 years to 63% in persons over 70 years of age (18,21). PVD occurs at an earlier age in myopes (1,71). The incidence is increased in persons who have had cataract extraction because the removal of the lens or opening of the lens capsule permits the hyaluronic acid to pass more easily into the anterior chamber and thence out of the eye (29,48). Inflammation, hemorrhage, and trauma also tend to promote vitreous liquefaction and PVD (54).

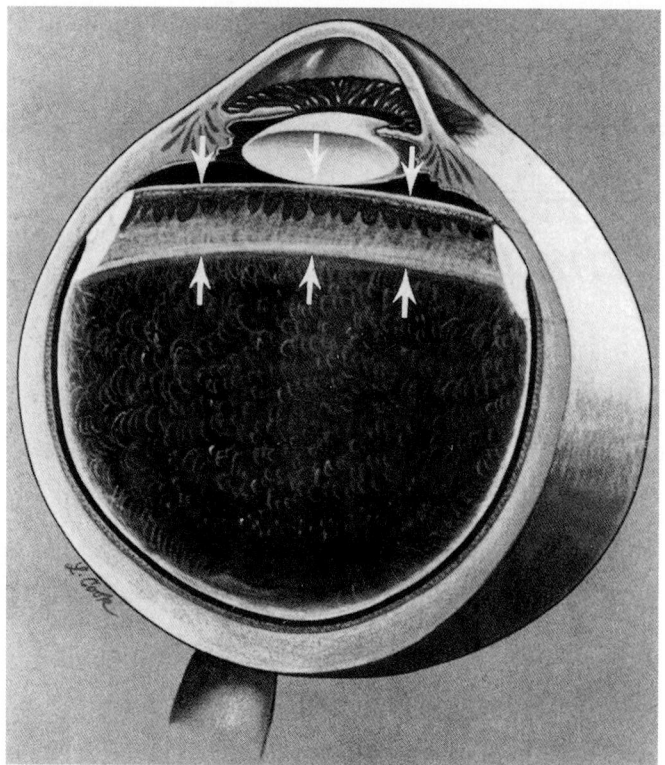

FIGURE 1-1. Vitreous base (between *arrows*) straddling the ora serrata.

Symptoms

In about one-third to one-half of the patients who present with acute PVD, traction on the peripheral retina causes photopsias, the subjective impression of flashing lights (8,38,44). The photopsias, which may even be colored, are most likely to be perceived in dim illumination and are reported more commonly by women than by men. In complete PVD, epipapillary glial tissue is torn from the optic disc. This condition is perceived by the patient as a floating complete or partial ring, called a Weiss ring (Fig. 1-2). In addition, the patient may notice cobwebs, "a shower of floaters," "reddish smoke," or simply blurred vision. These are all symptoms of vitreous hemorrhage, which is found in 13 to 19% of patients with acute PVD (38,63,64). The hemorrhage results when papillary or retinal vessels are torn by vitreous traction or when retinal vessels crossing retinal tears are avulsed. Fifty percent of patients with retinal detachment never experience flashes or floaters and instead present with the symptoms of detachment: visual field loss or decreased visual acuity (12,44).

Clinical Findings

Approximately 15% of all patients presenting with acute symptomatic PVD have a retinal tear (8,13,30,38,63,64). As many as one-half of these patients have more than one tear (43). Most of the tears are located superiorly. Although light flashes are believed to

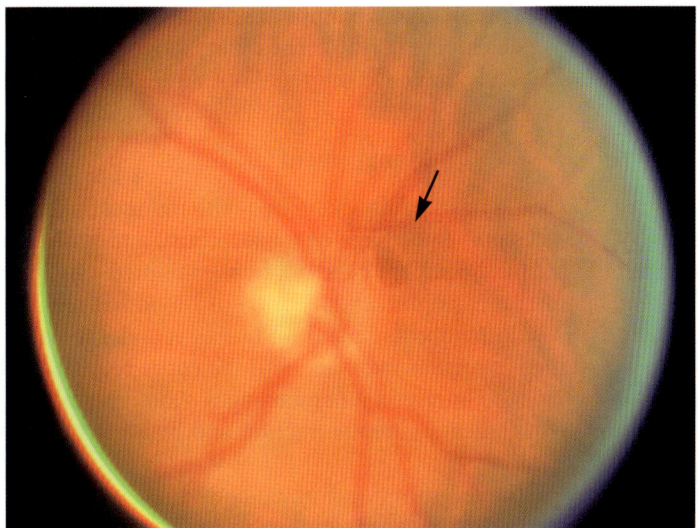

FIGURE 1-2. Epipapillary glial tissue *(arrow)* torn free by the collapsing vitreous.

be a sign of retinal traction, patients with flashes do not have a higher incidence of retinal tears than do patients without flashes (38).

Vitreous hemorrhage is an ominous sign. The incidence of retinal tears in acute PVD with vitreous hemorrhage is 70%, as opposed to a 2 to 4% incidence in acute PVD without hemorrhage (8,30,38,63,64). In nondiabetic patients, 44 to 86% of spontaneous vitreous hemorrhages are caused by PVD with or without a retinal tear (9,37,42,69).

The presence of pigment clumps in the anterior vitreous gel or anterior chamber ("tobacco dust") (Fig. 1-3) is another important sign to recognize. In eyes that have not un-

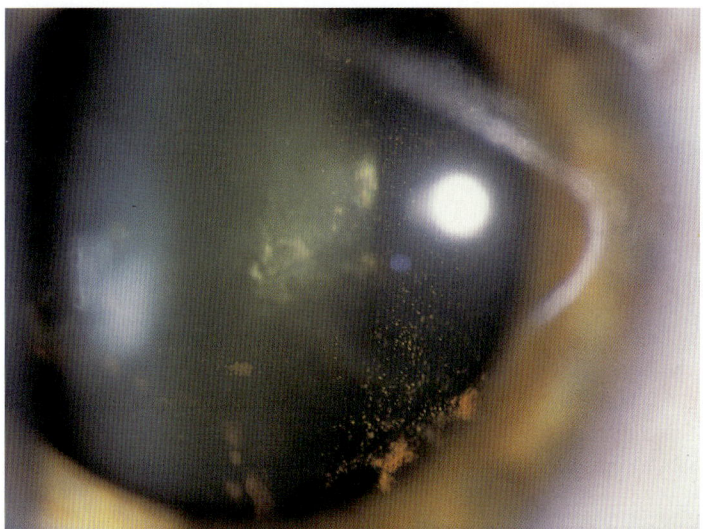

FIGURE 1-3. Pigment clumps ("tobacco dust") in the anterior chamber of a patient with long-standing retinal detachment.

dergone surgical procedures, these pigment clumps are practically pathognomonic for the presence of a retinal tear or detachment (27,56). The clumps represent aggregates of retinal pigment epithelial (RPE) cells that have migrated out through the retinal opening.

Management

All patients with PVD should be carefully examined with indirect ophthalmoscopy and scleral depression. If one sees no hemorrhage or tobacco dust, and symptoms have been present for more than 1 month, the patient need not be reexamined (8). If the patient has an acute PVD and no hemorrhage, a repeat examination in 1 month is recommended (11). If one sees an acute PVD with hemorrhage and no tear is found, the patient should be seen in 2 to 3 weeks and then at regular intervals until the entire retina can be examined. Patients with peripheral punctate intraretinal hemorrhages should be followed especially carefully. Such hemorrhages indicate vitreous traction and may mark the site of a later tear (63).

All patients should be instructed to return immediately if they notice an increase in floaters because this may indicate increased vitreous traction and a possible retinal tear. Patients with PVD should also be taught how to check their own peripheral vision and to report promptly if they perceive any defect.

Ultrasonography

A patient with a vitreous hemorrhage dense enough to obscure fundus details should undergo B-scan ultrasonography, which not only rules out retinal detachment, but also can make the diagnosis of PVD and, in some cases, can find the causative retinal break (14,46). If a break cannot be found, the patient should be patched bilaterally and should rest at home, either in a chair or in bed with extra pillows, for 2 to 4 days. In many cases, enough blood settles inferiorly to permit detection of superior retinal breaks. Until the entire periphery can be observed, reexamination with indirect ophthalmoscopy and, if necessary, ultrasonography should be done at 2- or 3-week intervals.

RETINAL BREAKS

Throughout this book, the following terminology is used: a retinal break is any full-thickness retinal defect; a tear is a break caused by vitreous traction; a hole is an atrophic round break.

Tears

When the vitreous body collapses, it usually separates easily from the retina except at the vitreous base. If no posterior vitreoretinal adhesions are present, a retinal tear is unlikely. On the other hand, the retina can be torn in areas of strong posterior vitreous adhesion (Figs. 1-4 and 1-5), such as may be present perivascularly (3,57), at posterior extensions of the vitreous base (19), at vitreoretinal tufts (Fig. 1-6) (7,19), at meridional folds (59), at enclosed ora bays (58), and in areas of lattice degeneration (Fig. 1-7) (62).

Traction on these adhesions may pull a strip of retina anteriorly, causing a flap (horseshoe) tear (Fig. 1-8). The posterior edge of the tear is called its apex. The area where the torn strip (flap) remains adherent to the retina is called its base. The horns are the ante-

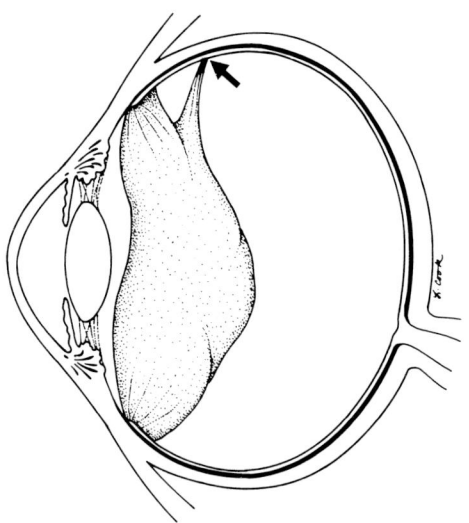

FIGURE 1-4. Posterior vitreous detachment with vitreoretinal adhesion *(arrow)* posterior to the vitreous base. The strong focal traction may cause a retinal tear.

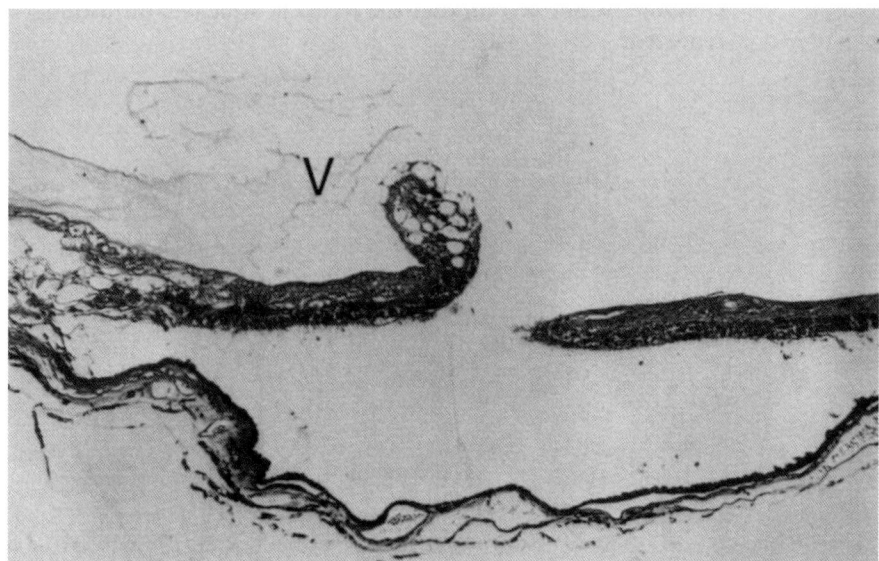

FIGURE 1-5. Flap (horseshoe) tear of the retina. Note vitreous *(V)* adherent to the flap (periodic acid–Schiff; 40× magnification). (From Yanoff M, Fine BS. *Ocular Pathology: A Text and Atlas.* Hagerstown, MD: Harper & Row, 1975.)

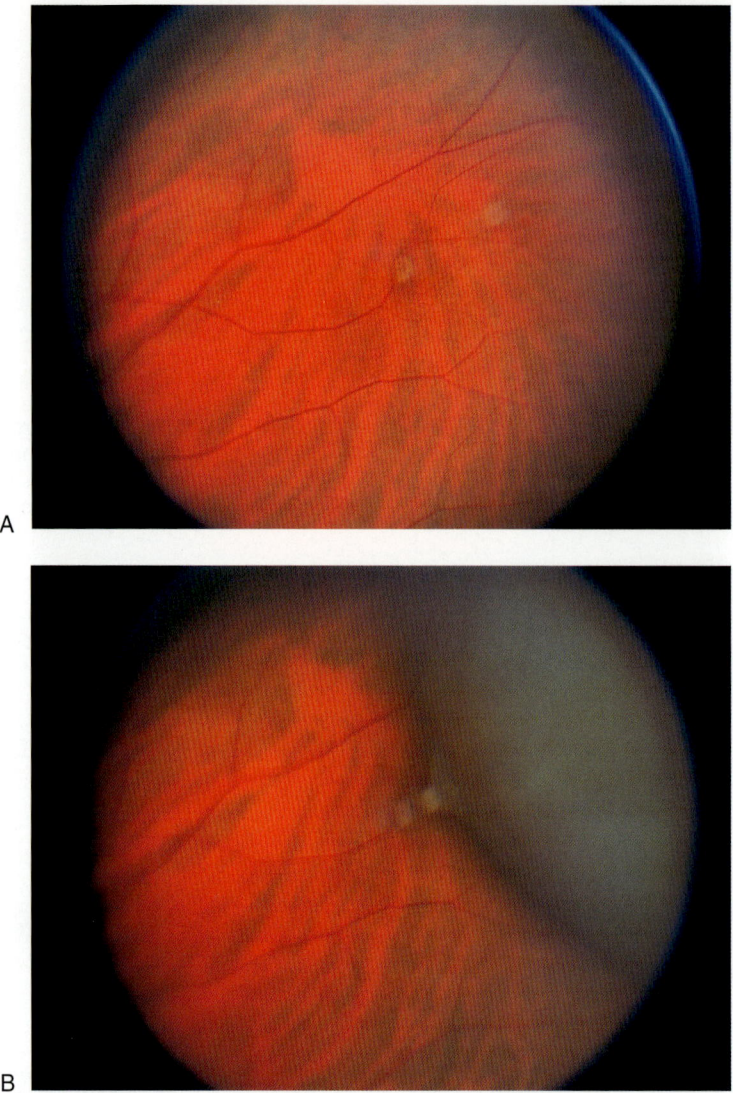

FIGURE 1-6. A: Two vitreoretinal traction tufts. They can be mistaken for flap tears. **B:** One of the tufts seen with scleral depression. A small traction retinal detachment is present at its base.

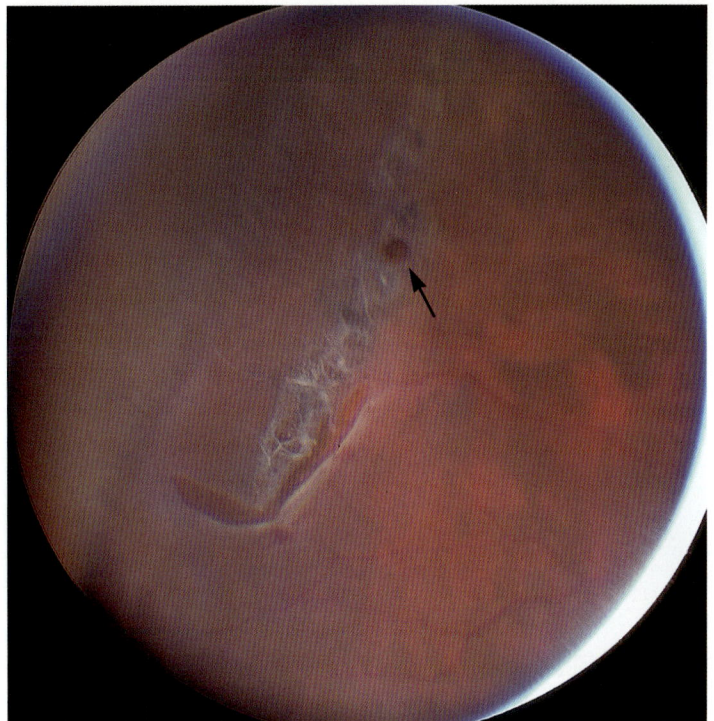

FIGURE 1-7. Crescentic tear caused by vitreous traction at the end of an area of lattice degeneration. An atrophic round hole is also present *(arrow)*.

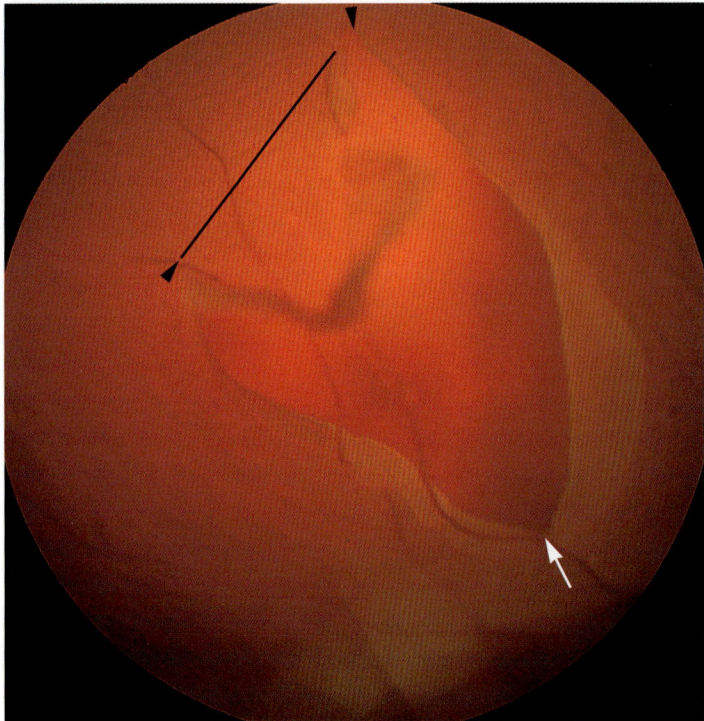

FIGURE 1-8. Flap (horseshoe) tear with two bridging vessels and a posteriorly rolled edge. *Arrow* indicates the apex; *solid line*, the base; and *arrowheads*, the horns.

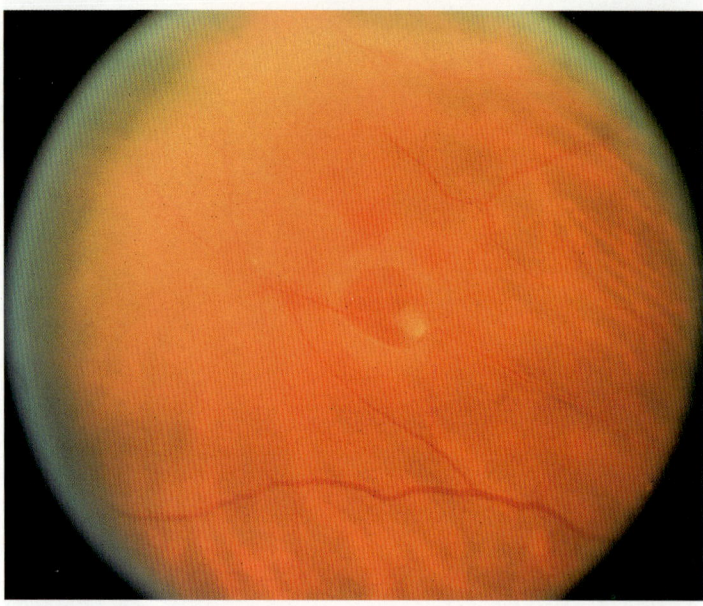

FIGURE 1-9. Operculated retinal tear. The retinal artery is attached to the operculum. (Courtesy of George W. Blankenship, M.D.)

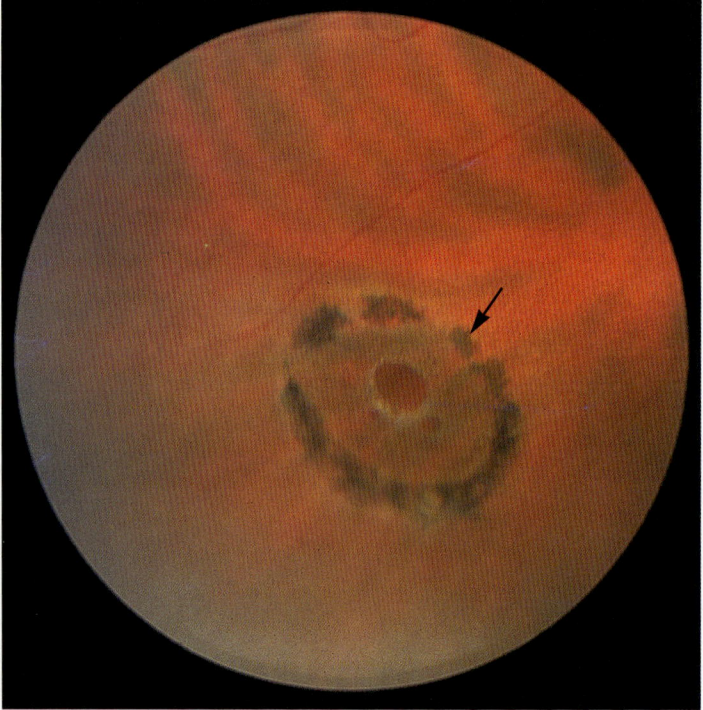

FIGURE 1-10. Atrophic round hole surrounded by a small rim of subretinal fluid and a pigmented demarcation line *(arrow)*.

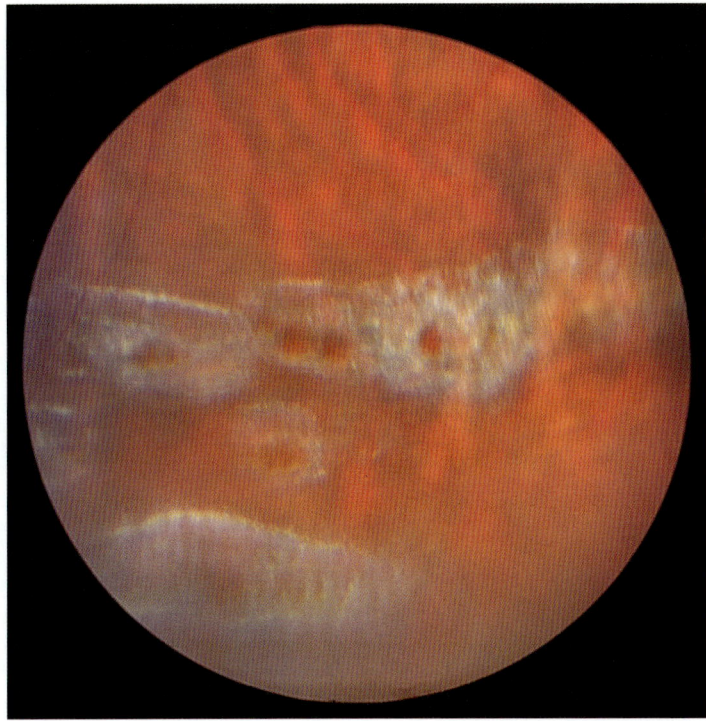

FIGURE 1-11. Multiple rows of lattice degeneration with atrophic round holes.

rior extensions of the tear. If a piece of the retina is torn completely free of the retinal surface, it is called an operculum, and the tear is said to be operculated (Fig. 1-9).

Round Holes

Focal retinal atrophy can result in a full-thickness retinal break (Fig. 1-10). Atrophic round holes are frequently found in areas of lattice degeneration (see Figs. 1-7 and 1-11). Round holes do not cause retinal detachment unless the overlying vitreous is liquefied. They are much less likely to cause a detachment than are tears (10) (see chapter 12, Prophylactic Therapy).

Degenerative Retinoschisis

Atrophic holes may develop in both walls of degenerative ("senile") retinoschisis cavities. Holes in the outer wall can give rise to retinal detachment even if the inner wall is intact (see chapter 3, Predisposing Conditions, and chapter 5, Differential Diagnosis).

Macular Holes

Idiopathic macular holes are caused by tangential traction of the overlying, adherent cortical vitreous (23,24). Other causes include trauma, various vascular occlusive dis-

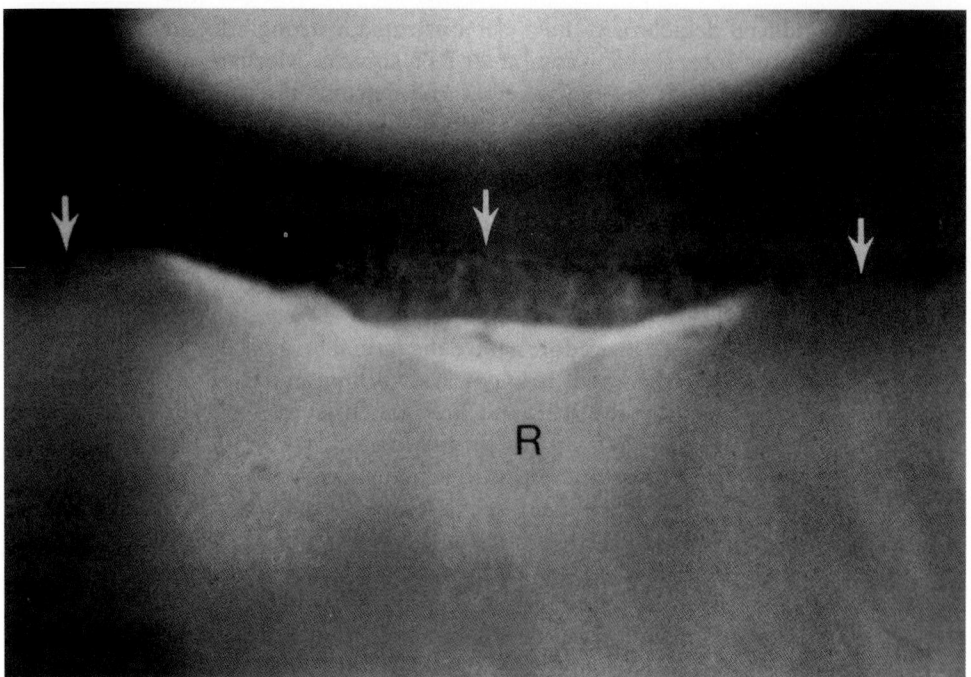

FIGURE 1-12. A retinal dialysis. The sensory retina *(R)* is separated from the nonpigmented epithelium of the pars plana at the ora serrata *(arrows)*. (Courtesy of W. Richard Green, M.D.)

eases, and, occasionally, chronic severe cystoid macular edema (CME). Macular holes rarely cause retinal detachment in eyes that are not highly myopic.

Dialysis (Disinsertion)

A retinal dialysis (Greek *dia*, apart; *lysis*, dissolution) is a separation of the sensory retina from the nonpigmented epithelium of the pars plana at the ora serrata (Fig. 1-12). Technically, dialyses are not retinal breaks, but they may cause a retinal detachment by exposing the subretinal space to liquid vitreous (see chapter 3, Predisposing Conditions, for a discussion of the causes of dialyses).

WHAT KEEPS THE RETINA ATTACHED?

Retinal detachment results when liquid vitreous passes through a retinal break to the potential space between the sensory retina and the RPE. Most persons with retinal breaks, however, never develop a retinal detachment. A few complementary mechanisms help the retina to remain attached, even in the presence of a break (40).

Active Mechanisms

Retinal Pigment Epithelial Cell Sheaths

In rabbits, the force required to peel the retina mechanically from the RPE is decreased within minutes of death (31,72), a finding indicating that active forces play a role in keeping the retina attached. Further, when peeling is performed *in vivo,* the RPE cell sheaths that surround and are closely apposed to the photoreceptor outer segments are stretched and deformed (60). When peeling is performed *in vitro,* they are not (72). This finding suggests that the actin-containing sheaths, whose contractile force is demonstrated by their ability to phagocytize outer segments, may actually hold the retina in place.

Retinal Pigment Epithelial Cell Pump

Removal of water from the subretinal space by the RPE pump lowers its hydrostatic pressure relative to that in the vitreous. Because the main resistance to diffusion of water from the vitreous to the choroid is the retina and not the RPE (47), the vitreous pressure then tends to keep the retina attached (4,15).

Passive Mechanisms

Interphotoreceptor Matrix

The proteins and glycosaminoglycans that make up the interphotoreceptor matrix between the sensory retina and the RPE may act as a "biologic glue," binding these surfaces together (25). Alternatively, they may help to prevent the liquid vitreous from gaining access to the potential subretinal space.

Hydrostatic and Osmotic Pressure

Subretinal fluid (SRF) is promptly absorbed once retinal breaks are closed by a scleral buckling (SB) procedure or by a gas bubble. Both oncotic pressure from the protein-rich choroid and metabolic transport across the RPE contribute to this rapid absorption (4,45). The finding that RPE is badly damaged by cryotherapy during retinal detachment surgery indicates that osmotic forces must play a large role. Further, experimental studies have shown that hyperosmotic solutions such as serum are absorbed up to ten times more slowly than isosmotic solutions (49,51). Finally, eyes that have had both the RPE and choroid removed as part of an eye wall resection for malignant melanoma rarely develop even a local retinal detachment. Clearly, water passes readily from the subretinal space to the outside of the eye (22).

Role of the Vitreous

Vitreous traction on a retinal break increases the likelihood of retinal detachment because it increases the exposure of the subretinal space to liquefied vitreous and to intraocular currents caused by eye movements (39). Another important factor is the availability of liquid vitreous. Retinal detachments tend to progress more slowly in young persons than in older ones because younger persons have less vitreous liquefaction, and intact cortical vitreous impedes movement of liquid vitreous through holes (50).

INCIDENCE AND EPIDEMIOLOGY

Phakic, nontraumatic retinal detachment occurs in approximately 5 to 12 persons per 100,000 population per year (5,26,28,35,53,61,66,68). The inclusion of traumatic retinal detachment only slightly increases this figure. Partly because boys and men are more likely to suffer trauma than are girls and women, they have a higher incidence of retinal detachment (61% versus 39%) (2). Although blacks have the same incidence of PVD and retinal lesions that predispose to retinal detachment as whites (20), for unknown reasons, black persons have a lower incidence of retinal detachment (6,67). The incidence of bilateral retinal detachment is about 10% (10,16,17,33,34,41,65,66). In patients under 20 years of age, the most common causes are trauma (44%), myopia (15%), aphakia (10%), and retinopathy of prematurity (8%) (52,70).

REFERENCES

1. Akiba J. Prevalence of posterior vitreous detachment in high myopia. *Ophthalmology* 1993;100:1384.
2. Ashrafzadeh MT, Schepens CL, Elzeneiny IH, et al. Aphakic and phakic retinal detachment. *Arch Ophthalmol* 1973;89:476.
3. Benson WE, Tasman W. Rhegmatogenous retinal detachments caused by paravascular vitreoretinal traction. *Arch Ophthalmol* 1984;102:669.
4. Bill A. Blood circulation and fluid dynamics in the eye. *Physiol Rev* 1975;55:383.
5. Bohringer HR. Statistisches zur Haufigkeit und Risiko der netzhautablosung. *Ophthalmologica* 1956;131:331.
6. Brown PR, Thomas RD. The incidence of primary retinal detachment in the Negro. *Am J Ophthalmol* 1965;60:109.
7. Byer NE. Cystic retinal tufts and their relationship to retinal detachment. *Arch Ophthalmol* 1981;99:1788.
8. Byer NE. Natural history of posterior vitreous detachment with early management as the premier line of defense against retinal detachment [see comments]. *Ophthalmology* 1994;101:1503.
9. Dana MR, Werner MS, Viana MA, et al. Spontaneous and traumatic vitreous hemorrhage. *Ophthalmology* 1993;100:1377.
10. Davis MD. Natural history of retinal breaks without detachment. *Arch Ophthalmol* 1974;92:183.
11. Dayan MR, Jayamanne DG, Andrews RM, et al. Flashes and floaters as predictors of vitreoretinal pathology: is follow-up necessary for posterior vitreous detachment? *Eye* 1996;10:456.
12. Delaney WV Jr, Oates RP. Retinal detachment in the second eye. *Arch Ophthalmol* 1978;96:629.
13. Diamond JP. When are simple flashes and floaters ocular emergencies? *Eye* 1992;6:102.
14. DiBernardo C, Blodi B, Byrne SF. Echographic evaluation of retinal tears in patients with spontaneous vitreous hemorrhage. *Arch Ophthalmol* 1992;110:511.
15. Fatt I, Shantinath K. Flow conductivity of retina and its role in retinal adhesion. *Exp Eye Res* 1971;12:218.
16. Folk JC, Arrindell EL, Klugman MR. The fellow eye of patients with phakic lattice retinal detachment. *Ophthalmology* 1989;96:72.
17. Folk JC, Burton TC. Bilateral phakic retinal detachment. *Ophthalmology* 1982;89:815.
18. Foos RY. Posterior vitreous detachment. *Trans Am Acad Ophthalmol Otolaryngol* 1972;76:480.
19. Foos RY. Vitreous base, retinal tufts, and retinal tears: pathogenic relationships. In: Pruett R, Regan C, eds. *Retina Congress*. New York: Appleton-Century-Crofts, 1972:259.
20. Foos RY, Simons KB, Wheeler NC. Comparison of lesions predisposing to rhegmatogenous retinal detachment by race of subjects. *Am J Ophthalmol* 1983;96:644.
21. Foos RY, Wheeler N. Vitreoretinal juncture: synchysis senilis and posterior vitreous detachment. *Ophthalmology* 1982;89:1502.
22. Foulds WS. Do we need a retinal pigment epithelium (or choroid) for the maintenance of retinal apposition? *Br J Ophthalmol* 1985;69:237.
23. Gass J. Reappraisal of biomicroscopic classification of stages of development of a macular hole. *Am J Ophthalmol* 1995;119:752.
24. Gass JDM. Idiopathic senile macular hole: its early stages and pathogenesis. *Arch Ophthalmol* 1988;106:629.
25. Hageman G, Marmor M, Yao X, et al. The interphotoreceptor matrix mediates primate retinal adhesion. *Arch Ophthalmol* 1995;113:655.
26. Haimann MH, Burton TC, Brown CK. Epidemiology of retinal detachment. *Arch Ophthalmol* 1982;100:289.
27. Hamilton AM, Taylor W. Significance of pigment granules in the vitreous. *Br J Ophthalmol* 1972;56:700.
28. Haut J, Massin M. Frequence des decollements de retine dans la population francise: pourcente des decollements bilateraux. *Arch Ophthalmol* 1975;35:533.
29. Heller MD, Straatsma BR, Foos RY. Detachment of the posterior vitreous in phakic and aphakic eyes. *Mod Probl Ophthalmol* 1972;10:23.
30. Hikichi T, Trempe CL. Relationship between floaters, light flashes, or both, and complications of posterior vitreous detachment [see comments]. *Am J Ophthalmol* 1994;117:593.
31. Kain HL. A new model for examining chorioretinal adhesion experimentally. *Arch Ophthalmol* 1984;102:608.
32. Kishi S, Demaria C, Shimizu K. Vitreous cortex remnants at the fovea after spontaneous vitreous detachment. *Int Ophthalmol* 1986;9:253.
33. Laatikainen L. The fellow eye in patients with unilateral retinal detachment: findings and prophylactic treatment. *Acta Ophthalmol* 1985;63:546.

34. Laatikainen L, Harju H. Bilateral rhegmatogenous retinal detachment. *Acta Ophthalmol* 1985;63:541.
35. Laatikainen L, Tolppanen EM, Harju H. Epidemiology of rhegmatogenous retinal detachment in a Finnish population. *Acta Ophthalmol* 1985;63:59.
36. Larsson L, Osterlin S. Posterior vitreous detachment: a combined clinical and physiochemical study. *Graefes Arch Clin Exp Ophthalmol* 1985;223:92.
37. Lincoff H, Kreissig I, Wolkstein M. Acute vitreous hemorrhage: a clinical report. *Br J Ophthalmol* 1976;60:454.
38. Lindner B. Acute posterior vitreous detachment. *Am J Ophthalmol* 1975;80:44.
39. Machemer R. The importance of fluid absorption, traction, intraocular currents, and chorioretinal scars in the therapy of rhegmatogenous retinal detachments. *Am J Ophthalmol* 1984;98:681.
40. Marmor MF. Control of subretinal fluid: experimental and clinical studies. *Eye* 1990;4:340.
41. Merin S, Feiler V, Hyams S, et al. The fate of the fellow eye in retinal detachment. *Am J Ophthalmol* 1971;71:477.
42. Morse PH, Aminlari A, Scheie HG. Spontaneous vitreous hemorrhage. *Arch Ophthalmol* 1974;92:297.
43. Morse PH, Scheie HG. Prophylactic cryoretinopexy of retinal breaks. *Arch Ophthalmol* 1974;92:204.
44. Morse PH, Scheie HG, Aminlari A. Light flashes as a clue to retinal disease. *Arch Ophthalmol* 1974;91:179.
45. Negi A, Marmor MF. Mechanisms of subretinal fluid resorption in the cat eye. *Invest Ophthalmol Visual Sci* 1986;27:1560.
46. Nischal KK, James JN, McAllister J. The use of dynamic ultrasound B-scan to detect retinal tears in spontaneous vitreous haemorrhage. *Eye* 1995;9:502.
47. Orr G, Goodnight R, Lean JS. Relative permeability of retina and retinal pigment epithelium to the diffusion of tritiated water from vitreous to choroid. *Arch Ophthalmol* 1986;104:1678.
48. Osterlin S. Vitreous changes after cataract extraction. In: Freeman H, Hirose T, Schepens C, eds. *Vitreous Surgery and Advances in Fundus Diagnosis and Treatment.* New York: Appleton-Century-Crofts, 1977:15.
49. Pederson JE, Cantrill HL. Experimental retinal detachment. V. Fluid movement through the retinal hole. *Arch Ophthalmol* 1984;102:136.
50. Pederson JE, Cantrill HL, Cameron JD. Experimental retinal detachment. II. Role of the vitreous. *Arch Ophthalmol* 1982;100:1155.
51. Pederson JE, MacLellan HM. Experimental retinal detachment. I. Effect of subretinal fluid composition on reabsorption rate and intraocular pressure. *Arch Ophthalmol* 1982;100:1150.
52. Rosner M, Treister G, Belkin M. Epidemiology of retinal detachment in childhood and adolescence. *J Pediatr Ophthalmol Strabismus* 1987;24:42.
53. Sasaki K, Ideta H, Yonemoto J, et al. Epidemiologic characteristics of rhegmatogenous retinal detachment in Kumamoto, Japan. *Graefes Arch Clin Exp Ophthalmol* 1995;233:772.
54. Sebag J. Aging of the vitreous. *Eye* 1987;1:254.
55. Sebag J. Vitreous biochemistry, morphology, and clinical examination. In: Tasman W, Jaeger EA, eds. *Duane's Clinical Ophthalmology.* Philadelphia: JB Lippincott, 1992:1.
56. Shafer D. Comment. In: Schepens C, Regan C, eds. *Controversial Aspects of the Management of Retinal Detachment.* Boston: Little, Brown, 1965:51.
57. Spencer LM, Foos RY. Paravascular vitreoretinal attachments: role in retinal tears. *Arch Ophthalmol* 1970;84:557.
58. Spencer LM, Foos RY, Straatsma BR. Enclosed bays of the ora serrata: relationship to retina tears. *Arch Ophthalmol* 1970;83:421.
59. Spencer LM, Foos RY, Straatsma BR. Meridional folds, meridional complexes, and associated abnormalities of the peripheral retina. *Am J Ophthalmol* 1970;70:679.
60. Spitznas M, Hogan MJ. Outer segments of photoreceptors and the retinal pigment epithelium: inter-relationship in the human eye. *Arch Ophthalmol* 1970;84:810.
61. Stein R, Feller-Ofry V, Romano A. The effect of treatment in the prevention of retinal detachment. In: Michaelson I, Berman E, eds. *Causes and Prevention of Blindness.* New York: Academic Press, 1972:409.
62. Straatsma BR, Zeegen PD, Foos RY, et al. Lattice degeneration of the retina: XXX Edward Jackson Memorial Lecture. *Am J Ophthalmol* 1974;77:619.
63. Tabotabo MD, Karp LA, Benson WE. Posterior vitreous detachment. *Ann Ophthalmol* 1980;12:59.
64. Tasman WS. Posterior vitreous detachment and peripheral retinal breaks. *Trans Am Acad Ophthalmol Otolaryngol* 1968;72:217.
65. Tornquist R. Bilateral retinal detachment. *Acta Ophthalmol* 1963;41:216.
66. Tornquist R, Stenkula S, Tornquist P. Retinal detachment: a study of a population-based patient material in Sweden 1971–1981. I. Epidemiology. *Acta Ophthalmol* 1987;65:213.
67. Weiss H, Tasman WS. Rhegmatogenous retinal detachments in blacks. *Ann Ophthalmol* 1978;10:799.
68. Wilkes SR, Beard CM, Kurland LT, et al. The incidence of retinal detachment in Rochester, Minnesota, 1970–1978. *Am J Ophthalmol* 1982;94:670.
69. Winslow RL. Spontaneous vitreous hemorrhage: etiology and management. *South Med J* 1980;73:1450.
70. Winslow RL, Tasman W. Juvenile rhegmatogenous retinal detachment. *Ophthalmology* 1978;85:607.
71. Yonemoto J, Ideta H, Sasaki K, et al. The age of onset of posterior vitreous detachment. *Graefes Arch Clin Exp Ophthalmol* 1994;232:67.
72. Zauberman H, deGuillebon H. Retinal traction in vivo and postmortem. *Arch Ophthalmol* 1972;87:549.

2
Pathophysiology

EARLY RETINAL DETACHMENT

As early as 2 to 4 days after retinal detachment, the photoreceptors show signs of irreversible necrosis, including extreme swelling of the inner segments and mitochondria, loss of the outer segments, and pyknotic and displaced nuclei (52). Apoptosis (intrinsically programmed cell death) plays an important role in this degeneration (12). Red and green cones are more resistant to degeneration than are blue cones and rods, a finding that explains blue–yellow color confusion in patients with successfully repaired retinas (52).

Because the retinal circulation remains intact, and because the degree of retinal degeneration is proportional to the height of the detachment, the foregoing changes are believed to be caused by separation of the retina from the retinal pigment epithelium (RPE) or choriocapillaris (41). As soon as the detachment is total, the electroretinogram is unrecordable (23).

Intraretinal edema, most pronounced in the inner nuclear layer, appears soon after detachment (Fig. 2-1). The edema causes decreased retinal transparency and, if severe, folding of the outer retina, which, on ophthalmoscopy, is manifested by irregular retinal corrugations (Fig. 2-2) (41,46).

Initially, the RPE cells under the detached retina become larger. Later, some cells undergo dedifferentiation, separate from Bruch's membrane, and float through the subretinal fluid (SRF) to reach all parts of the vitreous cavity and both retinal surfaces (33,41,46). Clumps of pigment epithelial cells proliferating on the outer surface of the retina are seen clinically as subretinal white dots (Fig. 2-3) (36).

LONG-STANDING RETINAL DETACHMENT

The longer the retina remains detached, the more all retinal layers atrophy (Fig. 2-4). If proliferative vitreoretinopathy (PVR) does not develop, the cell loss causes the retina to become semitransparent and smooth (Fig. 2-5). Occasionally, large intraretinal cystoid spaces develop (Fig. 2-6). Deterioration of the retina is reflected by a progressive decrease in opsin and outer segments of photoreceptors (24). The RPE gradually undergoes atrophy and depigmentation (28). In most long-standing detachments, "tobacco dust" is present (see Fig. 1-3).

In some retinal detachments of at least 3 months' duration, metaplastic RPE cells proliferate at the junction of attached and detached retina (28) and form what is clinically known as a demarcation line. The metaplastic cells may produce a firm, fibrous adhesion between the retina and the RPE. In 23% of cases with demarcation lines, the adhesion is

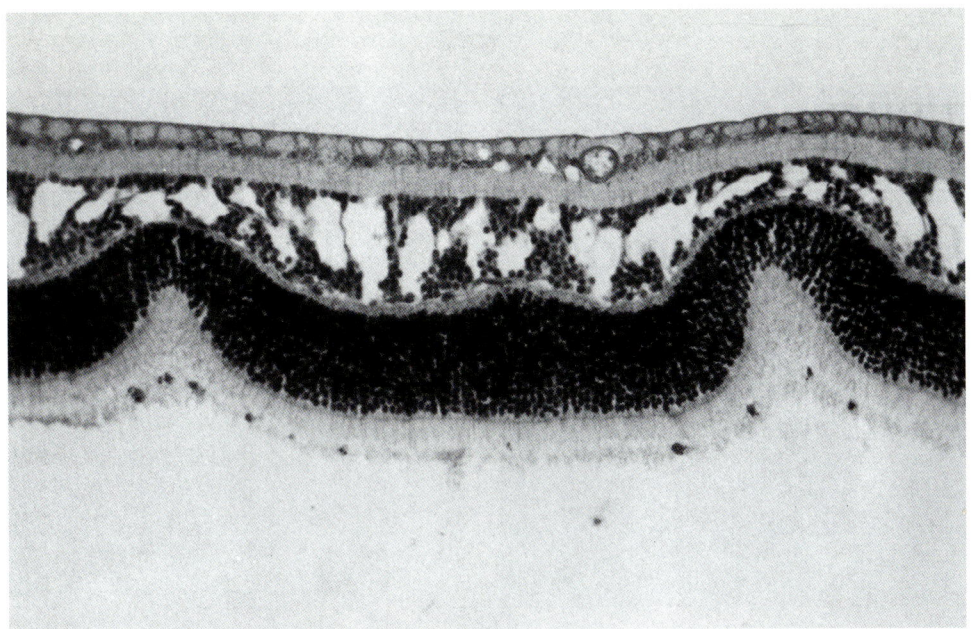

FIGURE 2-1. Detachment of 1 week's duration. Edema causes folding of the outer retina. The clinical result is the corrugated appearance seen in Figure 2-2 (periodic acid–Schiff; 190× magnification). (From Machemer R. Experimental retinal detachment in the owl monkey. II. Histology of retina and pigment epithelium. *Am J Ophthalmol* 1968;66:396. Copyright 1968, Ophthalmic Publishing Co.)

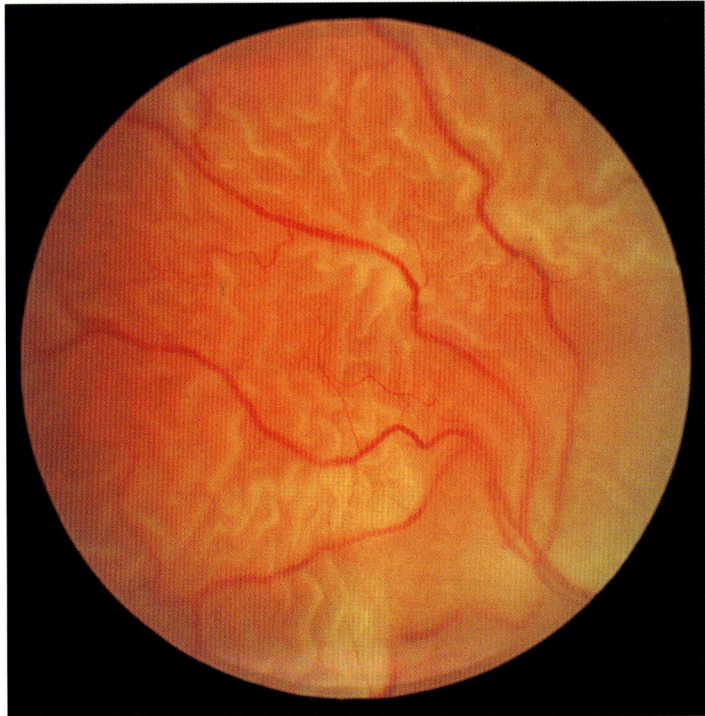

FIGURE 2-2. Rhegmatogenous retinal detachment. The corrugated appearance is caused by intraretinal edema.

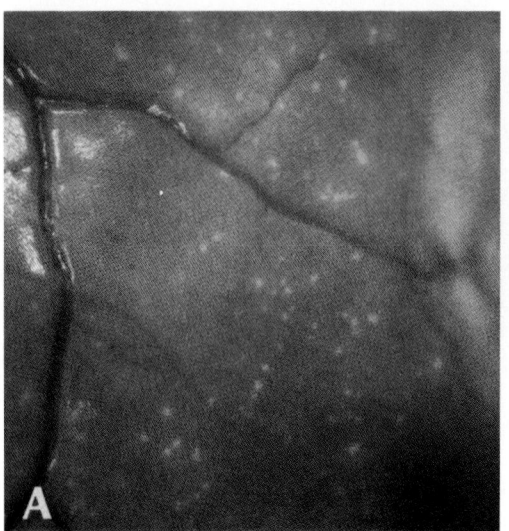
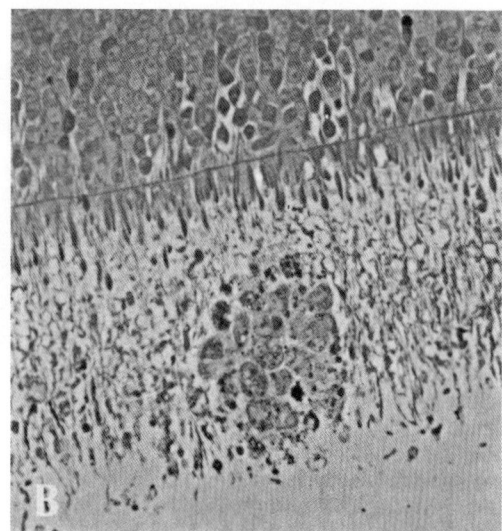

FIGURE 2-3. Four-week-old detachment. **A:** white retroretinal dots are visible through the retina (×25). **B:** dots consist of clusters of pigment epithelial macrophages (phase contrast; 250× magnification). (From Laqua H, Machemer R. Clinical-pathological correlation in massive periretinal proliferation. *Am J Ophthalmol* 1975;80:913. Copyright 1975, Ophthalmic Publishing Co.)

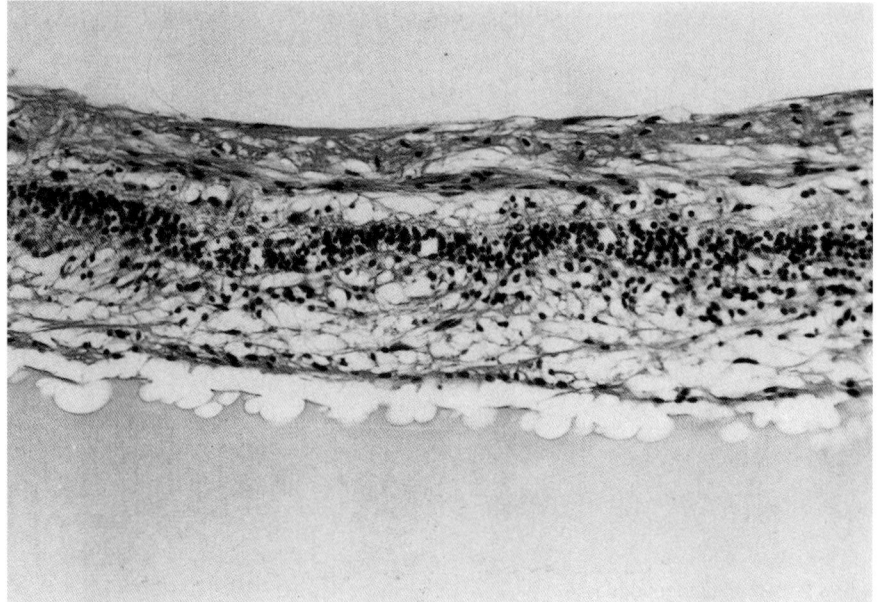

FIGURE 2-4. Chronic retinal detachment showing marked degeneration and thinning of outer retinal layers. (From Yanoff M, Fine BS. *Ocular Pathology: A Text and Atlas.* Hagerstown, MD: Harper & Row, 1975.)

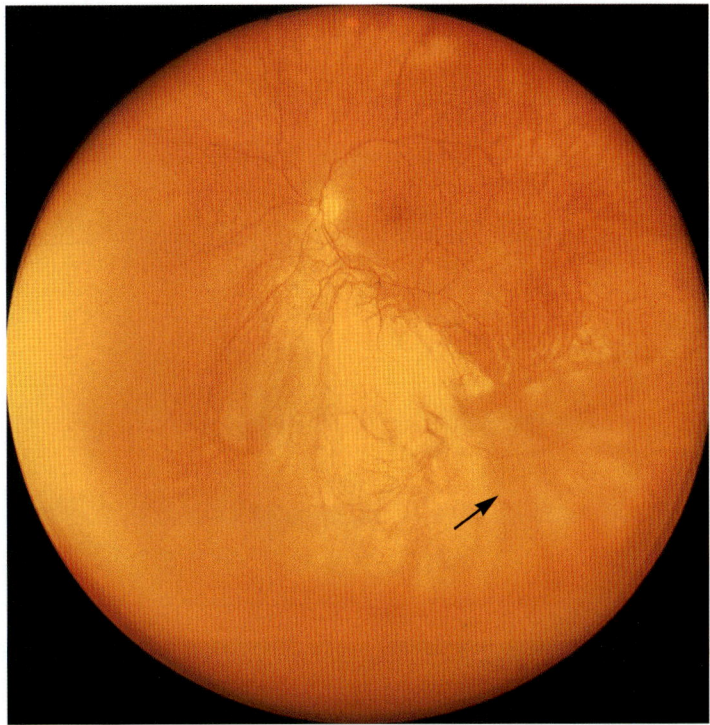

FIGURE 2-5. Long-standing inferotemporal retinal detachment without massive periretinal proliferation. The thin retina is semitransparent and smooth. The *arrow* indicates a round hole. A thin demarcation line is visible at the superior edge of the detachment.

strong enough to prevent progression of the detachment. In the other 77%, the detachment advances through the demarcation line (Fig. 2-7) (3). Why proliferative vitreoretinopathy does not develop in these eyes despite the long duration of detachment is not clear. The prognosis for surgical reattachment is excellent (3). In some long-standing retinal detachments, retinal neovascularization may develop (5,16).

SUBRETINAL FLUID

In an acute rhegmatogenous retinal detachment (RRD) the SRF is liquid vitreous which has passed through the retinal break. The protein concentration of the SRF is considerably lower than that of plasma and contains hyaluronic acid, which is a component of the vitreous but not of plasma (20,27).

With increasing duration of the retinal detachment, the composition of the SRF becomes more and more like that of plasma, a characteristic indicating breakdown of the blood–retinal barrier. The total protein content increases, as does the concentration of enzymes that are normally found only in plasma (4,31). As protein accumulates, the osmolality of the SRF increases. Fluid drained from a detachment of recent onset is watery, whereas fluid found in long-standing retinal detachments is viscous. Even when all the retinal holes are completely sealed, it may take months for this viscous fluid to be ab-

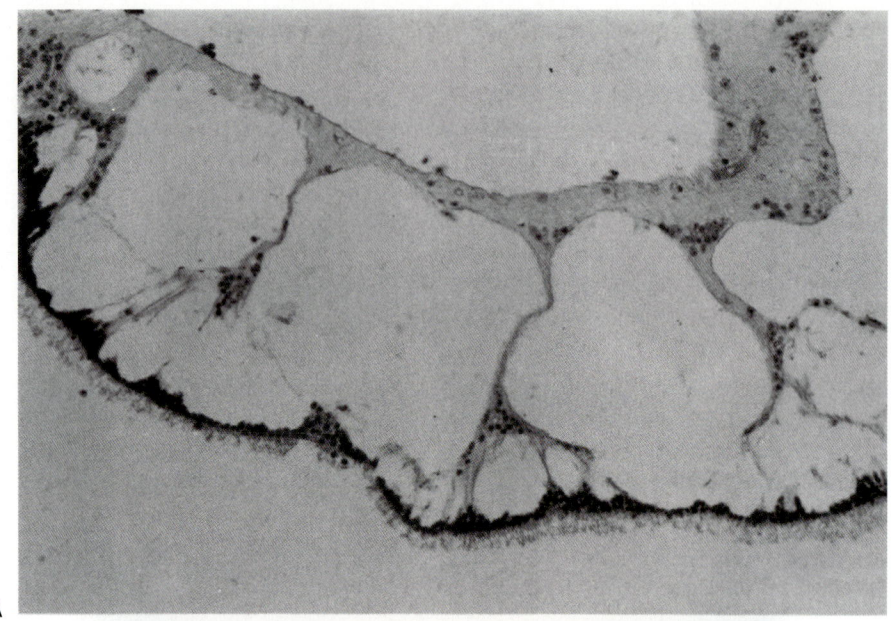

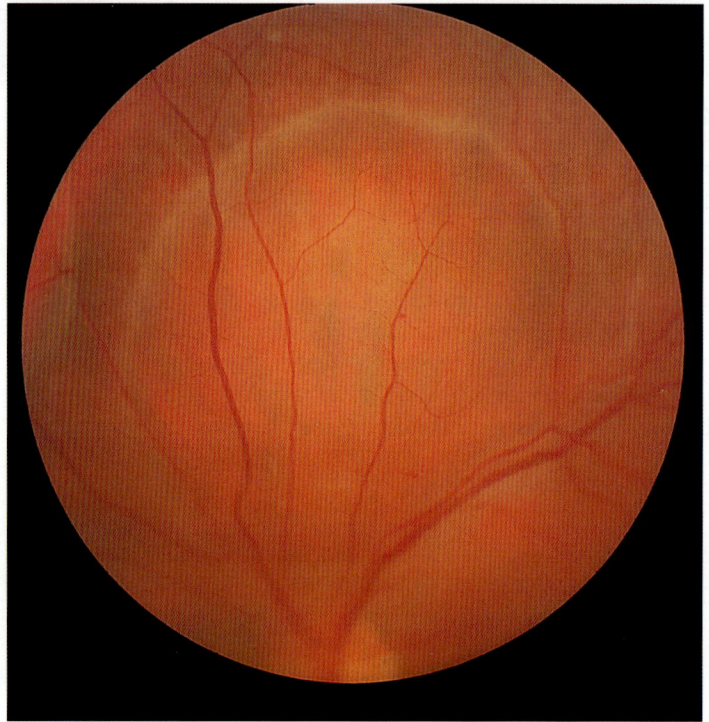

FIGURE 2-6. A: Fourteen-week-old detachment with large, cystoid spaces and loss of cells in inner and outer nuclear layer (periodic acid–Schiff; 190× magnification). (From Machemer, R. Experimental retinal detachment in the owl monkey. II. Histology of the retina and pigment epithelium. *Am J Ophthalmol* 1968;66:396. Copyright 1968, Ophthalmic Publishing Co.) **B:** Retinal macrocyst in a long-standing retinal detachment.

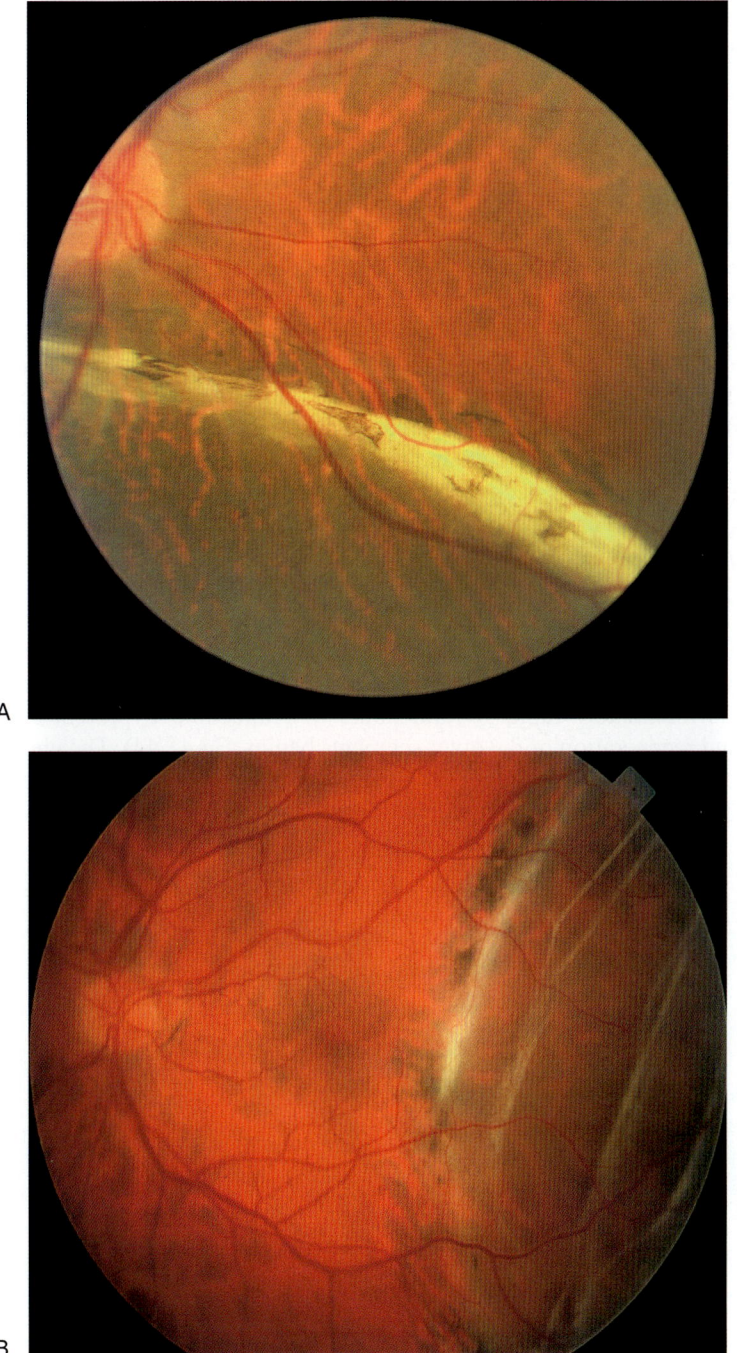

FIGURE 2-7. A: Thick demarcation line. It appears white because the metaplastic pigment epithelial cells have become depigmented and have also produced basement membrane material. Notice also the atrophic pigment epithelium inferior to the demarcation line. **B**: Retinal detachment that has broken through three demarcation lines before stopping at a thicker pigmented demarcation line.

sorbed. Although this delayed absorption of fluid is mostly caused by its increased viscosity and osmolarity, degeneration of the RPE or choriocapillaris probably also plays a role (see also the section in chapter 1, What Keeps the Retina Attached?).

INTRAOCULAR PRESSURE

In eyes with RRD, the intraocular pressure usually decreases in proportion to the extent and duration of the detachment (7). This relative hypotony is caused not by decreased aqueous secretion, but by misdirection of aqueous posteriorly, where it passes through the retinal break to be absorbed by the RPE and choroid (55,56,64–66). An important exception is sometimes encountered in eyes with long-standing retinal detachment (51,59). Here, the intraocular pressure may actually be elevated because of decreased aqueous outflow. The trabecular meshwork and aqueous outflow may be blocked either by small clumps of pigmented cells (38,59) ("tobacco dust") or by outer segments of photoreceptors (48). The intraocular pressure and the outflow facility usually return to normal after the retinal detachment has been repaired. In any case of unilateral glaucoma, long-standing retinal detachment must be ruled out; otherwise, the patient may be mistakenly treated for primary or uveitis-induced glaucoma.

RETINAL RECOVERY AFTER REATTACHMENT

After repair of experimental retinal detachments of less than 1 week's duration, retinal recovery is remarkably rapid. Within hours of reattachment, protein synthesis is increased, and regeneration of the outer segments begins (34,43,44). The electroretinogram may be recordable within 5 hours (23). Rod outer segments recover faster than do cone outer segments (35). Intraretinal edema begins to decrease within hours and is nearly

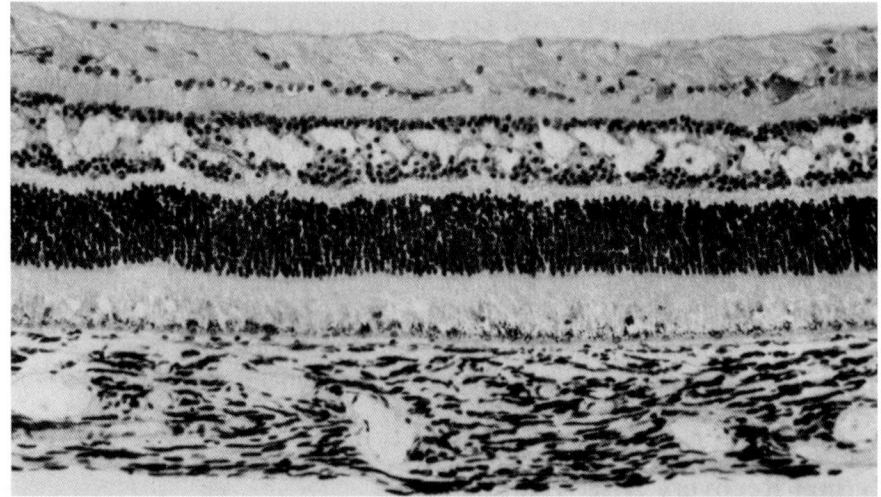

FIGURE 2-8. Residual edema in the inner nuclear layer of a 9-day-old reattached retina (periodic acid–Schiff; 590× magnification). (From Machemer R. Experimental retinal detachment in the owl monkey. 4. The reattached retina. *Am J Ophthalmol* 1968;66:1075. Copyright 1968, Ophthalmic Publishing Co.)

completely resolved within 9 days (Fig. 2-8). The electroretinogram continues to improve for 12 weeks, by which time the outer segments are histologically nearly normal (35). In humans, visual acuity may continue to improve for a year or longer. After repair of experimental retinal detachments of more than 1 month's duration, morphologic recovery is poor (1).

PROLIFERATIVE VITREORETINOPATHY

Definition

In some retinal detachments, cells proliferate on either or both surfaces of the retina and on vitreous strands and then contract, the process known as PVR (Figs. 2-9–2-11). (9,58) Contraction of focal membranes causes posteriorly rolled edges of flap tears (see Fig. 1-8) and fixed folds (Fig. 2-12). Diffuse contraction of membranes at the edge of the posterior surface of the detached vitreous causes equatorial traction folds with stretching of the anterior retina and its central displacement (Fig. 2-13). In severe cases, generalized retinal folding and stiffening give the detachment a funnel configuration (Fig. 2-14). The rigid retina and transvitreal traction hinder retinal reattachment (58,67,70). In some cases, subretinal proliferation causes linear bands, over which the retina is draped like sheets over a clothesline. For better comparison of papers on the prognosis and surgical management of detachments with PVR, the Retina Society developed a generally accepted classification (Table 2-1) (42).

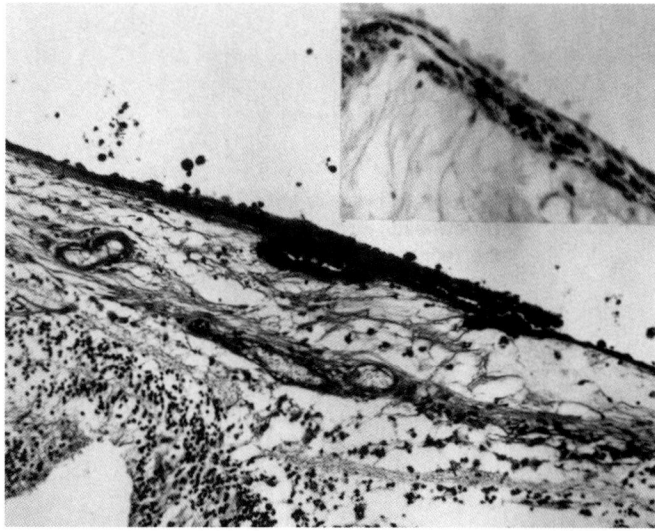

FIGURE 2-9. Densely pigmented preretinal membrane composed of retinal pigment epithelial cells (hematoxylin and eosin; 160× magnification). **Inset** illustrates the laminated appearance of the membrane with alternate areas of pigment epithelium and basement membrane (partially bleached, hematoxylin and eosin; 350× magnification). (From Clarkson JG, Green WR, Massof D. A histopathologic review of 168 cases of preretinal membrane. *Am J Ophthalmol* 1977;84:1. Copyright 1977, Ophthalmic Publishing Co.)

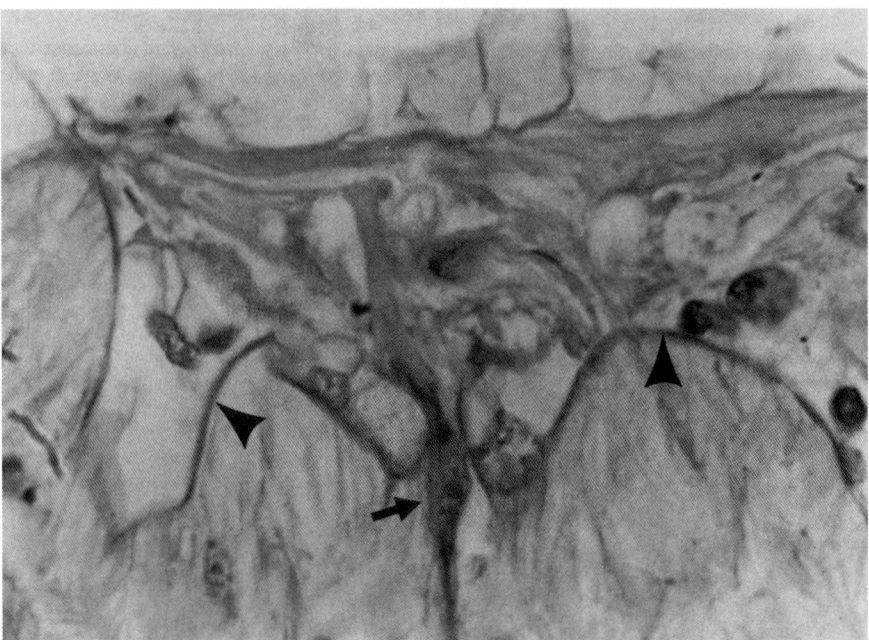

FIGURE 2-10. Small preretinal glial membrane connected to the retina by a thin bridge of tissue. (*Arrowheads* mark the internal limiting membrane of the retina.) A retinal cell is migrating out of the retina *(arrow)* (periodic acid–Schiff; 490× magnification). (From Laqua H, Machemer R. Glial cell proliferation in retinal detachment [massive periretinal proliferation]. *Am J Ophthalmol* 1975;80:602. Copyright 1975, Ophthalmic Publishing Co.)

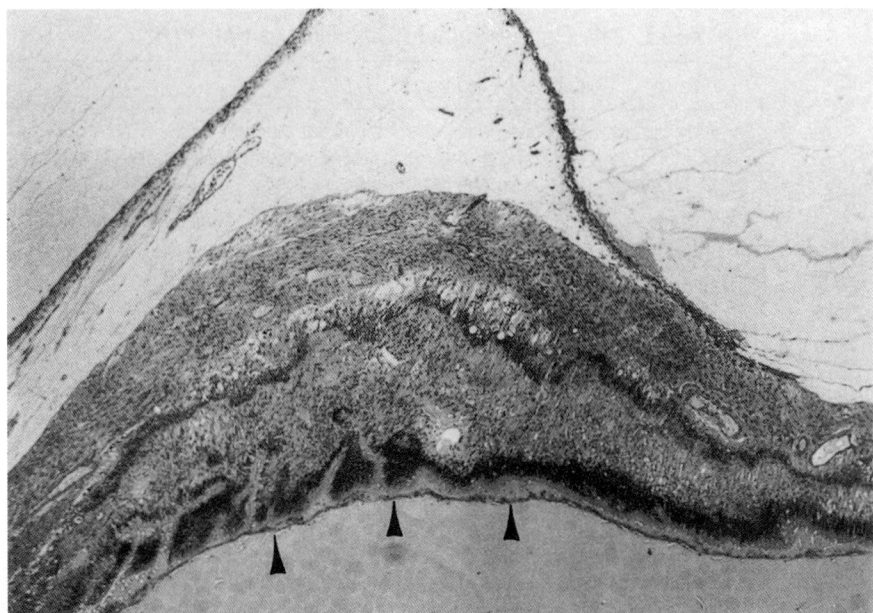

FIGURE 2-11. Fixed folds of outer retina caused by contraction of a membrane *(arrows)* on the outer retinal surface. Note folds in the external nuclear layer (hematoxylin and eosin; 16× magnification). (From Yanoff M, Fine BS. *Ocular Pathology: A Text and Atlas.* Hagerstown, MD: Harper & Row, 1975.)

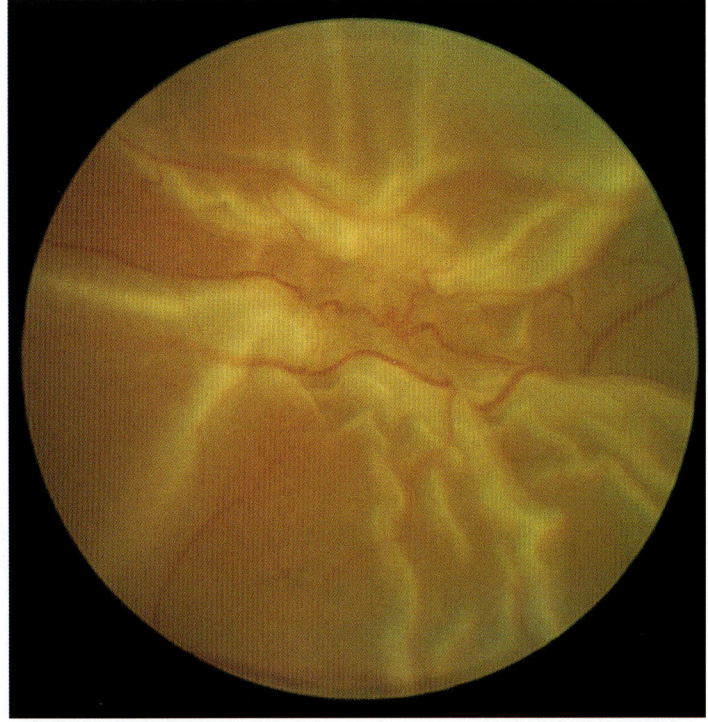

FIGURE 2-12. Clinical appearance of fixed fold caused by preretinal proliferation. The retinal fold is concave toward the pupil.

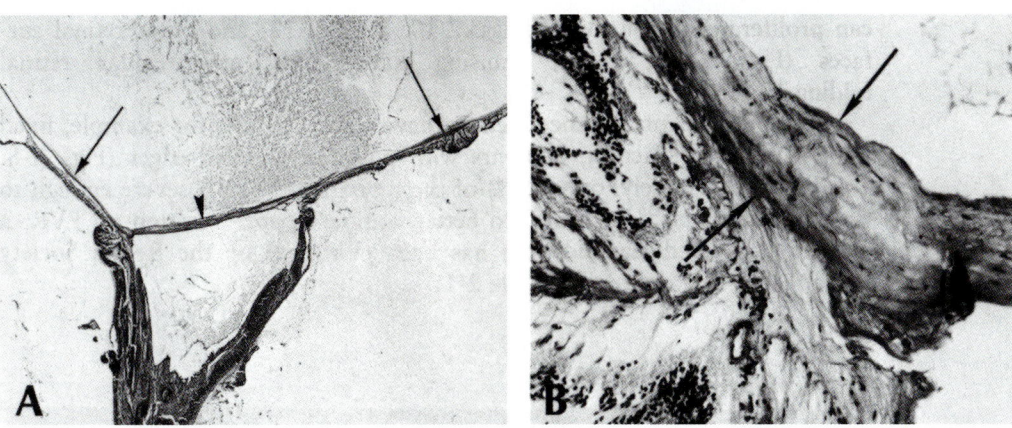

FIGURE 2-13. Eye with clinical diagnosis of massive periretinal proliferation after unsuccessful retinal detachment operation. **A:** The transvitreal portion of the membrane *(arrowhead)* holds the retina in a funnel shape. The preretinal portion *(arrows)* causes fixed folds (hematoxylin and eosin; 10× magnification). **B:** Higher power showing thick fibrous preretinal membrane (between *arrows*) (hematoxylin and eosin; 320× magnification). (From Clarkson JG, Green WR, Massof D. A histopathologic review of 168 cases of preretinal membrane. *Am J Ophthalmol* 1977;84:1. Copyright 1977, Ophthalmic Publishing Co.)

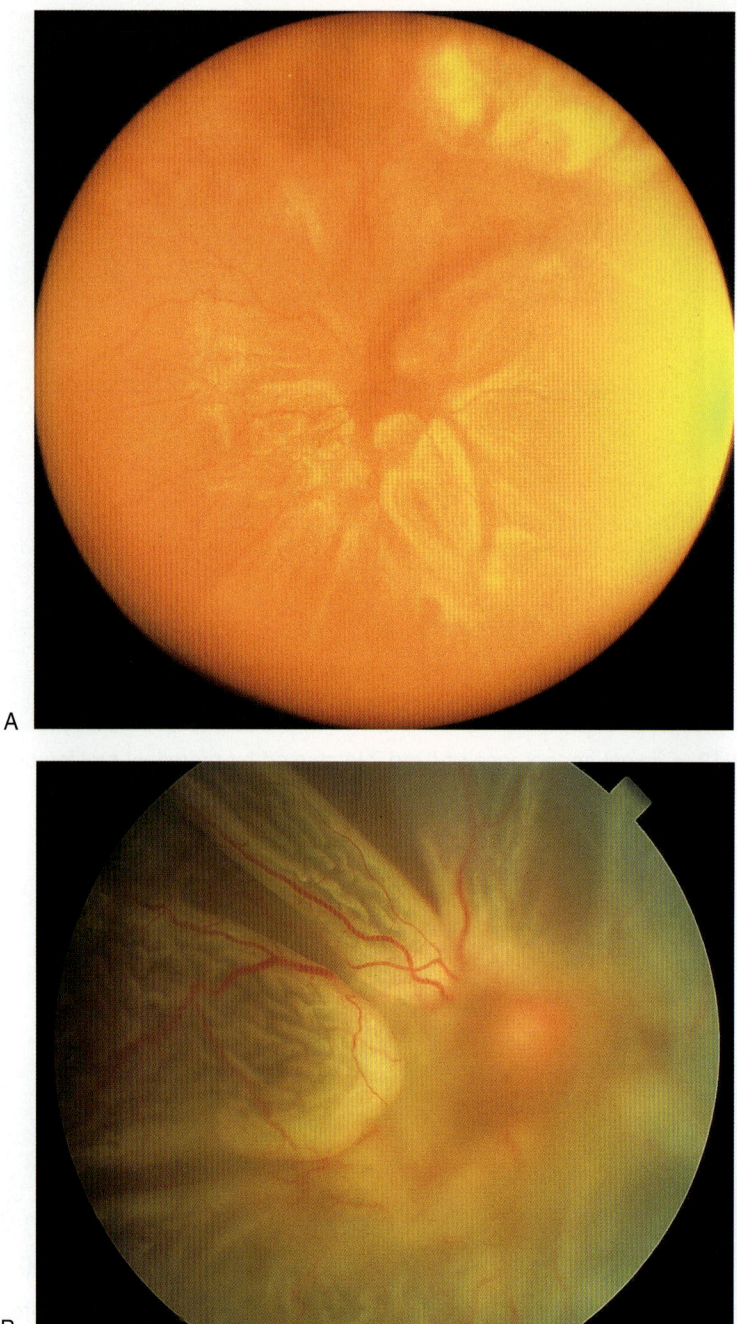

FIGURE 2-14. A: Equator-plus photograph of an eye with proliferative vitreoretinopathy (PVR). A scleral buckle is seen superiorly and a retinal break is seen inferiorly. **B:** Retinal detachment with advanced PVR. Visible are fixed retinal folds in all four quadrants and a narrow funnel configuration to the detachment.

TABLE 2-1. *Classification of proliferative vitreoretinopathy[a]*

Grade	Features
A	Vitreous haze, vitreous pigment clumps, pigment clusters on the inferior retina
B	Wrinkling of the inner retinal surface, retinal stiffness, vessel tortuosity, rolled and irregular edge of retinal break, decreased vitreous mobility
C P 1-12	Posterior to equator: focal, diffuse, or circumferential full-thickness folds,[b] subretinal strands[b]
C A 1-12	Anterior to equator: focal, diffuse, or circumferential full-thickness folds,[b] subretinal strands,[b] anterior displacement,[b] condensed vitreous with strands

[a]From Machemer, R, Aaberg, TM, Freeman, HM, et al. An updated classification of retinal detachment with proliferative vitreoretinopathy. *Am J Ophthalmol* 1991;112:159.
[b]Expressed in number of clock hours involved.

Histopathology

The membranes are mostly derived from dedifferentiated RPE cells, but they also include fibrocytes, glial cells, macrophages, and myofibroblasts (11,45,47,68). They grow on the inner (see Figs. 2-9–2-11) and outer retinal surfaces. The dedifferentiated cells produce collagen, which strengthens the membrane (49,63) (see Fig. 2-13). In addition to active forces generated by the myoblast-like cells (49), RPE cells pull collagen toward themselves, tightening the fibers and contributing to vitreoretinal traction (18). PVR has a predilection for the inferior retina, probably because gravity causes RPE cells floating in the vitreous to settle inferiorly, where they eventually are transformed into fibroblast-like cells (61).

Anterior Proliferative Vitreoretinopathy

Anterior proliferative vitreoretinopathy (APVR) refers to severe cellular proliferation at the vitreous base. It is mostly seen in eyes that have undergone vitrectomy. Residual vitreous gel at the vitreous base provides a scaffold on which the membranes grow. They extend anteriorly onto the pars plicata and iris. When they contract, the retina is displaced anteriorly (Fig. 2-15). In severe cases, the retina in the area of the posterior vitreous base is pulled far enough anteriorly to form a peripheral trough (14). Traction on the ciliary body pars plicata causes breakdown of the ciliary blood–aqueous barrier and results in chronic, intractable hypotony and the postvitrectomy fibrin syndrome (39).

Stimulus

Why only 10% of detached retinas have signs of PVR (26,50) or why only 25% of these progress to PVR severe enough to require vitrectomy is not known (50). Several factors that contribute to the excessive cellular proliferation in these cases have been implicated (9). Breakdown of the blood–retinal barrier releases growth factors into the vitreous (60). Dedifferentiated RPE cells contribute to their own proliferation by producing diffusible substances (autokines) such as platelet-derived growth factor (8,25). Monocytes enter the vitreous, where they not only induce RPE cells to produce cytokines (29), but also are transformed into macrophages with fibroblast-like properties (57). The cytokines, such as transforming growth factor beta and interleukins, stimulate cellular proliferation and the production of fibronectin, a chemoattractant for RPE and glial cells. A vicious cycle is set up with growth of dense membranes (2,10,15,30,32,37,40,53,54,69,71,72).

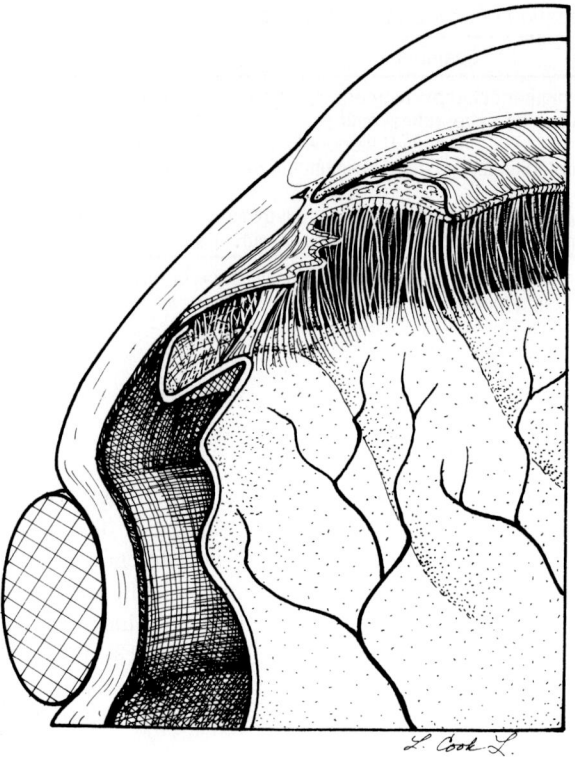

FIGURE 2-15. Drawing of an eye with anterior proliferative vitreoretinopathy. Membranes extend anteriorly onto the pars plicata and iris, pull the retina anteriorly, and create a peripheral trough.

Risk Factors

Eyes with any degree of preoperative PVR are more likely to progress to clinically significant PVR postoperatively than are eyes without preoperative PVR. Other predictors of PVR are factors that cause breakdown of the blood–retinal barrier, such as vitreous hemorrhage, large tears, choroidal detachment, long duration of retinal detachment, total detachment, and inflammation (17,21), and factors that allow release of RPE cells into the vitreous, such as large tears and extensive cryotherapy (6,22). Scleral indentation during cryotherapy contributes to the release of RPE cells (19,62). Finally, the surgical procedure itself may accelerate the process (13).

REFERENCES

1. Anderson DH, Guerin CJ, Erickson PA, et al. Morphological recovery in the reattached retina. *Invest Ophthalmol Vis Sci* 1986;27:168.
2. Baudouin C, Fredj-Reygrobellet D, Brignole F, et al. Growth factors in vitreous and subretinal fluid cells from patients with proliferative vitreoretinopathy. *Ophthalmic Res* 1993;25:52.
3. Benson WE, Nantawan P, Morse PH. Characteristics and prognosis of retinal detachments with demarcation lines. *Am J Ophthalmol* 1977;84:641.
4. Berrod JP, Kayl P, Rozot P, et al. Proteins in the subretinal fluid. *Eur J Ophthalmol* 1993;3:132.
5. Bonnet M. Peripheral neovascularization complicating rhegmatogenous retinal detachments of long duration. *Graefes Arch Clin Exp Ophthalmol* 1987;225:59.
6. Bonnet M, Guenoun S. Surgical risk factors for severe postoperative proliferative vitreoretinopathy (PVR) in retinal detachment with grade B PVR. *Graefes Arch Clin Exp Ophthalmol* 1995;233:789.
7. Burton TC, Arafat NI, Phelps CD. Intraocular pressure in retinal detachment. *Int Ophthalmol* 1979;1:147.

8. Campochiaro P, Hackett SF, Vinores SA, et al. Platelet-derived growth factor is an autocrine growth stimulator in retinal pigmented epithelial cells. *J Cell Sci* 1994;107:2459.
9. Campochiaro PA. Pathogenic mechanisms in proliferative vitreoretinopathy. *Arch Ophthalmol* 1997;115:237.
10. Charteris DG, Hiscott P, Grierson I, et al. Proliferative vitreoretinopathy: lymphocytes in epiretinal membranes. *Ophthalmology* 1992;99:1364.
11. Clarkson JG, Green WR, Massof D. A histopathologic review of 168 cases of preretinal membrane. *Am J Ophthalmol* 1977;84:1.
12. Cook B, Lewis GP, Fisher SK, et al. Apoptotic photoreceptor degeneration in experimental retinal detachment. *Invest Ophthalmol Vis Sci* 1995;36:990.
13. Cowley M, Conway BP, Campochiaro PA, et al. Clinical risk factors for proliferative vitreoretinopathy. *Arch Ophthalmol* 1989;107:1147.
14. Elner SG, Elner VM, Diaz-Rohena R, et al. Anterior proliferative vitreoretinopathy: clinicopathologic, light microscopic, and ultrastructural findings. *Ophthalmology* 1988;95:1349.
15. Elner SG, Elner VM, Jaffe GJ, et al. Cytokines in proliferative diabetic retinopathy and proliferative vitreoretinopathy. *Curr Eye Res* 1995;14:1045.
16. Felder KS, Brockhurst RJ. Retinal neovascularization complicating rhegmatogenous retinal detachment of long duration. *Am J Ophthalmol* 1982;93:773.
17. Girard P, Mimoun G, Karpouzas I, et al. Clinical risk factors for proliferative vitreoretinopathy after retinal detachment surgery. *Retina* 1994;14:417.
18. Glaser BM, Cardin A, Biscoe B. Proliferative vitreoretinopathy: the mechanism of development of vitreoretinal traction. *Ophthalmology* 1987;94:327.
19. Glaser BM, Vidaurri-Leal J, Michels RG, et al. Cryotherapy during surgery for giant retinal tears and intravitreal dispersion of viable retinal pigment epithelial cells. *Ophthalmology* 1993;100:466.
20. Godtfredsen E. Investigations into hyaluronic acid and hyaluronidase in the subretinal fluid in retinal detachment, partly due to ruptures and partly secondary to malignant choroidal melanoma. *Br J Ophthalmol* 1949;33:721.
21. Grizzard WS, Hilton GF, Hammer ME, et al. A multivariate analysis of anatomic success of retinal detachments treated with scleral buckling. *Graefes Arch Clin Exp Ophthalmol* 1994;232:1.
22. Hackett SF, Conway BP, Campochiaro PA. Subretinal fluid stimulation of retinal pigment epithelial cell migration and proliferation is dependent on certain features of the detachment or its treatment [see comments]. *Arch Ophthalmol* 1989;107:391.
23. Hamasaki DI, Machemer R, Norton EW. Experimental retinal detachment in the owl monkey. VI. The ERG of the detached and reattached retina. *Graefes Arch Clin Exp Ophthalmol* 1969;177:212.
24. Hara S, Ishiguro S, Hayasaka S, et al. Immunoreactive opsin content in subretinal fluid from patients with rhegmatogenous retinal detachments. *Arch Ophthalmol* 1987;105:260.
25. Hardwick C, Morris R, Witherspoon D, et al. Pathologic human vitreous promotes contraction by fibroblasts: implications for proliferative vitreoretinopathy. *Arch Ophthalmol* 1995;113:1545.
26. Havener WH. Massive vitreous retraction. *Ophthalmic Surg* 1973;4:22.
27. Hayasaka S, Shiono T, Hara S, et al. Lysosomal hyaluronidase in the subretinal fluid of patients with rhegmatogenous retinal detachments. *Am J Ophthalmol* 1982;94:58.
28. Hogan MJ, Zimmerman LE. *Ophthalmic Pathology.* Philadelphia: WB Saunders, 1962:549.
29. Jaffe GJ, Roberts WL, Wong HL, et al. Monocyte-induced cytokine expression in cultured human retinal pigment epithelial cells. *Exp Eye Res* 1995;60:533.
30. Kauffmann DJ, van Meurs JC, Mertens DA, et al. Cytokines in vitreous humor: interleukin-6 is elevated in proliferative vitreoretinopathy. *Invest Ophthalmol Vis Sci* 1994;35:900.
31. Kaufman PL, Podos SM. Subretinal fluid butyrylcholinesterase. 1. Source of the enzyme and factors affecting its concentration in subretinal fluid from primary rhegmatogenous retinal detachments. *Am J Ophthalmol* 1973;75:627.
32. Kirchhof B, Sorgente N. Pathogenesis of proliferative vitreoretinopathy: modulation of retinal pigment epithelial cell functions by vitreous and macrophages. *Dev Ophthalmol* 1989;16:1.
33. Kroll AJ, Machemer R. Experimental retinal detachment in the owl monkey. 3. Electron microscopy of retina and pigment epithelium. *Am J Ophthalmol* 1968;66:410.
34. Kroll AJ, Machemer R. Experimental retinal detachment in the owl monkey. 8. Photoreceptor protein renewal in early retinal reattachment. *Am J Ophthalmol* 1971;72:356.
35. Kroll AJ, Machemer R. Experimental retinal detachment in the owl monkey. 5. Electron microscopy of the reattached retina. *Am J Ophthalmol* 1969;67:117.
36. Laqua H, Machemer R. Clinical-pathological correlation in massive periretinal proliferation. *Am J Ophthalmol* 1975;80:913.
37. Limb GA, Earley O, Jones SE, et al. Expression of mRNA coding for TNF alpha, IL-1 beta and IL-6 by cells infiltrating retinal membranes. *Graefes Arch Clin Exp Ophthalmol* 1994;232:646.
38. Linner E. Intraocular pressure in retinal detachment. *Arch Ophthalmol* 1966;84:101.
39. Lopez PF, Grossniklaus HE, Aaberg TM, et al. Pathogenetic mechanisms in anterior proliferative vitreoretinopathy. *Am J Ophthalmol* 1992;114:257.
40. MacDonald IM, Pannu R, Kovithavongs K, et al. Effect of retinoic acid on expression of transforming growth factor-beta by retinal pigment epithelial cells in culture. *Can J Ophthalmol* 1995;30:301.

41. Machemer R. Experimental retinal detachment in the owl monkey. II. Histology of retina and pigment epithelium. *Am J Ophthalmol* 1968;66:396.
42. Machemer R, Aaberg TM, Freeman HM, et al. An updated classification of retinal detachment with proliferative vitreoretinopathy. *Am J Ophthalmol* 1991;112:159.
43. Machemer R, Buettner H. Experimental retinal detachment in the owl monkey. IX. Radioautographic study of protein metabolism. *Am J Ophthalmol* 1972;73:377.
44. Machemer R, Kroll AJ. Experimental retinal detachment in the owl monkey. 7. Photoreceptor study of protein metabolism. *Am J Ophthalmol* 1971;73:337.
45. Machemer R, Laqua H. Pigment epithelium proliferation in retinal detachment (massive periretinal proliferation). *Am J Ophthalmol* 1975;80:1.
46. Machemer R, Norton EW. Experimental retinal detachment in the owl monkey. I. Methods of production and clinical picture. *Am J Ophthalmol* 1968;66:388.
47. Machemer R, van Horn D, Aaberg TM. Pigment epithelial proliferation in human retinal detachment with massive periretinal proliferation. *Am J Ophthalmol* 1978;85:181.
48. Matsuo N, Takabatake M, Ueno H, et al. Photoreceptor outer segments in the aqueous humor in rhegmatogenous retinal detachment. *Am J Ophthalmol* 1986;101:673.
49. Mietz H, Stodtler M, Wiedemann P, et al. Immunohistochemistry of cellular proliferation in eyes with long-standing retinal detachment. *Int Ophthalmol* 1994;18:329.
50. Morse PH. Fixed retinal star folds in retinal detachment. *Am J Ophthalmol* 1974;77:760.
51. Netland PA, Mukai S, Covington HI. Elevated intraocular pressure secondary to rhegmatogenous retinal detachment. *Surv Ophthalmol* 1994;39:234.
52. Nork TM, Millecchia LL, Strickland BD, et al. Selective loss of blue cones and rods in human retinal detachment. *Arch Ophthalmol* 1995;113:1066.
53. Ohsato M, Shiga S, Kato H, et al. Immunohistochemical study of cellular fibronectin in preretinal membranes. *Retina* 1994;14:430.
54. Osusky R, Soriano D, Ye J, et al. Cytokine effect on fibronectin release by retinal pigment epithelial cells. *Curr Eye Res* 1994;13:569.
55. Pederson JE. Experimental retinal detachment. IV. Aqueous humor dynamics in rhegmatogenous detachments. *Arch Ophthalmol* 1982;100:1814.
56. Pederson JE, Cantrill HL. Experimental retinal detachment. V. Fluid movement through the retinal hole. *Arch Ophthalmol* 1984;102:136.
57. Reuter U, Champion C, Kain HL. Transdifferentiation of human monocytes into fibroblast-like cells in vitro. *Ger J Ophthalmol* 1995;4:182.
58. Ryan SJ. Traction retinal detachment. XLIX Edward Jackson Memorial Lecture [see comments]. *Am J Ophthalmol* 1993;115:1.
59. Schwartz A. Chronic open-angle glaucoma secondary to rhegmatogenous retinal detachment. *Am J Ophthalmol* 1973;75:205.
60. Sen H, Robertson T, Conway B, et al. The role of breakdown of the blood–retinal barrier in cell-injection models of proliferative vitreoretinopathy. *Arch Ophthalmol* 1988;106:1291.
61. Singh AK, Glaser BM, Lemor M, et al. Gravity-dependent distribution of retinal pigment epithelial cells dispersed into the vitreous cavity. *Retina* 1986;6:77.
62. Singh AK, Michels RG, Glaser BM. Scleral indentation following cryotherapy and repeat cryotherapy enhance release of viable retinal pigment epithelial cells. *Retina* 1986;6:176.
63. Stodtler M, Mietz H, Wiedemann P, et al. Immunohistochemistry of anterior proliferative vitreoretinopathy: report of 11 cases. *Int Ophthalmol* 1994;18:323.
64. Toris CB, Pederson JE. Experimental retinal detachment. VIII. Retinochoroidal horseradish peroxidase diffusion across the blood–retinal barrier. *Arch Ophthalmol* 1985;103:266.
65. Tsuboi S, Pederson JE. Permeability of the blood–retinal barrier to carboxyfluorescein in eyes with rhegmatogenous retinal detachment. *Invest Ophthalmol Vis Sci* 1987;28:96.
66. Tsuboi S, Taki-Noie J, Emi K, et al. Fluid dynamics in eyes with rhegmatogenous retinal detachments. *Am J Ophthalmol* 1985;99:673.
67. Van Horn DL, Aaberg TM, Machemer R, et al. Glial cell proliferation in human retinal detachment with massive periretinal proliferation. *Am J Ophthalmol* 1977;84:383.
68. Walshe R, Esser P, Wiedemann P, et al. Proliferative retinal diseases: myofibroblasts cause chronic vitreoretinal traction. *Br J Ophthalmol* 1992;76:550.
69. Wiedemann P. Growth factors in retinal diseases: proliferative vitreoretinopathy, proliferative diabetic retinopathy, and retinal degeneration. *Surv Ophthalmol* 1992;36:373.
70. Wilson DJ, Green WR. Histopathologic study of the effect of retinal detachment surgery on 49 eyes obtained post mortem. *Am J Ophthalmol* 1987;103:167.
71. Wilson-Holt N, Khaw P, Savage F, et al. The chemoattractant activity of the vitreous to human scleral fibroblasts following retinal detachment and proliferative vitreoretinopathy. *Br J Ophthalmol* 1992;76:159.
72. Yang CM, Cousins SW. Quantitative assessment of growth stimulating activity of the vitreous during PVR. *Invest Ophthalmol Vis Sci* 1992;33:2436.

3
Predisposing Conditions

Chapter 1 discussed the basic mechanism of primary or spontaneous rhegmatogenous retinal detachment (RRD). This chapter discusses specific events and conditions that predispose to retinal breaks and subsequent detachment.

LATTICE DEGENERATION

Lattice degeneration is a condition of the peripheral retina characterized by thinning of the inner retinal layers and localized liquefaction of the overlying vitreous (Fig. 3-1A). It is called lattice because, on ophthalmoscopy, the characteristically elliptical areas of degeneration are often marked by a criss-crossing lattice work of white lines (hyalinized-appearing blood vessels). In pigmented lattice (see Fig. 3-1B), retinal pigment epithelial cells proliferate into the retina. A typical area of lattice degeneration parallels the ora serrata (see Figs. 1-7 and 1-11). Less common is radial lattice, which parallels retinal blood vessels (Fig. 3-2).

Lattice is found in 6% to 10% of the population and is bilateral in 33% of affected persons (17,18,89). It is more common in myopic than in hyperopic eyes; its incidence rises as axial length increases (16,51,96). In 31% of affected patients, the retina is thinned sufficiently to allow the formation of atrophic round holes (15).

Lattice is the direct cause of 21% of all retinal detachments and is present in 41% (3). In 30% to 45% of retinal detachments caused by lattice, the detachment results from atrophic holes in the lattice (8,15). Seventy percent of such detachments are seen in myopic eyes, and 70% occur in patients younger than 40 years of age. These detachments typically progress slowly, and demarcation lines are often present. Almost 100% can be successfully reattached (9,95).

Although the incidence of posterior vitreous detachment (PVD) in eyes with lattice is the same as it is in eyes without (34), the strong vitreoretinal adhesions that surround lattice increase the risk of tears. In some cases, these adhesions are made still stronger by glial proliferation along the overlying vitreal surface (76,90). In 55% to 70% of detachments caused by lattice, the causative break is a tear beginning posterior to or at the end of a patch of lattice (8,15). Ninety percent of these detachments are in patients 50 years of age or older, and only 43% of the affected eyes are myopic (8). The detachments progress more rapidly than do those arising from atrophic holes. Demarcation lines are rarely present.

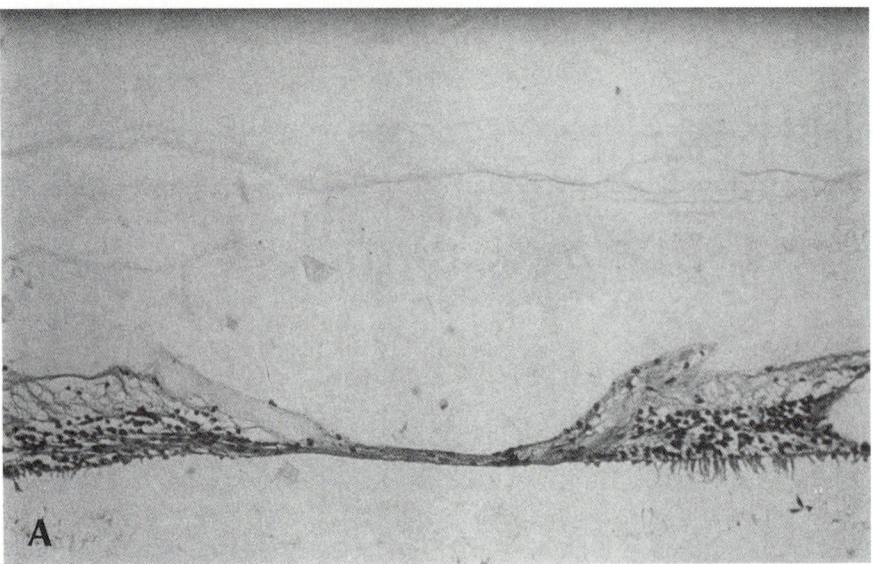
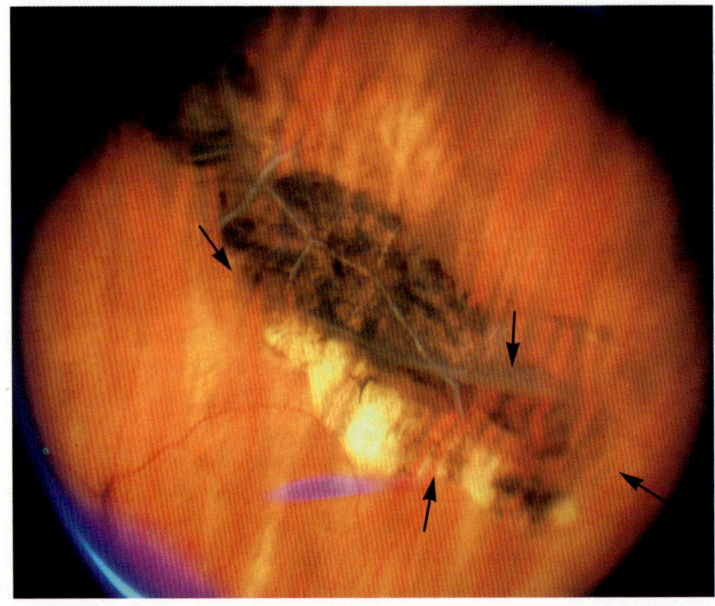

FIGURE 3-1. A: Lattice degeneration. Notice thinning of the inner retinal layers and liquefaction of the overlying vitreous (hematoxylin and eosin; 10× magnification; Armed Forces Institute of Pathology Accession No. 1319686). **B:** Pigmented lattice degeneration with lattice work of hyalinized retinal blood vessels. At the right end of the lattice, a crescentic tear *(arrows)* is present.

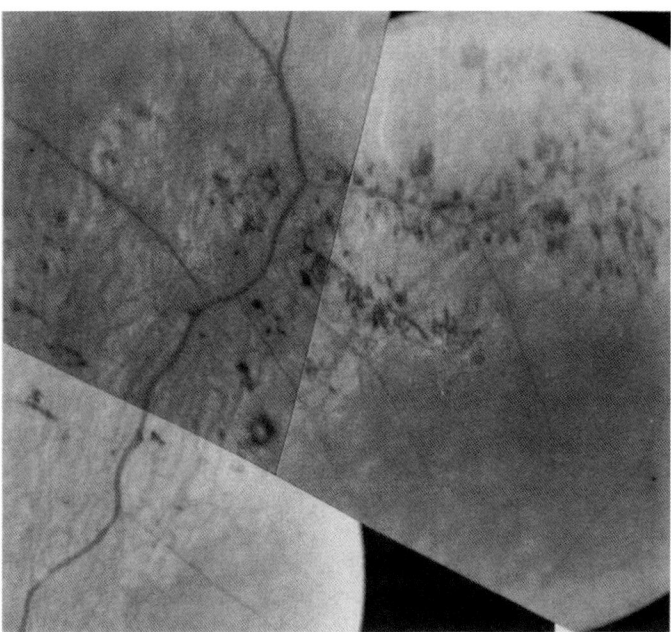

FIGURE 3-2. Radial (or meridional) lattice degeneration, which characteristically straddles retinal blood vessels and extends far posteriorly.

MYOPIA

In eyes that have not undergone intraocular surgical procedures or trauma, myopia is by far the largest risk factor. Three reasons exist for this morbidity. First, myopic eyes have an increased incidence of lattice degeneration (16,51,96). Second, they have a higher incidence of PVD (42). Third, the thin retina of a myopic eye is prone to develop spontaneous or traumatic retinal breaks. Indeed, 18% of eyes with 6 or more diopters of myopia have full-thickness retinal breaks (41), as compared with a 7% incidence for the population at large.

When compared with nonmyopic eyes, eyes with a spherical refractive error of −1 to −3 diopters have a fourfold increased risk of retinal detachment (32). High myopia increases this risk to as much as tenfold (32,56,78). High myopes have 42% of all retinal detachments (3), but they make up only 10% of the population at large (10). Myopes with a refractive error of greater than 8 diopters account for 10% of all retinal detachments (3), though they comprise only 1% of the general population (10).

CATARACT SURGERY

Intracapsular Cataract Extraction

One of the reasons that intracapsular cataract extraction (ICCE) is rarely done anymore in the United States is that the risk of retinal detachment is less with expression or phacoemulsification extracapsular cataract extraction (ECCE). In one report, the incidence of retinal detachment after ICCE was 2% to 5% (104). In high myopes, ICCE has been particularly risky, with 6% to 8% developing retinal detachment (59,87). Patients who had an aphakic retinal detachment in one eye had a risk of 26% to 41% of retinal detachment if they underwent ICCE in the fellow eye (7,19). If a patient had successful repair of a phakic retinal detachment and then underwent ICCE, the risk of redetachment was about 5% to 10% (1).

Extracapsular Cataract Extraction

The incidence of retinal detachment after ECCE by either expression or phacoemulsification approach is about 1% (46,67,68). Even though the risk is now relatively low, enough cataract operations are performed annually that it is still the second largest risk factor for retinal detachment. The risk is lowest if the posterior capsule remains intact, but, unfortunately, the advantage of ECCE is partially negated by neodymiun:yttrium aluminum garnet posterior capsulotomy. Although one study failed to demonstrate a causal relationship, three large series showed that capsulotomy caused a four- to fivefold increase in the risk of retinal break or detachment (45,67,68,94). Furthermore, intraoperative capsular disruption with vitreous loss increases the risk of retinal detachment to about 5% (46).

Eyes with high myopia have a lower risk of retinal detachment after ECCE (about 1% at 4 years) than after ICCE (67,68), but they still have a higher risk than do emmetropic and hyperopic eyes (33,58,67,68). One study found that the odds ratio for retinal detachment increased by 1.21 per millimeter of axial length (94). With regard to bilaterality, a patient who has pseudophakic retinal detachment in one eye has a 6% risk of having one in the fellow eye if he or she undergoes ECCE (24). The incidence of redetachment of previously successfully attached retinas after ECCE is lower than it is after ICCE. One study reported that no patient who had successful repair of a phakic retinal detachment and then underwent phacoemulsification had a redetachment (52).

Detachments after ECCE typically have small flap tears along the posterior vitreous base similar to those found after ICCE (105). Not only is the risk of aphakic retinal detachment reduced by ECCE, but also when detachment does occur, it is much less likely to be total, to have macular detachment, or to have signs of proliferative vitreoretinopathy (PVR) than does detachment after ICCE. The prevalence of these findings actually approximates that of phakic retinal detachments (25,40,69,105). The rate of successful reattachment of the retina after ECCE is approximately the same as that in phakic retinal detachment (higher than 95%) (25,40,105).

Congenital Cataract Extraction

No recent studies have been conducted on the incidence of retinal detachment in patients who undergo congenital cataract surgery using current techniques. In 1984, a study found the incidence to be 1.5% (20). The true incidence is probably higher, because the mean length of follow-up was only 5.5 years. Earlier studies found that the average interval between congenital cataract surgery and the onset of detachment is 22.8 years (97). The rate of successful reattachment in these cases is only approximately 50% to 75%, probably because the diagnosis is often delayed and PVR develops (43,50). Another problem is poor visualization of the retina because of capsular opacification. Vitrectomy is often necessary to remove remaining lens material and to manage the PVR. Patients with congenital cataracts who have retinal detachment in one eye must be watched carefully, because 70% develop retinal detachment in their fellow eye (43).

GLAUCOMA

A genetic relationship appears to exist between chronic open-angle glaucoma and retinal detachment. A study of fellow eyes in patients who had unilateral retinal detachment, but did not have open-angle glaucoma, found a significant percentage of decreased aqueous outflow facility, large cup-to-disc ratio, and marked elevation of intraocular pressure after administration of topical steroids (83). Moreover, eyes in patients with open-angle glaucoma are prone to develop retinal detachment. Clinical studies have reported that although chronic open-angle glaucoma is present in less than 1% of the general population, it is present in 4% to 9% of patients with retinal detachment (6,73). Patients with the pigmentary dispersion syndrome seem to be especially prone to retinal detachment, probably because of their increased incidence of myopia and lattice degeneration (103).

Investigators have suggested that the miotic drugs used in glaucoma therapy can cause retinal detachment; this suggestion is based on many reports of retinal detachment in glaucoma patients who are treated with parasympathomimetics or anticholinesterases (54). However, because thousands of patients have used miotic drugs without developing a retinal detachment, some investigators believe that miotic-induced retinal detachment probably does not occur in patients free of retinal disease (5).

Because glaucoma patients are more likely to develop retinal detachment than the population at large, they should have a careful peripheral retinal examination at regular intervals. Should they experience a sudden uniocular decrease in intraocular pressure, or should they have a sudden decrease in visual field despite adequate glaucoma control, retinal detachment should be suspected.

Congenital glaucoma also predisposes to retinal detachment, probably because of thinning of the retina induced by the progressive enlargement of the eye. Visualization of the breaks in such detachments is difficult because of a cloudy cornea, a cataract, or both (23,106).

TRAUMA

Blunt Trauma

Because men and boys are most likely to be engaged in fighting or contact sports, it is not surprising that they comprise at least three-fourths of the patients with traumatic retinal detachment (27,28), and blunt trauma is the leading cause of retinal detachment in children and adolescents (27,28,106). Boxers have an especially high risk (60).

Blunt trauma can cause retinal breaks by several mechanisms. Blunt trauma compresses the eye along its anteroposterior diameter and expands it in the equatorial plane. Because the vitreous body is relatively elastic, slow compression of the eye usually has no deleterious effect on the retina. However, when the eye is rapidly compressed, the vitreous does not have sufficient time to stretch, and resultant severe traction occurs at the vitreous base. This most commonly causes linear retinal tears at the posterior border of the vitreous base or linear tears of the nonpigmented epithelium of the pars plana at the anterior border of the vitreous base, or both (28,102). Severe traction can avulse a section of the vitreous base from the retina, a finding pathognomonic of ocular contusion (Fig. 3-3) (28). Generally, but not always, when the vitreous base is avulsed, the peripheral retina and the pars plana are torn. Occasionally, the trauma causes a true retinal dialysis.

Traumatic breaks at the vitreous base are most commonly located in the inferotemporal quadrant (37,47). Although some authors believe that all inferotemporal dialyses are

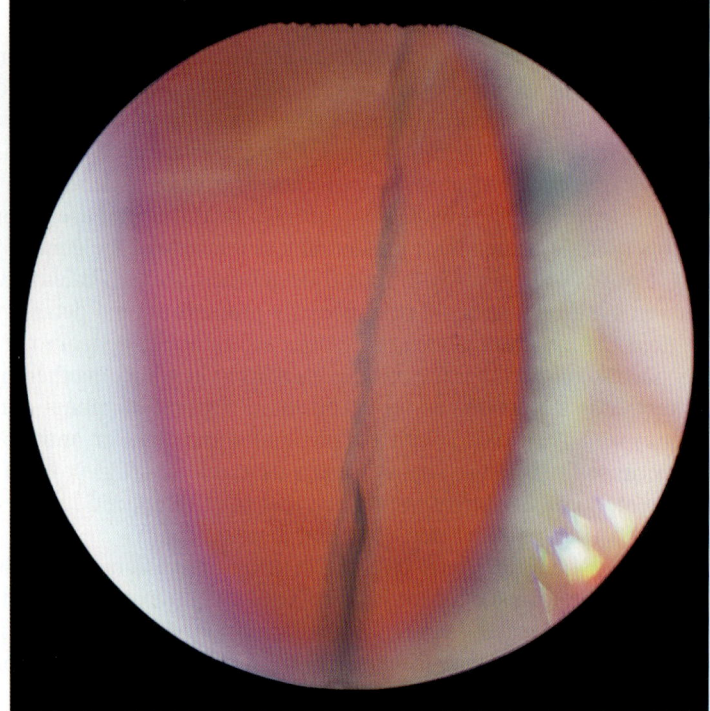

FIGURE 3-3. Pigmented avulsed vitreous base.

traumatic (77), many such dialyses are familial, bilateral, or found in patients with no history or histopathologic evidence of injury (85,99–101,107). These patients probably have a developmental abnormality of the inferotemporal peripheral retina and vitreous base. No controversy exists about superonasal dialyses. They are believed to be pathognomonic of blunt trauma.

Most retinal breaks caused by blunt trauma probably occur at the time of impact. In two studies, patients with traumatic hyphema underwent a careful retinal examination as soon as the media were clear (82,91). Four percent to 18% of the eyes had either tears along the posterior vitreous base or dialyses. Four percent had posterior breaks. No eyes developed late tears.

Blunt trauma can also cause posterior breaks, although these are rarer sequelae of trauma than tears along the vitreous base. A posterior flap tear can occur if the vitreous is strongly adherent to a focal area of retina. A direct blow to the eye can cause retinal necrosis, which may give rise to irregular breaks with ragged edges. Shock waves (contrecoup) from anterior trauma may cause enough macular damage to result in a macular hole. Finally, in rare cases, horizontal stretching of the eye can cause a retinal stretch tear.

Because most traumatic retinal breaks are in young persons, whose vitreous is still mostly in a gel-like state, traumatic detachments characteristically progress slowly and often bear the signs of long-standing detachment: demarcation lines, clumps of pigmented cells ("tobacco dust") (see Fig. 1-3), smooth, transparent retina, and intraretinal cysts (37). Therefore, even though the tears occur at the time of impact, the interval between the trauma and the diagnosis of retinal detachment exceeds 8 months in 50% of

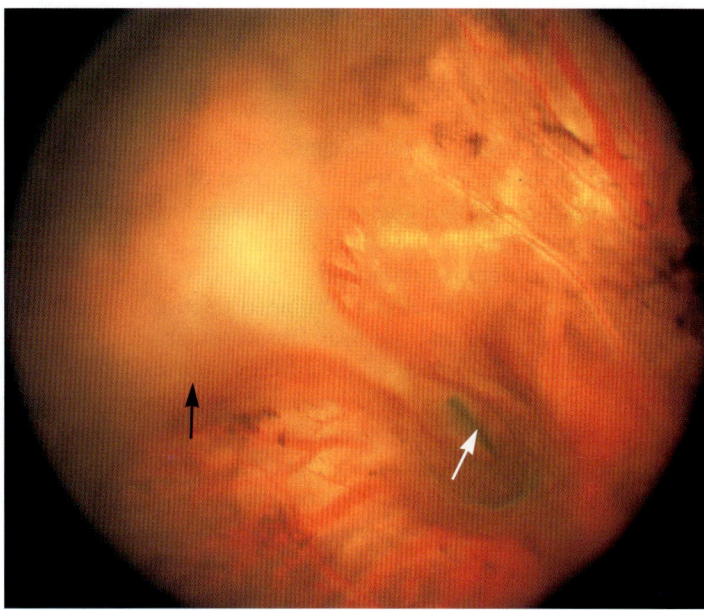

FIGURE 3-4. Fibrovascular proliferation *(black arrow)* from the entry site of a foreign body to where it is now embedded *(white arrow)*. Contraction of such tissue can cause retinal detachment.

cases (28). The prognosis for successful reattachment is excellent (37), unless a giant tear is involved (see chapter 10, Surgery of Complicated Cases).

Whether indirect trauma can cause retinal tears is controversial. Sudden acceleration of the vitreous by a blow to the head seems likely to produce a retinal tear in an eye predisposed to retinal detachment, such as an eye with high myopia or lattice degeneration. However, a study of 247 patients who had suffered severe head trauma failed to reveal any retinal breaks (29).

Penetrating Injuries

Penetrating injuries involving the posterior segment have a high risk of subsequent retinal detachment. Detachment is much more likely if vitreous hemorrhage is present and if the wound is large or posterior (72,74). Late retinal breaks are usually caused by contraction of fibrovascular tissue, which proliferates from the entry wound along vitreous fibers (Fig. 3-4). The tears are usually located 90 to 180 degrees from the wound (26,57,72). Even with vitrectomy techniques, the prognosis is guarded (74) (see chapter 10, Surgery of Complicated Cases).

PROLIFERATIVE RETINOPATHIES

Diabetes

In diabetes, retinal ischemia stimulates the proliferation of new blood vessels that are accompanied by fibroglial tissue. Posterior vitreous detachment in the eyes of persons who do not have diabetes is characterized by a clean separation of the posterior cortical vitreous from the retina. In diabetic patients, however, the vitreous is often strongly adherent to the retina or to fibrovascular proliferation. Therefore, as the vitreous body slowly collapses and moves forward, traction is placed on the posterior retina. The most common type of retinal detachment in diabetic patients is nonrhegmatogenous traction retinal detachment. In these cases, the retina characteristically has a smooth surface and is immobile. The detachment is concave toward the front of the eye and rarely extends to the ora serrata. In many cases, a small traction retinal detachment remains unchanged for years. In others, progression into the macula is relentless.

Diabetic patients with proliferative retinopathy rarely develop a typical RRD with peripheral flap tears. When they do develop a combined traction–rhegmatogenous detachment, the breaks are usually oval and are near fibrovascular vitreoretinal proliferations (49,92) (Fig. 3-5). Vitreous hemorrhage or the proliferation itself may block the examiner's view of the hole. However, even if the break cannot be located, the correct diagnosis can be made because the retina is mobile and has the irregular corrugations characteristic of RRD (see chapter 2, Pathophysiology). The detachment is convex toward the front of the eye and may extend to the ora serrata. Vitrectomy is required for repair of both traction and combined traction–RRDs (see chapter 10, Surgery of Complicated Cases).

Branch Retinal Vein Occlusion

Branch retinal vein occlusion is a rare cause of RRD (48). As in proliferative diabetic retinopathy, retinal ischemia stimulates the proliferation of new blood vessels, which usually adhere to the posterior cortical vitreous. When the vitreous body collapses, traction on the neovascularization can tear a hole in the retina, and a RRD may result (Fig. 3-6).

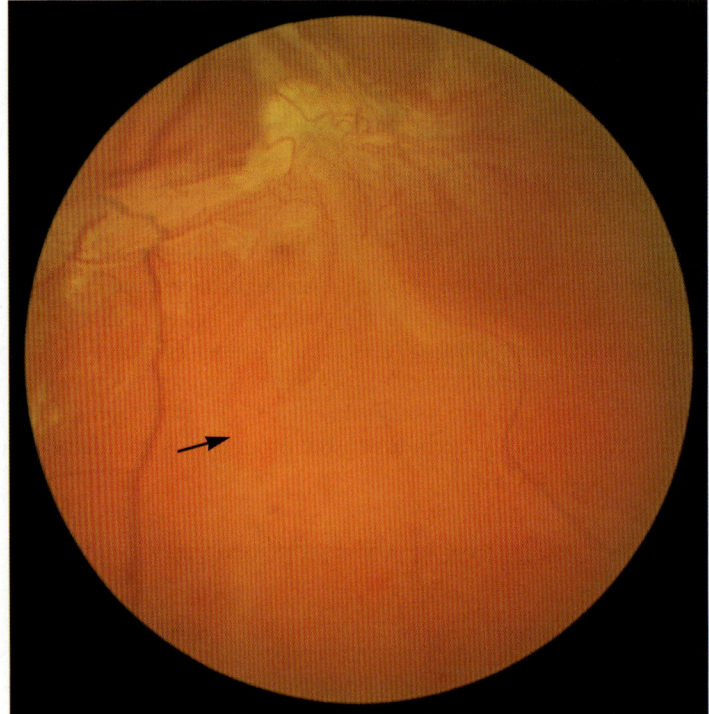

FIGURE 3-5. Oval retinal break *(arrow)* caused by diabetic fibrovascular proliferations.

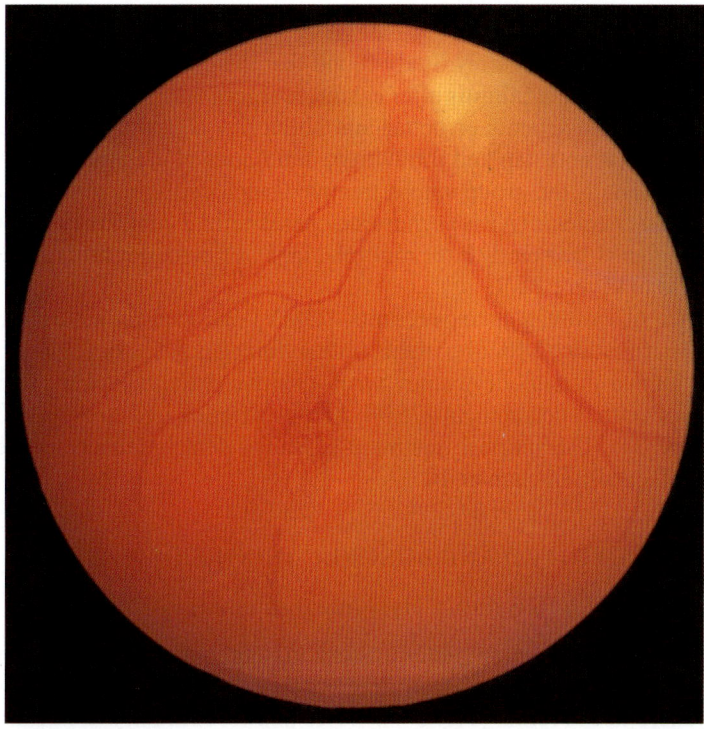

FIGURE 3-6. Rhegmatogenous retinal detachment caused by vitreous traction on neovascularization from branch retinal vein occlusion. Note the rolled edge of the break.

Sickle Cell Retinopathy

Traction on proliferative fronds initially causes peripheral traction retinal detachment. In some cases, the thin, ischemic retina tears, giving rise to a combined traction–RRD similar to that seen in proliferative diabetic retinopathy. The prognosis for repair is good (44) because the anterior location of the breaks allows these cases to be treated successfully with a scleral buckling (SB) procedure alone. Anterior segment necrosis may complicate surgical repair, so the surgeon must attempt to avoid maneuvers known to predispose to this condition (79) (see chapter 11, Postoperative Complications of Primary Retinal Detachment Repair). Occasionally, patients have vitreous hemorrhage and traction–RRDs. Then, vitrectomy is needed to clear the hemorrhage and to find the breaks. The overall results in these patients are not as good (50% reattached) (21) because of complications such as iatrogenic breaks (33%), repeated postoperative hemorrhages, and glaucoma (44). Finally, because patients with sickle trait alone may have occlusion of the central retinal artery at an intraocular pressure as low as the midthirties, careful monitoring of the intraocular pressure during and after any operation is essential.

Retinopathy of Prematurity

Rhegmatogenous retinal detachment is an uncommon late complication of cicatricial retinopathy of prematurity (93). Intravitreal proliferation of fibrovascular tissue may make it difficult to find the retinal breaks, which, in some cases, are in an extremely posterior location.

INFECTIONS

The Endophthalmitis Vitrectomy Study found that the incidence of retinal detachment in patients who had endophthalmitis after cataract surgery was 1.4% if their vision before treatment was hand movements or better and about 5% if it was light perception. The group treated with vitreous tap and intravitreal antibiotics alone had the same incidence of retinal detachment as the group whose treatment included vitrectomy (31).

The acute retinal necrosis (ARN) syndrome causes retinal detachment in 50% of cases (30). The detachments frequently have multiple, large, or posterior retinal breaks and frequently progress to severe PVR.

The incidence of cytomegalovirus retinitis (CMV)–induced retinal detachment is increasing. In Great Britain, 28% of patients with cytomegalovirus develop retinal detachment (80). In human immunodeficiency virus–positive patients, cytomegalovirus is the leading cause of retinal detachment (75%); herpes simplex and toxoplasmosis are less common causes (84). The surgical treatment of retinal detachments caused by necrotizing retinitis is discussed in chapter 10.

INHERITED AND MISCELLANEOUS DISEASES

Hereditary Hyaloideoretinopathies

The hallmark of this group of conditions is early and extensive vitreous liquefaction, which results in an optically empty vitreous cavity, except for whitish bands and membranes that adhere to the retina (Fig. 3-7). Other possible findings are cataract, myopia, optic atrophy, choroidal and pigment epithelial atrophy, radial and circumferential lattice degeneration, peripheral retinoschisis, retinal detachment, and glaucoma (39,53,62,63). The electroretinogram is often subnormal. The lattice degeneration, retinoschisis, and vitreous membranes predispose to retinal detachments, which may be difficult to repair because the retinal breaks are often large, multiple, and at different distances from the ora serrata. Moreover, the vitreous membranes may prevent settling of the retina, often necessitating vitrectomy techniques with or without a scleral buckle (14,39).

The classification of the hereditary hyaloideoretinopathies is controversial. In general, they can be classified into two main groups (62,63). The first group is characterized by ocular signs and symptoms only and includes Wagner's disease, erosive vitreoretinopathy, and Jansen's disease. Patients with Wagner's disease do not have an increased risk of retinal detachment (39). Patients with erosive vitreoretinopathy and Jansen's disease have a high risk of retinal detachment. Erosive vitreoretinopathy is allelic to Wagner's disease (11).

The second group, of which Stickler's syndrome is the most common, has associated systemic abnormalities (88). Orofacial findings include midfacial flattening, cleft palate, and the Pierre Robin malformation complex, which is characterized by micrognathia, cleft palate (which may be submucosal), and glossoptosis. The generalized skeletal abnormalities include joint hyperextensibility and enlargement, arthritis, and mild spondyloepiphyseal dysplasia. A genetic defect in the type II procollagen (COL2A1) has been identified (2,12,86).

Congenital Optic Disc Abnormalities

Eyes in patients with the morning glory syndrome can develop a total bullous retinal detachment, in which the subretinal fluid (SRF) passes from the vitreous through defects in the tissue over the disc into the subretinal space (81). The currently recommended

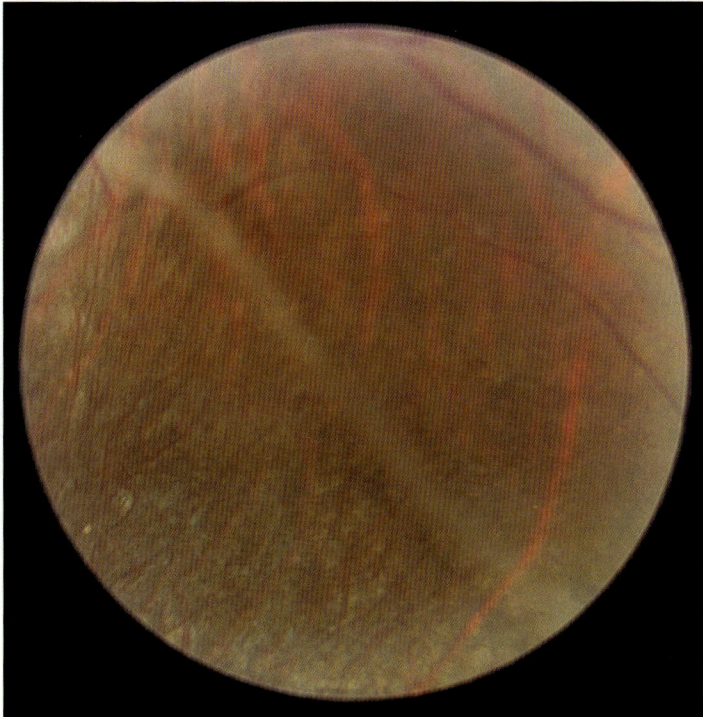

FIGURE 3-7. Vitreous band in Stickler's syndrome. Aside from the bands, the vitreous is optically empty.

treatment is pars plana vitrectomy, endolaser photocoagulation, and use of long-lasting gases (see chapter 10, Surgery of Complicated Cases) (4,13,22).

Congenital Choroidal Colobomas

In detachments caused by choroidal colobomas, the breaks are often small and atrophic and are found in the base of the coloboma. The treatment is the same as for the morning glory syndrome. Vitrectomy and internal tamponade with long-lasting gas or silicone oil are usually necessary (see chapter 10, Surgery of Complicated Cases) (36,38,64).

Congenital Retinoschisis

In this X-linked recessive condition, also called juvenile retinoschisis, the nerve fiber layer is separated from the other layers of the retina. This results in a characteristic spoke-wheel "cystoid" macula (Fig. 3-8). In the periphery, especially inferotemporally, the nerve fiber layer may be elevated into the vitreous. Holes in this elevated "inner wall" (Fig. 3-9) are common but do not cause retinal detachment. The rarer "outer wall" holes, which are holes through the remaining retinal layers, can cause full-thickness retinal detachment. The prognosis for successful repair is good, but advanced vitreoretinal surgical techniques may be necessary (see chapter 10, Surgery of Complicated Cases) (35,75). If macular traction is present, removal of the inner wall of the peripheral schisis cavity by vitrectomy can be helpful (98).

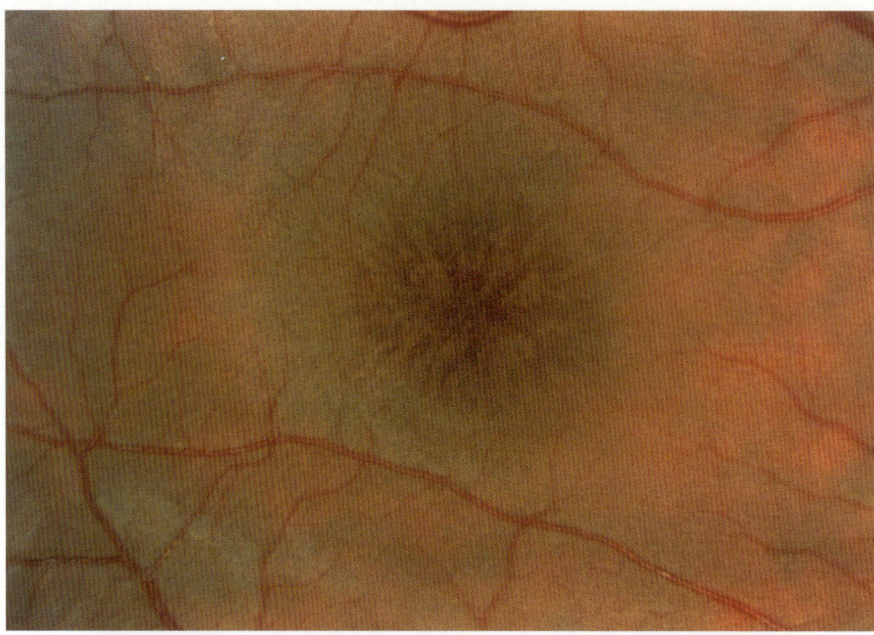

FIGURE 3-8. Juvenile retinoschisis, with a typical cystoid spoking pattern in fovea.

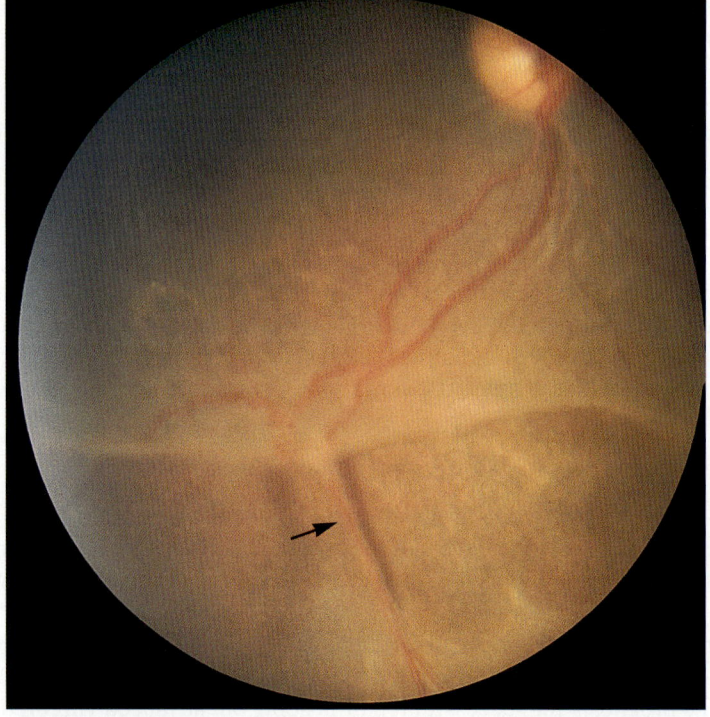

FIGURE 3-9. Juvenile retinoschisis, with a large hole in the inner wall with a bridging vessel *(arrow).*

Ehlers–Danlos Syndrome

Myopia and retinal detachment may accompany this autosomal dominant condition in which collagen fibrils throughout the body are not organized into a strong supporting network. Repair of retinal detachment is hazardous because the sclera, which is largely composed of collagen, does not hold sutures well. In addition, fragile choroidal blood vessels bleed easily when drainage of SRF is attempted (71).

Goldmann–Favre Syndrome

This autosomal recessive ocular condition is characterized by cataract, peripheral and macular retinoschisis, retinal changes resembling those of retinitis pigmentosa, radial lattice degeneration, and an optically empty vitreous cavity with vitreous membranes. Patients suffer from night blindness and progressive visual loss. The electroretinogram is severely depressed. As in Stickler's syndrome, retinal detachments may be difficult to repair.

Marfan's Syndrome and Homocystinuria

In these conditions, the risk of retinal detachment is related to high myopia, lattice degeneration, and ectopia lentis, which are common. Removal of the lens is frequently complicated by vitreous loss, further increasing the chances of retinal detachment (66).

Atopic Dermatitis

In Japan, 10% of all patients younger than 30 years who have retinal detachment have atopic dermatitis (65). The detachments are characterized by tears at the anterior and posterior borders of the vitreous base and suggest a self-induced traumatic origin (55,70). Another possibility is that the detachments are caused by an abnormal vitreous base; during vitrectomies, this structure appears to be abnormally condensed, like fluffy cotton (61).

REFERENCES

1. Ackerman AL, Seelenfreund MH, Freeman HM, et al. Cataract extraction following retinal detachment surgery. *Arch Ophthalmol* 1970;84:41.
2. Ahmad NN, Dimascio J, Knowlton RG, et al. Stickler syndrome: a mutation in the nonhelical 3' end of type II procollagen gene. *Arch Ophthalmol* 1995;113:1454.
3. Ashrafzadeh MT, Schepens CL, Elzeneiny IH, et al. Aphakic and phakic retinal detachment. *Arch Ophthalmol* 1973;89:476.
4. Bartz-Schmidt KU, Heimann K. Pathogenesis of retinal detachment associated with morning glory disc. *Int Ophthalmol* 1995;19:35.
5. Beasley H, Fraunfelder FT. Retinal detachments and topical ocular miotics. *Ophthalmology* 1979;86:95.
6. Becker B. Discussion of retinal detachment and glaucoma by Smith JL. *Trans Am Acad Ophthalmol Otolaryngol* 1963;67:731.
7. Benson WE, Grand MG, Okun E. Aphakic retinal detachment: management of the fellow eye. *Arch Ophthalmol* 1975;93:245.
8. Benson WE, Morse PH. The prognosis of retinal detachment due to lattice degeneration. *Ann Ophthalmol* 1978;10:1197.
9. Benson WE, Nantawan P, Morse PH. Characteristics and prognosis of retinal detachments with demarcation lines. *Am J Ophthalmol* 1977;84:641.
10. Bohringer HR. Statistisches zur Haufigkeit und Risiko der netzhautablosung. *Ophthalmologica* 1956;131:331.
11. Brown DM, Graemiger RA, Hergersberg M, et al. Genetic linkage of Wagner disease and erosive vitreoretinopathy to chromosome 5q13-14. *Arch Ophthalmol* 1995;113:671.
12. Brown DM, Nichols BE, Weingeist TA, et al. Procollagen II gene mutation in Stickler syndrome. *Arch Ophthalmol* 1992;110:1589.

13. Brown GC, Brown MM. Repair of retinal detachment associated with congenital excavated defects of the optic disc. *Ophthalmic Surg* 1995;26:11.
14. Brown GC, Tasman W. Vitrectomy in Wagner's vitreoretinal degeneration. *Am J Ophthalmol* 1978;86:485.
15. Byer NE. Changes in and prognosis of lattice degeneration of the retina. *Trans Am Acad Ophthalmol Otolaryngol* 1974;78:OP114.
16. Byer NE. Clinical study of lattice degeneration of the retina. *Trans Am Acad Ophthalmol Otolaryngol* 1965;69:1064.
17. Byer NE. Lattice degeneration of the retina. *Surv Ophthalmol* 1979;23:213.
18. Byer NE. Long-term natural history of lattice degeneration of the retina. *Ophthalmology* 1989;96:1396.
19. Campbell CJ, Rittler MC. Cataract extraction in the retinal detachment prone patient. *Am J Ophthalmol* 1972;73:17.
20. Chrousos GA, Parks MM, O'Neill JF. Incidence of chronic glaucoma, retinal detachment and secondary membrane surgery in pediatric aphakic patients. *Ophthalmology* 1984;91:1238.
21. Cohen SB, Fletcher ME, Goldberg MF, et al. Diagnosis and management of ocular complications of sickle hemoglobinopathies. Part V. *Ophthalmic Surg* 1986;17:369.
22. Coll GE, Chang S, Flynn TE, et al. Communication between the subretinal space and the vitreous cavity in the morning glory syndrome. *Graefes Arch Clin Exp Ophthalmol* 1995;233:441.
23. Cooling RJ, Rice NS, McLeod D. Retinal detachment in congenital glaucoma. *Br J Ophthalmol* 1980;64:417.
24. Coonan P, Fung WE, Webster RG, et al. The incidence of retinal detachment following extracapsular cataract extraction: a ten-year study. *Ophthalmology* 1985;92:1096.
25. Cousins S, Boniuk I, Okun E, et al. Pseudophakic retinal detachments in the presence of various IOL types. *Ophthalmology* 1986;93:1198.
26. Cox MS, Freeman HM. Retinal detachment due to ocular penetration. *Arch Ophthalmol* 1976;96:1354.
27. Cox MS, Freeman HM. Traumatic retinal detachment. In: Freeman HM, ed. *Ocular Trauma*. New York: Appleton-Century-Crofts, 1979:285.
28. Cox MS, Schepens CL, Freeman HM. Retinal detachment due to ocular contusion. *Arch Ophthalmol* 1966;76:678.
29. Doden W, Stark N. Retina and vitreous findings after serious indirect eye trauma. *Klin Monatsbl Augenheilkd* 1974;614:32.
30. Duker JS, Blumenkranz MS. Diagnosis and management of the acute retinal necrosis (ARN) syndrome. *Surv Ophthalmol* 1991;35:327.
31. Endophthalmitis Vitrectomy Study Group. Results of the Endophthalmitis Vitrectomy Study: a randomized trial of immediate vitrectomy and of intravenous antibiotics for the treatment of postoperative bacterial endophthalmitis: Endophthalmitis Vitrectomy Study Group. *Arch Ophthalmol* 1995;113:1479.
32. Eye Disease Case-Control Study Group. Risk factors for idiopathic rhegmatogenous retinal detachment. *Am J Epidemiol* 1993;137:749.
33. Ficker LA, Vickers S, Capon MR, et al. Retinal detachment following Nd:YAG posterior capsulotomy. *Eye* 1987;1:86.
34. Foos RY, Simons KB. Vitreous in lattice degeneration of retina. *Ophthalmology* 1984;91:452.
35. George ND, Yates JR, Moore AT. Clinical features in affected males with X-linked retinoschisis. *Arch Ophthalmol* 1996;114:274.
36. Gopal L, Kini MM, Badrinath SS, et al. Management of retinal detachment with choroidal coloboma. *Ophthalmology* 1991;98:1622.
37. Hagler WS, North AW. Retinal dialyses and retinal detachment. *Arch Ophthalmol* 1968;79:376.
38. Hanneken AM, Michels RG. Vitrectomy and scleral buckling methods for proliferative vitreoretinopathy. *Ophthalmology* 1988;95:865.
39. Hirose T, Lee KY, Schepens CL. Wagner's hereditary vitreoretinal degeneration and retinal detachment. *Arch Ophthalmol* 1973;89:176.
40. Ho PC, Tolentino FI. Pseudophakic retinal detachment: surgical success rate with various types of intraocular lenses. *Ophthalmology* 1984;91:847.
41. Hyams SW, Neumann E, Friedman Z. Myopia-aphakia. II. Vitreous and peripheral retina. *Br J Ophthalmol* 1975;59:483.
42. Jaffe N. *Vitreous Detachments*. St Louis: CV Mosby, 1969.
43. Jagger JD, Cooling RJ, Fison LG, et al. Management of retinal detachment following congenital cataract surgery. *Trans Ophthalmol Soc U K* 1983;103:103.
44. Jampol LM, Green JL Jr, Goldberg MF, et al. Update of vitrectomy surgery and retinal detachment repair in sickle cell disease. *Arch Ophthalmol* 1982;100:591.
45. Javitt JC, Tielsch JM, Canner JK, et al. National outcomes of cataract extraction: increased risk of retinal complications associated with Nd:YAG laser capsulotomy. The Cataract Patient Outcomes Research Team [see comments]. *Ophthalmology* 1992;99:1487.
46. Javitt JC, Vitale S, Canner JK, et al. National outcomes of cataract extraction. I. Retinal detachment after inpatient surgery. *Ophthalmology* 1991;98:895.
47. Johnston PB. Traumatic retinal detachment. *Br J Ophthalmol* 1991;75:18.
48. Joondeph HC, Goldberg MF. Rhegmatogenous retinal detachment after tributary vein occlusion. *Am J Ophthalmol* 1975;80:253.

49. Kakehashi A, Trempe CL, Fujio N, et al. Retinal breaks in diabetic retinopathy: vitreoretinal relationships. *Ophthalmic Surg* 1994;25:695.
50. Kanski JJ, Elkington AR, Daniel R. Retinal detachment after congenital cataract surgery. *Br J Ophthalmol* 1974;58:92.
51. Karlin DB, Curtin BJ. Peripheral chorioretinal lesions and axial length of the myopic eye. *Am J Ophthalmol* 1976;81:625.
52. Kerrison JB, Marsh M, Stark WJ, et al. Phacoemulsification after retinal detachment surgery. *Ophthalmology* 1996;103:216.
53. Knobloch WH, Layer JM. Clefting syndromes associated with retinal detachment. *Am J Ophthalmol* 1972;73:517.
54. Kraushar MF, Steinberg JA. Miotics and retinal detachment: upgrading the community standard. *Surv Ophthalmol* 1991;35:311.
55. Kusaka S, Kodama T, Ohashi Y. Condensation of silicone oil on the posterior surface of a silicone intraocular lens during vitrectomy. *Am J Ophthalmol* 1996;121:574.
56. Laatikainen L, Tolppanen EM, Harju H. Epidemiology of rhegmatogenous retinal detachment in a Finnish population. *Acta Ophthalmol* 1985;63:59.
57. Labelle P, Brunet M, Basmadjian G, et al. Retinal detachment following intraocular foreign body. *Can J Ophthalmol* 1974;9:2.
58. Lindstrom RL. Retinal detachment in axial myopia. *Dev Ophthalmol* 1987;14:37.
59. Lusky M, Weinberger D, Ben-Sira I. The prevalence of retinal detachment in aphakic high myopic patients. *Ophthalmic Surg* 1987;18:444.
60. Maguire JI, Benson WE. Retinal injury and detachment in boxers. *JAMA* 1986;255:2451.
61. Matsuo T, Shiraga F, Matsuo N. Intraoperative observation of the vitreous base in patients with atopic dermatitis and retinal detachment. *Retina* 1995;15:286.
62. Maumenee IH. Vitreoretinal degeneration as a sign of generalized, connective tissue diseases. *Am J Ophthalmol* 1979;88:432.
63. Maumenee IH, Stoll HU, Mets MB. The Wagner syndrome versus hereditary arthroophthalmopathy. *Trans Am Ophthalmol Soc* 1982;80:349.
64. McDonald HR, Lewis H, Brown G, et al. Vitreous surgery for retinal detachment associated with choroidal coloboma. *Arch Ophthalmol* 1991;109:1399.
65. Nakatsu A, Wada Y, Kondo T. Retinal detachment in patients with atopic dermatitis: 5-year retrospective survey. *Ophthalmologica* 1995;209:160.
66. Nelson L, Maumenee I. Ectopia lentis. *Surv Ophthalmol* 1982;27:143.
67. Nielsen NE, Naeser K. Epidemiology of retinal detachment following extracapsular cataract extraction: a follow-up study with an analysis of risk factors. *J Cataract Refract Surg* 1993;19:675.
68. Ninn-Pedersen K, Bauer B. Cataract patients in a defined Swedish population, 1986 to 1990. V. Postoperative retinal detachments. *Arch Ophthalmol* 1996;114:382.
69. Ober RR, Wilkinson CP, Fiore JV Jr, et al. Rhegmatogenous retinal detachment after neodymium-YAG laser capsulotomy in phakic and pseudophakic eyes. *Am J Ophthalmol* 1986;101:81.
70. Oka C, Ideta H, Nagasaki H, et al. Retinal detachment with atopic dermatitis similar to traumatic retinal detachment. *Ophthalmology* 1994;101:1050.
71. Pemberton JW, Freeman HM, Schepens CL. Familial retinal detachment and the Ehlers–Danlos syndrome. *Arch Ophthalmol* 1966;76:817.
72. Percival SPB. Late complications from posterior segment intraocular foreign bodies. *Br J Ophthalmol* 1972;56:462.
73. Phelps CD, Burton TC. Glaucoma and retinal detachment. *Arch Ophthalmol* 1977;95:418.
74. Pieramici D, MacCumber M, Humayan M, et al. Open-globe injury: update on types of injury and visual results. *Ophthalmology* 1996;103:1798.
75. Regillo CD, Tasman WS, Brown GC. Surgical management of complications associated with X-linked retinoschisis. *Arch Ophthalmol* 1993;111:1080.
76. Robinson MR, Streeten BW. The surface morphology of retinal breaks and lattice retinal degeneration: a scanning electron microscopic study. *Ophthalmology* 1986;93:237.
77. Ross WH. Retinal dialysis: lack of evidence for a genetic cause. *Can J Ophthalmol* 1991;26:309.
78. Ruben M, Rajpurohit P. Distribution of myopia in aphakic retinal detachments. *Br J Ophthalmol* 1976;60:517.
79. Ryan SJ, Goldberg MF. Anterior segment ischemia following scleral buckling in sickle cell hemoglobinopathy. *Retina* 1986;6:146.
80. Sandy CJ, Bloom PA, Graham EM, et al. Retinal detachment in AIDS-related cytomegalovirus retinitis. *Eye* 1995;9:277.
81. Schubert HD. Schisis-like rhegmatogenous retinal detachment associated with choroidal colobomas. *Graefes Arch Clin Exp Ophthalmol* 1995;233:74.
82. Sellors PJ, Mooney D. Fundus changes after traumatic hyphaema. *Br J Ophthalmol* 1973;57:600.
83. Shammas HF, Halasa AH, Faris BM. Intraocular pressure, cup-disc ratio, and steroid responsiveness in retinal detachment. *Arch Ophthalmol* 1976;94:1108.
84. Sidikaro Y, Silver L, Holland GN, et al. Rhegmatogenous retinal detachments in patients with AIDS and necrotizing retinal infections. *Ophthalmology* 1991;98:129.

85. Smiddy WE, Green WR. Retinal dialysis: pathology and pathogenesis. *Retina* 1982;2:94.
86. Snead MP, Payne SJ, Barton DE, et al. Stickler syndrome: correlation between vitreoretinal phenotypes and linkage to COL 2A1. *Eye* 1994;8:609.
87. Stein R, Pinchas A, Treister G. Prevention of retinal detachment by a circumferential barrage prior to lens extraction in high myopic eyes. *Ophthalmologica* 1972;165:125.
88. Stickler GB, Belau PG, Farrell FJ, et al. Hereditary progressive arthro-ophthalmopathy. *Mayo Clin Proc* 1965;40:433.
89. Straatsma BR, Zeegen PD, Foos RY, et al. Lattice degeneration of the retina: XXX Edward Jackson Memorial Lecture. *Am J Ophthalmol* 1974;77:619.
90. Streeten BW, Bert M. Retinal surface in lattice degeneration of the retina. *Am J Ophthalmol* 1972;74:1201.
91. Tasman W. Peripheral retinal changes following blunt trauma. *Trans Am Ophthalmol Soc* 1972;70:190.
92. Tasman W. Retinal detachment secondary to proliferative diabetic retinopathy. *Arch Ophthalmol* 1972;87:286.
93. Tasman W. Vitreoretinal changes in cicatricial retrolental fibroplasia. *Trans Am Ophthalmol Soc* 1970;68:548.
94. Tielsch J, Legro M, Cassard S, et al. Risk factors for retinal detachment after cataract surgery: a population-based case control study. *Ophthalmology* 1996;103:1537.
95. Tillery WV, Lucier AC. Round atrophic holes in lattice degeneration: an important cause of phakic retinal detachment. *Trans Am Acad Ophthalmol Otolaryngol* 1976;81:509.
96. Tornquist R, Stenkula S, Tornquist P. Retinal detachment: a study of a population-based patient material in Sweden 1971–1981. I. Epidemiology. *Acta Ophthalmol* 1987;65:213.
97. Toyofuku H, Hirose T, Schepens CL. Retinal detachment following congenital cataract surgery. I. Preoperative findings in 114 eyes. *Arch Ophthalmol* 1980;98:669.
98. Trese MT, Ferrone PJ. The role of inner wall retinectomy in the management of juvenile retinoschisis. *Graefes Arch Clin Exp Ophthalmol* 1995;233:706.
99. Vaiser A, Jost BF. Bilateral inferotemporal dialysis in identical twins. *Ann Ophthalmol* 1992;24:378.
100. Verdaguer J. Juvenile retinal detachment. *Am J Ophthalmol* 1982;93:145.
101. Verdaguer TJ, Rojas B, Lechuga M. Genetical studies in nontraumatic retinal dialysis. *Mod Probl Ophthalmol* 1975;15:34.
102. Weidenthal DT, Schepens CL. Peripheral fundus changes associated with ocular contusion. *Am J Ophthalmol* 1966;62:465.
103. Weseley P, Liebmann J, Walsh JB, et al. Lattice degeneration of the retina and the pigment dispersion syndrome. *Am J Ophthalmol* 1992;114:539.
104. Wilkes SR, Beard CM, Kurland LT, et al. The incidence of retinal detachment in Rochester, Minnesota, 1970–1978. *Am J Ophthalmol* 1982;94:670.
105. Wilkinson CP. Pseudophakic retinal detachments. *Retina* 1985;5:1.
106. Winslow RL, Tasman W. Juvenile rhegmatogenous retinal detachment. *Ophthalmology* 1978;85:607.
107. Zion VM, Burton TC. Retinal dialysis. *Arch Ophthalmol* 1980;98:1971.

4
History

The history of the diagnosis and management of retinal detachment begins, for all practical purposes, with the invention of the ophthalmoscope by von Helmholtz in 1851 (87). He thereby provided not only the means for accurate clinical descriptions of retinal detachment but also an impetus for its cure.

Numerous ingenious, but incorrect, theories of etiology and inventive, but misguided, attempts at treatment preceded the postulation of the rhegmatogenous theory by de Wecker, Leber, and Gonin. The Gonin Era started in 1919, when Gonin performed the first operation in which the goal of surgery was to cure the detachment by closing the breaks and includes many advances in techniques to create a chorioretinal scar. The Schepens-Custodis-Lincoff Era began in 1947 when Schepens invented the electric binocular ophthalmoscope and includes the introduction of scleral buckling (SB) and cryotherapy. The invention of pars plana vitrectomy in 1971 ushered in the Machemer Era.

THE EARLY PERIOD (1851–1918)

Instruments for Examination

Shortly after the invention of the direct ophthalmoscope by von Helmholtz in 1851, accurate clinical descriptions of retinal detachment were reported by von Graefe (85) and von Arlt (83). In 1852, Ruete introduced the monocular indirect ophthalmoscope (66). This instrument was later improved by an electric bulb light source upon and remained popular in Europe for many years. In 1861, Giraud-Teulon invented a binocular indirect ophthalmoscope (20).

It is amazing what the early ophthalmoscopists were able to see with reflected candle or lamp light. Better illumination was provided in 1885 by the first electric ophthalmoscope (14). In 1900, Trantas, with the aid of the direct ophthalmoscope, examined the anterior portion of the retina using his thumb to depress the sclera (81). Gullstrand's invention of the slit lamp in 1911 was another important advance (27). In conjunction with either the pre-corneal lenses of Lemoine and Valois (82) or Hruby (30), or with Koeppe's corneal contact lens (34), the slit lamp provided a binocular view of the posterior portions of the eye.

Incorrect Theories of Etiology

Theory of Distension

It was soon recognized that retinal detachment was much more frequent in myopic than in emmetropic and hyperopic eyes. Von Graefe proposed that the retina detached because

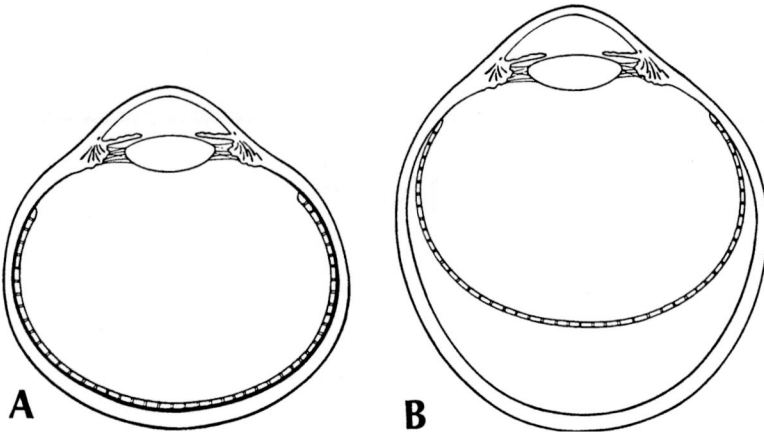

FIGURE 4-1. Theory of distension. **A:** Normal eye. **B:** As the eye enlarges in high myopia the "less elastic" retina detaches.

it was less elastic than the choroid and the sclera, which stretched as the globe became larger (Fig. 4-1) (84).

Theory of Hypotony

Because eyes with retinal detachment often have decreased intraocular pressure, and because many eyes which suffer vitreous loss during cataract surgery later develop retinal detachment, some physicians hypothesized that a reduction of "vitreous pressure" induced detachment. They held that the formed vitreous gel, in its normal state, helped to counter-balance "hydrostatic pressure" exerted by the choroid (21). Iwanoff supplied histopathological evidence for this theory when he found vitreous liquefaction and posterior vitreous detachment (PVD) in most eyes with retinal detachment (31). Supposedly, the liquid vitreous did not exert as much pressure as did the normal vitreous gel (Fig 4-2).

Theory of Exudation

Recognizing that severe nephritis and toxemia of pregnancy, conditions in which generalized edema is common, are both causes of retinal detachment, certain ophthalmologists postulated that exudation of fluid from the choroid caused detachment (Fig. 4-3). We now know, of course, that the retinal detachment in these conditions is non-rhegmatogenous in nature and is reversible with treatment of the underlying disease state. A variant of the exudation theory, taking into consideration the inflammation noted in many eyes with retinal detachment, proposed that the inflamed choroid exuded a highly albuminous fluid under the retina (Fig. 4-4A) (64). Osmotic pressure exerted by this exudate purportedly drew water from the vitreous through the retina, thereby elevating it from the choroid (see Fig. 4-4B). Supporters of this theory felt that retinal breaks noted on clinical examination were secondary to the force of this exudative fluid. Since the edges of many tears were noted to be rolled outward, it seemed likely that fluid was passing from the subretinal space into the vitreous cavity.

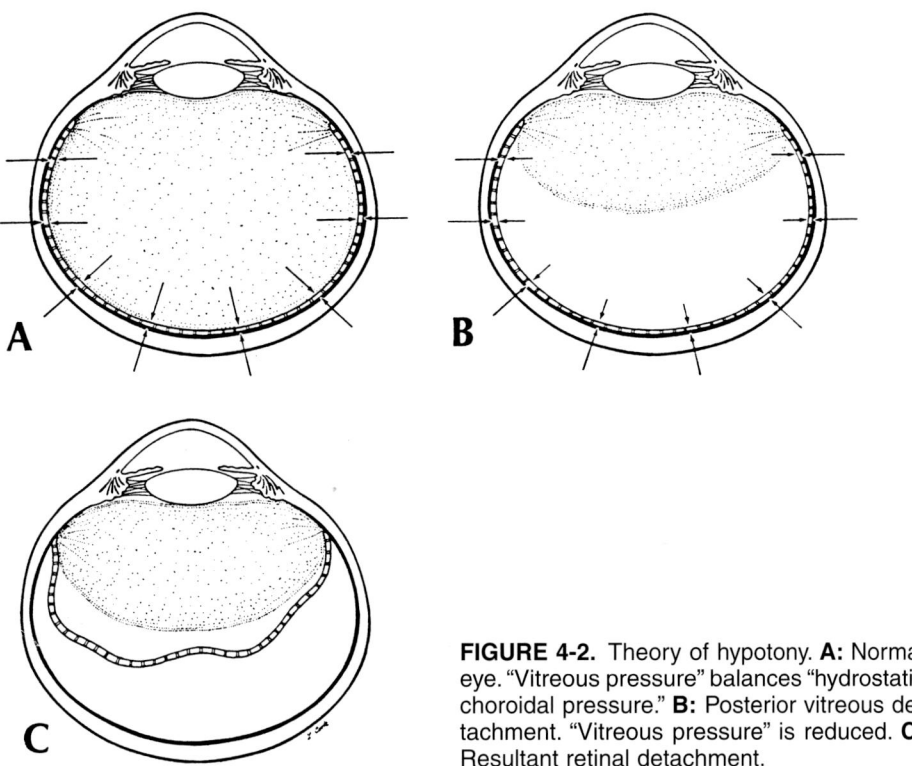

FIGURE 4-2. Theory of hypotony. **A:** Normal eye. "Vitreous pressure" balances "hydrostatic choroidal pressure." **B:** Posterior vitreous detachment. "Vitreous pressure" is reduced. **C:** Resultant retinal detachment.

Attempts at Treatment

Since the main problem in retinal detachment appeared to be fluid under the retina, it is not surprising that the earliest attempted treatment was simple drainage of the fluid (86). Very few cures resulted, as the fluid quickly reaccumulated postoperatively.

A different approach was taken by those who felt that retinal detachment was caused by exudation. These surgeons deliberately slashed holes in the retina to allow the subretinal fluid (SRF) to pass into the vitreous (86). The same tactic was tried by those who felt that the stiff retina would not reattach unless relaxing incisions were made (78). An-

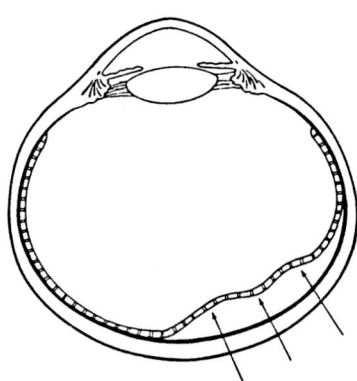

FIGURE 4-3. Theory of exudation. An outpouring of fluid from the choroid elevates the retina.

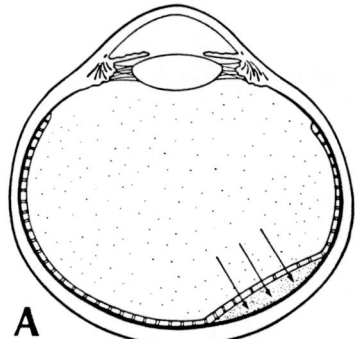 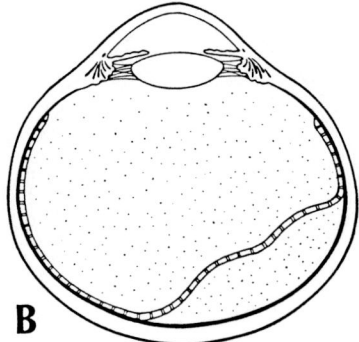

FIGURE 4-4. Theory of exudation. Diffusion variant. **A:** The osmotic pressure of the protein-rich choroidal exudate draws water from the protein-poor vitreous through the retina. **B:** Diffusion continues until the osmotic pressure is equal on both sides of the retina.

other futile attempt to counteract exudation was the injection of hypertonic (30%) saline under the conjunctiva to draw out the SRF.

Some surgeons attempted to create scars between the retina and pigment epithelium to hold the retina in place (13). Thermocautery and direct current electricity (galvanocautery) were two early treatment modalities. The treatment was not directed at retinal breaks but was randomly applied in the area of the detachment. Other surgeons tried to suture the retina to the choroid (18). On histopathological examination, Müller found vitreoretinal fibrous bands which he felt were pulling the retina forward and causing the detachment (60). His finding led Deutschmann to postulate that the retina could be reattached only if the vitreous bands were sectioned (15). He introduced a fine knife into the vitreous and slashed backwards and forwards in an effort to sever them. The retinal tears which were sometimes produced in the process were not felt to be a complication, on the contrary, it was believed that the holes would help the retina to settle.

The theory of distension suggested another form of therapy. Since the retina was too short for the size of the globe, it seemed necessary to make the globe smaller. Müller introduced the scleral resection operation in 1903. He excised a full-thickness wedge of sclera and then sewed the edges together (61).

THE GONIN ERA (1919–1947)

Rhegmatogenous Theory

Coccius was the first to find retinal breaks on clinical examination (9), but deWecker first suggested that they were the cause of what was then called spontaneous retinal detachment (12). He felt that liquid vitreous forced holes in the retina. Leber found retinal breaks in 70% of recent retinal detachments and noted that there was nearly always a retinal break in the area where the retinal detachment started (40). His own clinical and histopathological findings led him to conclude that vitreous traction, caused by degeneration and collapse of the vitreous body, tore holes in the retina. Liquefied vitreous passed through these holes and under the retina, causing the detachment.

It is apparent that at this point Leber understood the etiology of retinal detachment. In 1908, however, influenced more by histopathological than by clinical findings, he abandoned his initial theory in favor of an incorrect one (38,39). He now postulated that retinitis stimulated the growth of preretinal membranes which later contracted, tearing holes in the retina. He still recognized the importance of retinal breaks in the genesis of retinal detachment, but he now maintained that vitreous degeneration was secondary to the detachment, and not its precipitating event. It is apparent from Leber's drawings that his error stemmed from studying cases of retinal detachment with proliferative vitreoretinopathy (PVR).

Ignipuncture (Thermocautery) Operation

Jules Gonin, the father of retinal detachment surgery, revived Leber's first theory (16,67), stressing that contraction of the vitreous body tore holes in the retina. The tears occurred at sites of abnormal vitreoretinal adhesion caused by either a previous chorioretinitis or by chorioretinal degeneration. Once Gonin realized that the breaks found in retinal detachment were the cause of the detachment, he knew that a permanent cure depended on sealing them. In 1919, he performed the first operation designed to close the breaks (22,23). After careful localization of the break, he made a radial incision down to the choroid with a Graefe knife. The same knife was then used to drain the SRF. Next, a red-hot cautery was inserted 2 to 3 mm into the wound and held in place for 2 to 3 seconds to insure that the retina had been directly cauterized (Fig. 4-5). It was not until 1929 that the world became convinced that Gonin's operation would cure retinal detachment (23).

Gonin had achieved a miracle. Retinal detachment, which had previously been considered inoperable, now had a surgical success rate of 40% to 50%. Gonin's two principles have remained the basis for all successful retinal detachment surgery. The first is that all breaks must be found. He emphasized careful clinical examination to this end. The second principle is that all breaks must be accurately localized so that they can be sealed by the treatment. Gonin recognized that a surgical failure meant either that the retinal break was not properly closed or that another break existed which had not yet been found. Once it was recognized that sealing the hole would cure a detachment, others quickly improved upon Gonin's original operation. Its complications included intraocular hemorrhage and vitreous loss with retinal incarceration. Retinal folds often prevented reattachment of the retina. Fibrous ingrowth caused late redetachment. Another problem was that an essential part of the operation, exact localization of the break on the sclera, was extremely difficult. Because of the severe hypotony

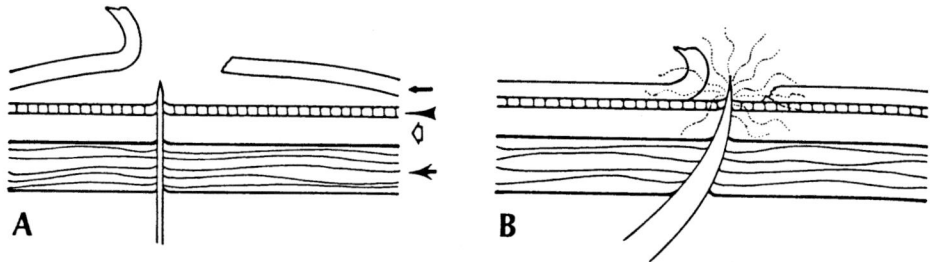

FIGURE 4-5. Gonin's operation. **A:** Drainage of subretinal fluid by a Graefe knife. *Small arrow* indicates the retina; *arrowhead*, the pigment epithelium; *open arrow*, the choroid, and *large arrow*, the sclera. **B:** Coagulation of the choroid by thermocautery.

which followed removal of the cautery, only one puncture could be performed in a single operation. Therefore, if the localization were incorrect and the retinal break inadequately treated, a second operation became necessary. Furthermore, since only one break could be treated at a time, cases with multiple breaks required multiple operations.

Early Improvements on Ignipuncture

Guist's Operation (Multiple Trephination)

Guist trephined out multiple plugs of sclera surrounding the retinal tear(s) and treated the bare choroid with a potassium hydroxide stick (26). Once the SRF had been drained, chorioretinal scars formed and walled off the retinal break (Fig. 4-6).

Larsson's Operation (Surface Diathermy)

When electric current flows in a resistive conductor such as the tissues of the eye, the heat generated causes localized coagulation. Larsson used this principle to surround the retinal break with a firm chorioretinal scar (36,37). He found that applications of diathermy (radio frequency electric current) to full-thickness sclera coagulated the choroid (Fig. 4-7). Drainage of the SRF then brought the retina into contact with the treated choroid. If no tears could be found, he scattered treatment in the area which he felt had detached first.

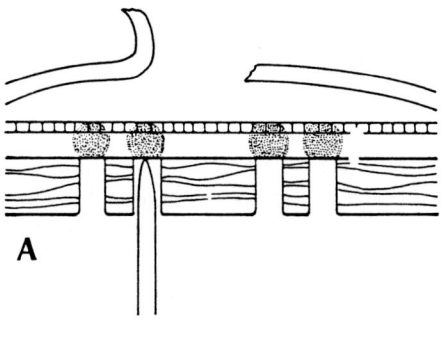

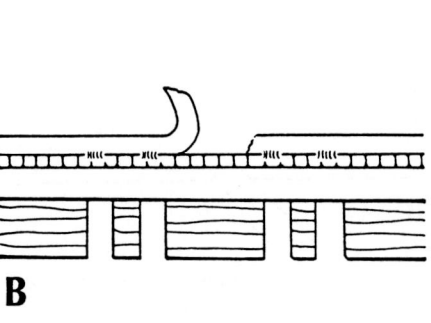

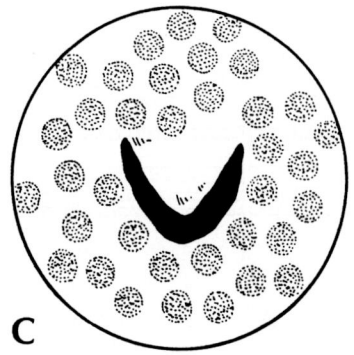

FIGURE 4-6. Guist's operation. **A:** Multiple plugs of sclera have been trephined out to allow cautery of the choroid by a potassium hydroxide stick. **B:** Chorioretinal scars after drainage of subretinal fluid. **C:** The scars surround the retinal break.

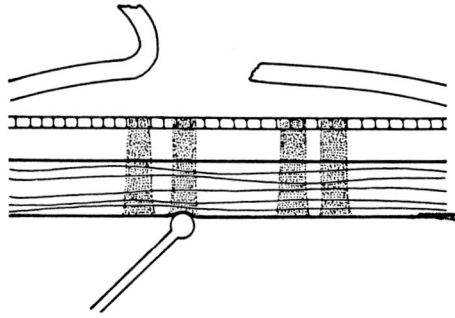

FIGURE 4-7. Larsson's operation. Applications of full-thickness diathermy surround the break.

Weve's Operation (Penetrating Diathermy)

Weve improved upon Gonin's procedure by substituting penetrating diathermy for heat cautery (89). A fine needle electrode introduced into the eye coagulated the choroid and the retina. Gonin's procedure allowed only a single application of cautery, whereas Weve's operation made multiple applications of treatment possible. His rate of success was therefore higher because his chances of sealing the break were better. Coagulation of the retina appeared as a white mark which could be observed with an ophthalmoscope and used as a guide in positioning the next penetration. Each time the needle was removed form the sclera, there was some drainage of SRF. The procedure was continued until the tear was completely surrounded by treatment. The major advantage of this procedure was that at the end of the procedure the retinal break was completely treated and no SRF was present. As in Gonin's operation, however, vitreous was occasionally lost and the punctures sometimes produced new retinal holes.

Šafář's Operation (Simultaneous Multiple Puncture)

Šafář mounted fine needles on small conducting plates (68). He inserted the needles around the break piercing the sclera, choroid, and pigment epithelium. No needles were removed until diathermy had been applied to all of the plates (Fig. 4-8). Therefore, there was neither premature drainage of SRF nor vitreous loss. When the needles were removed, the SRF slowly oozed out. This operation was popularized in the United States by Walker and Pischel (88).

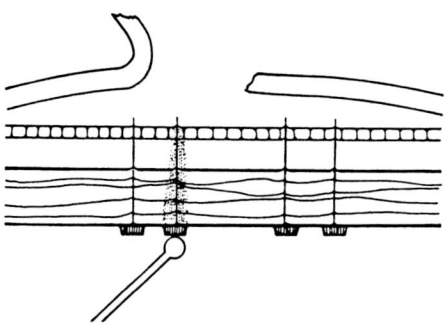

FIGURE 4-8. Šafář's operation. Diathermy is applied to multiple fine needles which perforate the sclera, choroid, and pigment epithelium.

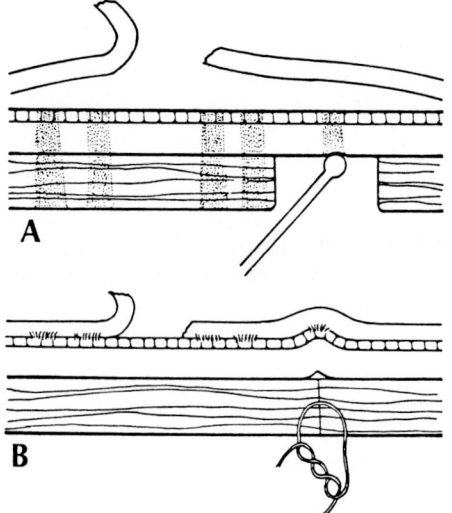

FIGURE 4-9. Lindner's operation. **A:** The bar choroid is cauterized by potassium hydroxide after a strip of full-thickness sclera has been removed. **B:** The edges are sutured together. Shortening the sclera was the goal of the operation. The location of the resection did not necessarily correspond to the location of the break(s).

Lindner's Operation (Scleral Resection)

In 1931, Lindner revived Müller's scleral resection operation, i.e., removal of a full-thickness strip of sclera (49–52). The bare choroid was coagulated by potassium hydroxide (Fig. 4-9). This operation had two theoretical benefits. First, it reduced the volume of the eye so that the retina could more easily fall into place; and second, multiple holes could be treated. However, the operation was dangerous and difficult. Deep lamellar resection, a safer and easier variation, had been abandoned by Lindner as ineffectual, but Shapland (77) and Paufique (63) revived it as an improvement in the early 1950s (Fig. 4-10). They recognized that this procedure, in which a very thin layer of sclera was left over the choroid, had the additional benefit of causing a broad area of inflammation which could treat unseen retinal tears.

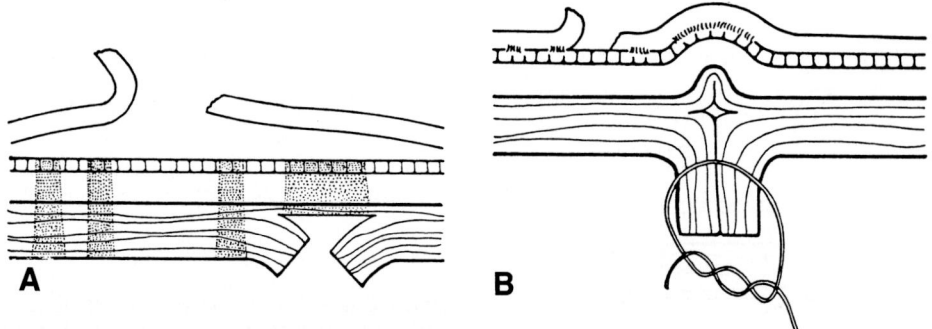

FIGURE 4-10. Shapland and Paufique's operation. **A:** Diathermy or potassium hydroxide coagulation is applied in the bed of the lamellar dissection. Diathermy surrounds the break. **B:** The scleral flaps are closed, shortening the sclera.

THE CUSTODIS–SCHEPENS–LINCOFF ERA (1947–1971)

Instruments for Examination

The current high rate of reattachment is due not only to improvements in surgical technique but also to improved methods of ocular examination. Two significant advances in fundus examination were made in the late 1940s. Charles Schepens' electrically illuminated binocular indirect ophthalmoscope is, by far, the most valuable instrument currently available for evaluation of the detached retina (see chapter 6, Fundus Examination and Preoperative Management) (69). Additional important information is obtained with the Goldmann three-mirror lens, which permits stereoscopic slit lamp examination of almost the entire retina if the pupil can be widely dilated and if the ocular media are clear. It is especially useful for finding small breaks and for evaluating the vitreous. More recently, wide-angle contact lenses combined with scleral depression have been found to be useful in patients with small pupils (43).

Intravitreal Air Injection

In 1938, Rosengren (65) increased the rate of reattachment by injecting air into the vitreous to tamponade the retinal break after diathermy treatment and drainage of SRF. Postoperatively, the patient had to be positioned so that the air rose against the hole (Fig. 4-11). Using this technique, Rosengren was able to achieve successful reattachment in 76% of his cases (65).

Scleral Buckling Explants

In the history of retinal detachment surgery, scleral indentation ("buckling"), introduced by Ernst Custodis in 1953, is second in importance only to the contributions of Jules Gonin. Custodis called his procedure plombenaufnähung, literally, the sewing on of a seal (10,11). He first treated all breaks with surface diathermy and then closed them by sewing a polyviol explant (the plombe) onto the overlying sclera. The indenting explant reduced vitreous traction and closed the break, allowing a firm chorioretinal scar to form

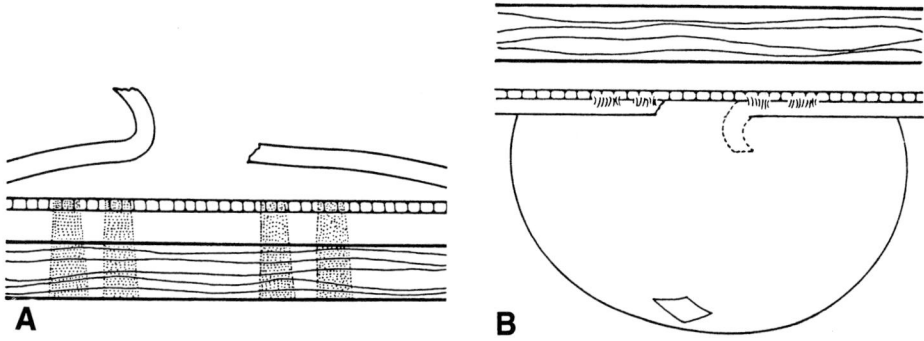

FIGURE 4-11. Rosengren's operation. **A:** Application of full-thickness diathermy to surround the break. **B:** After drainage of the subretinal fluid, air is injected in to the vitreous cavity. The patient is positioned so that air tamponades the break and pushes it toward the choroid.

(Fig. 4-12). Custodis emphasized that the explant must be large enough to close the entire retinal break, since a misplaced explant can keep the break open (80).

In addition to permanently reducing vitreous traction, Custodis' explant technique made drainage of SRF unnecessary in many cases. He found that even if the break remained open at the end of the operation, a properly placed and correctly sized explant would result in successful reattachment of the retina. He was able to cure 84% of his cases.

A major complication of Custodis' operation was that the surface diathermy caused scleral necrosis. If a reoperation became necessary, it was difficult to place sutures in the thinned sclera. Photocoagulation, invented by Meyer-Schwickerath, eliminated this complication (59). The explant was placed, and, either immediately or 1 to 2 days later, the breaks were treated with photocoagulation (3,19,29). Unfortunately, because xenon arc photocoagulation requires anesthesia, the patient was often subjected to 2 operative procedures. Moreover, successful treatment is dependent upon wide dilation of the pupil, which is sometimes impossible immediately after a SB procedure.

Lincoff made the next major advance in explant technique by adapting cryotherapy for retinal surgery (47). This was a more benign treatment than its predecessors, as it did not cause scleral necrosis. Lincoff also introduced a soft silicone sponge material (41) for use as an explant, and a spatula needle (48) for safe scleral suturing. His latest contribution is the temporary balloon buckling device (see below and chapter 9, Alternative Techniques) (46).

Scleral Buckling Implants

One of the main problems in the use of diathermy was judging the effect on the choroid of applications made on full-thickness sclera. If the applications were not heavy enough, the retinal seal was inadequate. If the applications were too heavy, there was excessive scleral necrosis. Schepens, Black, and Clark realized independently that Shapland's lamellar scleral resection could be used to thin the sclera so that the diathermy could be evenly and accurately applied to the choroid around the break (2,8,73). Then, when the

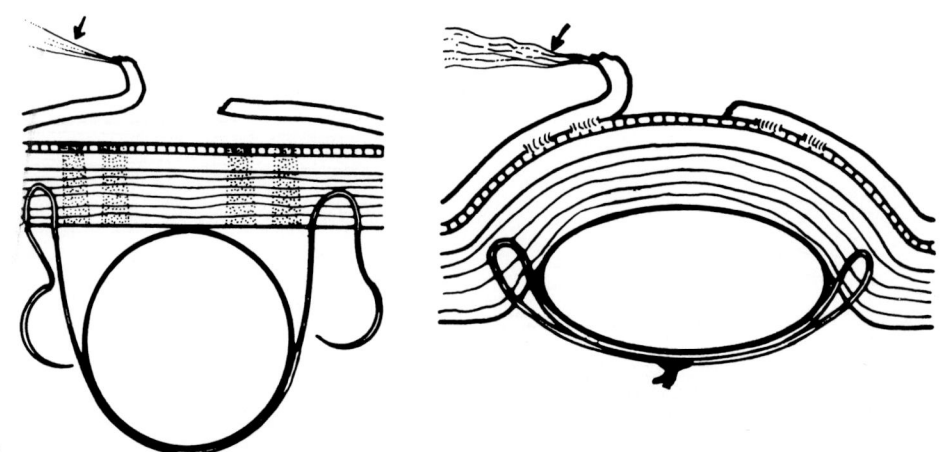

FIGURE 4-12. Custodis operation. **A:** Applications of full-thickness diathermy to surround the break. Explant and sutures are positioned. Note vitreous traction (*arrow*). **B:** The retinal break is closed by the indented ("buckled") sclera. The vitreous traction (*arrow*) is released.

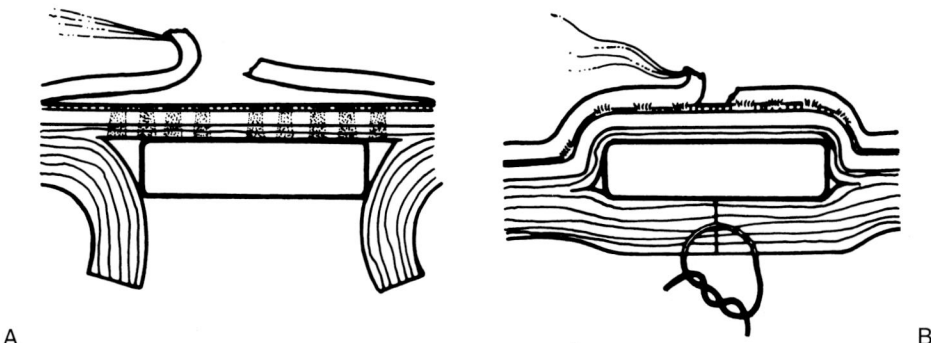

FIGURE 4-13. Schepens' operation. **A:** Diathermy is applied in the bed of the lamellar scleral dissection. Implant is positioned. **B:** Sutured scleral flaps enclose the implant. Vitreous traction is reduced.

scleral flaps were closed, the sclera was nearly restored to its original strength. Schepens pioneered the use of implants (various materials buried in the bed of a lamellar scleral dissection) to reduce vitreous traction and to prevent posterior progression of the detachment (73). Originally, he buried polyethylene tubing at the posterior end of the most posterior break and drained the SRF. The implant was intended to act as a postoperative "dyke," preventing posterior leakage of SRF from any open anterior break. He later used implants made of solid silicone to completely close all retinal breaks (Fig. 4-13) (74). Another of Schepens' important contributions was the introduction of the encircling procedure to permanently reduce vitreous traction (70,71,72,74). Dr. Schepens' remarkable career has seen the success rate for surgery at the Massachusetts Eye and Ear Infirmary improve from 40% in 1947 to 90% in 1960, to close to 98% today (28).

THE MACHEMER ERA

Pars Plana Vitrectomy

The first rational attempts at vitreous surgery were made by Cibis (6,7). He realized that in eyes with PVR, preretinal and vitreous membranes prevented settling of the retina. He slowly injected liquid silicone under these membranes to strip them from the retinal surface. Although many of these eyes had complications from the silicone or subsequent redetachment of the retina, some otherwise hopelessly lost eyes were saved.

Kasner performed the first planned open-sky vitrectomy in 1966 (32). Shortly thereafter, Robert Machemer made a great advance in retinal surgery with the invention of the vitreous infusion suction cutter (VISC) and the development of pars plana vitrectomy (53). Modern pars plana vitrectomy techniques have dramatically increased the surgical success rate for retinal detachment caused by giant tears, macular holes, proliferative retinopathies, and penetrating injuries and for those complicated by PVR (see chapter 10, Surgery of Complicated Cases).

Pneumatic Retinopexy (PR)

Fineberg and Norton were the first to use sulfur hexafluoride gas (SF_6) as an adjunct to scleral buckles to help close the breaks. This relatively insoluble gas has major advantages over air. If undiluted, it expands within the eye, so that a small injection volume results in a large bubble. Further, it is absorbed slowly, remaining for two weeks (62). Kreissig and Lincoff were the first to report the use of SF_6, without drainage, curing detachments with large retinal breaks (35,42,45). In the mid-1980s, Dominguez and Hilton independently described the use of gas to treat and cure a much larger number of retinal detachments.

The procedure, called pneumocausis by Dominguez and PR by Hilton, is quite simple. The break is treated with cryotherapy and then tamponaded with gas injected into the vitreous cavity. Postoperatively, the patient is positioned so that the gas bubble rises against the retinal break. The SRF is absorbed and a chorioretinal adhesion forms around the break (see chapter 8, Pneumatic Retinopexy, for further details).

Silicone Oil

Recent progress has concentrated on treating retinal detachments complicated by PVR. Until we have pharmacological means of preventing this proliferation, cures will depend on their mechanical removal and on the ability to tamponade the retinal breaks until a firm chorioretinal scar can form. Long-lasting gases often are sufficient, but in some cases, when they are absorbed, the detachment recurs. After Cibis, the use of silicone oil fell into disfavor for years, but its use was revived by Scott (75,76) and others (24,25,55–58,79). Although many more complicated retinal detachments can now be repaired with advanced vitrectomy techniques and indefinite internal tamponade with silicone oil, the visual results are not always good and such surgery in patients with a good fellow eye has been questioned (1,54).

Perfluorocarbon Liquids

Even with all the refinements in vitrectomy techniques and the availability of gases and silicone oil, the repair of giant tears, especially those with rolled-over retina, was very difficult until the relatively recent introduction of the heavier-than-water perfluorocarbon liquids (PFCL). Now, retinal detachments caused by giant tears can be easily reattached in most cases. In addition, these liquids have been found to be useful in the management of other complicated retinal detachments such as those associated with trauma or PVR (see chapter 10, Surgery of Complicated Cases) (4,5).

Primary Vitrectomy

Pars plana vitrectomy without SB was introduced in Europe by Kloti and in the United States by Escoffrey (17,33). Currently, the procedure consists of a pars plana vitrectomy with careful excision of the vitreous base. Subretinal fluid is removed during an air-liquid exchange through a posterior drainage retinotomy or through the original retinal break. The breaks are treated with laser photocoagulation. In addition, some surgeons place several rows of laser posterior to the entire circumference of the vitreous base.

Temporary Balloon Device

Lincoff and Kreissig have long been champions of non-drainage SB procedures. Their development of a balloon catheter advances this technique another degree. It is an inflatable device that is placed under Tenon's capsule and under the retinal break so that it temporarily buckles it, promoting absorption of the SRF (44,46). Further, since the balloon is removed after a week or so and since no foreign material is sutured to the eye, many complications of permanent SB are avoided (see chapter 9, Alternative Techniques).

REFERENCES

1. Andenmatten R, Gonvers M. Sophisticated vitreoretinal surgery in patients with a healthy fellow eye: an 11-year retrospective study. *Graefes Arch Clin Exp Ophthalmol* 1993;231:495.
2. Black G. The role of the sclera in operations upon simple detachment of the retina. *Trans Ophthalmol Soc U K* 1957;77:89.
3. Böke W. Über die Kombination der Plombenaufnähung mit der Lichtkoagulation zur Behandlung der Netzhautablösung. *Klin Monatsbl Augenheilkd* 1960;136:355.
4. Chang S, Coleman DJ, Lincoff H, et al. Perfluoropropane gas in the management of proliferative vitreoretinopathy. *Am J Ophthalmol* 1984;98:180.
5. Chang S, Lincoff HA, Coleman DJ, et al. Perfluorocarbon gases in vitreous surgery. *Ophthalmology* 1985;92:651.
6. Cibis P. *Vitreoretinal Pathology and Surgery in Retinal Detachments.* St. Louis: CV Mosby, 1960.
7. Cibis PA, Becker B, Oakum E, et al. The use of liquid silicone in retinal detachment surgery. *Arch Ophthalmol* 1962;68:590.
8. Clark G. The importance and employment of diathermy in retinal detachment surgery of today. *Arch Ophthalmol* 1958;60:251.
9. Coccius E. *Uber die Anwendung des Augenspiegels nebst Angabe eines neuen Instruments.* Leipzig: Immanuel Muller, 1853.
10. Custodis E. Bedeutet die Plombenaufnähung auf die Sklera eine Fortschritt im der operativen Behandlung der Netzhautablösung? *Ber Dtsch Ophthalmol Ges* 1953;58:102.
11. Custodis E. Scleral buckling without excision and with polyviol implant. In: Schepens C, ed. *Importance of the Vitreous Body in Retina Surgery with Special Emphasis on Reoperations.* St. Louis: CV Mosby, 1960:175.
12. de Wecker L, de Jaeger E. *Traité des maladies du fond de l'oeil et atlas d'ophtalmoscopie.* Paris: Adrian Delahaye, 1870:151.
13. de Wecker L, Masselon J. Emploi de la galvanocaustique en chirurgie oculaire. *Ann Oculist* 1882;87:39.
14. Dennett W. The electric light ophthalmoscope. *Trans Am Ophthalmol Soc* 1885;4:156.
15. Deutschmann R. Ueber ein neues Heilverfahren bei Netzhautablösung. *Beitr Augenheilkd* 1895;2:849.
16. Dufour M, Gonin J. Décollement rétinien. In: Lagrange F, Valude E, eds. *Encyclopédie française d'ophtalmologie.* Paris: Octave Doin, 1906:975.
17. Escoffery RF, Olk RJ, Grand MG, et al. Vitrectomy without scleral buckling for primary rhegmatogenous retinal detachment. *Am J Ophthalmol* 1985;99:275.
18. Galezowski X. Des différentes variétés des décollements de la rétine at leur traitement. *Recueil Ophtal* 1883–1884;5:669.
19. Girard LJ, McPherson AR. Scleral buckling: full thickness and circumferential, using silicone rubber rodding and photocoagulation. *Arch Ophthalmol* 1962;67:409.
20. Giraud-Teulon M. Note sur un nouvel ophtalmoscope binoculaire. *Bull Acad Med (Paris)* 1860–1861;26:510.
21. Gonin J. Décollement idiopathique: le processus pathogenique. In: *Le Décollement de la rétine.* Lausanne: Librairie Payot, 1934:82.
22. Gonin J. Guérisons operatoires des décollements rétiniens. *Rev Gen Ophthalmol* 1923;37:337.
23. Gonin J. Le traitement opératoire. In: *Le Décollement de la rétine.* Lausanne: Librairie Payot, 1934:138.
24. Gonvers M. Temporary silicone oil tamponade in the management of retinal detachment with proliferative vitreoretinopathy. *Am J Ophthalmol* 1985;100:239.
25. Gonvers M, Thresher R. Temporary use of silicone oil in the treatment of proliferative vitreoretinopathy: an experimental study with a new animal model. *Graefes Arch Clin Exp Ophthalmol* 1983;221:46.
26. Guist G. Eine neue Ablatiooperation. *Z Augenheilkdl* 1931;74:232.
27. Gullstrand A. Demonstration der Nernstspaltlampe. *Ber Dtsch Ophthalmol Ges* 1911;37:374.
28. Guyer D. Interview with Dr. Schepens. *Ophthalmol Times* 1997;22(5):50.
29. Höpping W. Kombination von Lichtkoagulation mit operativen Verfahren bei Netzhautablösung. *Ber Dtsch Ophthalmol Ges* 1961;64:512.
30. Hruby K. Spaltlampenmikroskopie des hinteren Augenabschnittes ohne Kontaktglas. *Klin Montatsbl Augenheilkd* 1942;108:195.
31. Iwanoff A. Beitrage zur normalen und pathologischen Anatomie des Auges. I. Beitrage zur Ablösung des Glaskorpers. *Arch Ophthalmol* 1869;15:1.
32. Kasner D, Miller GF, Sever R, et al. Surgical treatment of amyloidosis of the vitreous. *Trans Am Acad Ophthalmol Otolaryngol* 1968;72:410.
33. Kloti R. Amotio-chirurgie ohne Skleraeindellung: primare Vitrektome. *Klin Monatsbl Augenheilkd* 1983;182:474.

34. Koeppe L. *Die Mikroskopie des lebenden Auges.* Berlin: J. Springer, 1921.
35. Kreissig I. Bisherige Erfahrungen mit SF6-Gas in der Ablatio-chirurgie. *Ber Dtsch Ophthalmol Ges* 1979; 76:553.
36. Larsson S. Electro-endothermy in detachment of the retina. *Arch Ophthalmol* 1932;7:661.
37. Larsson S. Operative Behandlung von Netzhautablösung mit Elektro endothermie und Trepanation. *Acta Ophthalmol* 1930;8:172.
38. Leber T. Die Netzhautablosung. In: Graefe-Saemisch, ed. *Handbuch der gesamten Augenheilkunde,* 2nd ed. Leipzig: Wilheim Englemann, 1916:1374.
39. Leber T. Ueber die Enstehung der Netzhautablösung. *Ber Dtsch Ophthalmol Ges* 1908;35:120.
40. Leber T. Ueber die Entstehung der Netzhautablösung. *Ber Dtsch Ophthalmol Ges* 1882;14:18.
41. Lincoff HA, Baras I, McLean J. Modifications to the Custodis procedure for retinal detachment. *Arch Ophthalmol* 1965;73:160.
42. Lincoff HA, Coleman J, Kreissig I, et al. The perfluorocarbon gases in the treatment of retinal detachment. *Ophthalmology* 1983;90:546.
43. Lincoff HA, Kreissig I. Finding the retinal hole in the pseudophakic eye with detachment. *Am J Ophthalmol* 1994;117:442.
44. Lincoff HA, Kreissig I. Results with a temporary balloon buckle for the repair of retinal detachment. *Am J Ophthalmol* 1981;92:245.
45. Lincoff HA, Kreissig I, Coleman D, et al. Use of an intraocular gas tamponade to find retinal breaks. *Am J Ophthalmol* 1983;96:510.
46. Lincoff HA, Kreissig I, Hahn YS. A temporary balloon buckle for the treatment of small retinal detachments. *Ophthalmology* 1979;86:586.
47. Lincoff HA, McLean JM, Nano H. Cryosurgical treatment of retinal detachment. *Trans Am Acad Ophthalmol Otolaryngol* 1964;68:412.
48. Lincoff HA, Nano H. A new needle for scleral surgery. *Am J Ophthalmol* 1965;60:146.
49. Lindner K. Ein Beitrage zur Entstehung und Behandlung der idiopatischen und der traumatischen Netzhautabhebung. *Graefes Arch Klin Exp Ophthalmol* 1931;127:177.
50. Lindner K. Heilungsversuche bein prognostisch ungunstigen Fallen von Netzhautabhebung. *Z Augenheilkd* 1933;81:277.
51. Lindner K. Shortening of the eyeball for detached retina. *Arch Ophthalmol* 1949;42:635.
52. Lindner K. Unsere bisherigen Erfahrungen mit der Unterminierung Methode bei Operation von Netzhautabhebungen. *Ber Dtsch Ophthalmol Ges* 1932;49:83.
53. Machemer R, Buettner H, Norton EW, et al. Vitrectomy: a pars plana approach. *Trans Am Acad Ophthalmol Otolaryngol* 1971;75:813.
54. McCormack P, Simcock PR, Charteris D, et al. Is surgery for proliferative vitreoretinopathy justifiable? *Eye* 1994;8:75.
55. McCuen BWD, de Juan E Jr, Landers MBD, et al. Silicone oil in vitreoretinal surgery. Part 2. Results and complications. *Retina* 1985;5:198.
56. McCuen BWD, de Juan E Jr, Machemer R. Silicone oil in vitreoretinal surgery. Part 1. Surgical techniques. *Retina* 1985;5:189.
57. McCuen BWD, Landers MBD, Machemer R. The use of silicone oil following failed vitrectomy for retinal detachment with advanced proliferative vitreoretinopathy. *Graefes Arch Clin Exp Ophthalmol* 1986;224:38.
58. McCuen BWD, Landers MBD, Machemer R. The use of silicone oil following failed vitrectomy for retinal detachment with advanced proliferative vitreoretinopathy. *Ophthalmology* 1985;92:1029.
59. Meyer-Schwickerath G. Light coagulation. St. Louis, CV Mosby; 1960, pp. 1–113.
60. Müller H. Anatomische Beitrage zur Ophthalmologie 7: Beschreibung einiger von Prof. v. Graefe exstirpieter Augapfel. *Graefes Arch Klin Exp Ophthalmol* 1858;4:363.
61. Müller L. Eine neue operative Behandlung der Netzhautabhebung. *Klin Monatsbl Augenheilkd* 1903;41:459.
62. Norton EW. Intraocular gas in the management of selected retinal detachments. *Trans Am Acad Ophthalmol Otolaryngol* 1973;77:OP85.
63. Paufique L, Hugonnier R. Traitement du décollement de la rétine par la résection sclerale: technique personnelle, indications et résultats. *Bull Soc Ophtalmol Fr* 1951;64:435.
64. Raehlmann E. A critical comparison of Leber's theory of detachment of the retina, with the diffusion theory. *Arch Ophthalmol* 1894;23:92.
65. Rosengren B. Über die Behandlung der Netzhautablösung mittelst Diathermie und Luftijektionen in den Glaskörper. *Acta Ophthalmol (Copenh)* 1938;16:3.
66. Ruete CGT. *Der Augenspiegel und das Optometer fur practische Aerzte.* Gottingen: Dieterichschen Bechhandlung, 1852.
67. Rumpf J. Jules Gonin: inventor of the surgical treatment for retinal detachment. *Surv Ophthalmol* 1976;21:276.
68. Šafář K. Detachment of the retina: treatment with multiple diathermic puncture and its results. *Arch Ophthalmol* 1934;11:933.
69. Schepens CL. A new ophthalmoscope demonstration. *Trans Am Acad Ophthalmol Otolaryngol* 1947;51:298.
70. Schepens CL. Management of retinal detachment. *Ophthalmic Surg* 1994;25:427.
71. Schepens CL. Scleral buckling with circling element. *Trans Am Acad Ophthalmol Otolaryngol* 1964;68:959.
72. Schepens CL, Acosta F. Scleral implants: an historical perspective. *Surv Ophthalmol* 1991;35:447.

73. Schepens CL, Okamura ID, Brockhurst RJ. The scleral buckling procedures. I. Surgical techniques and management. *Arch Ophthalmol* 1957;58:797.
74. Schepens CL, Okamura ID, Brockhurst RJ, et al. Scleral buckling procedures. IV. Synthetic sutures and silicone implants. *Arch Ophthalmol* 1960;64:868.
75. Scott JD. A rationale for the use of liquid silicone. *Trans Ophthalmol Soc U K* 1977;97:235.
76. Scott JD. Treatment of massive vitreous retraction. *Trans Ophthalmol Soc U K* 1975;95:429.
77. Shapland CD. Scleral resection: lamellar. *Trans Ophthalmol Soc U K* 1951;71:29.
78. Sourdille G. Une méthode de traitement de décollement de la rétine. *Arch Ophthalmol* 1923;40:419.
79. Stilma JS, Koster R, Zivojnovic R. Radical vitrectomy and silicone-oil injection in the treatment of proliferative vitreoretinopathy following retinal detachment. *Doc Ophthalmol* 1986;64:109.
80. Teichmann K. History of scleral buckling. *Surv Ophthalmol* 1992;36:323.
81. Trantas A. Moyens d'explorer par l'ophtalmoscope et par translucidité la partie antérieure du fond oculaire, le circle ciliaire y compris. *Arch Ophthalmol* 1900;20:314.
82. Valois G, Lemoine P. Ophtalmoscopie microscopique du fonde d'oeil vivant (sans verre de contact). *Bull Soc Fr Ophtalmol* 1923;36:36.
83. von Arlt C. *Die Krankheiten des Auges, für protische Äerzte Geschildert.* Prague: FA Credner, 1858.
84. von Graefe A. Cited by Gonin in: *Le décollement de la rétine.* Lausanne: Librarie Pavot, 1934:82.
85. von Graefe A. Notiz über die Ablösungen der Netzhaut von der Chorioidea. *Arch Ophthalmol* 1854;1:362.
86. von Graefe, A. Perforation von Abgelösten Netzhauten und Glaskorpermembranen. *Arch Ophthalmol* 1863;9:85.
87. von Helmholtz H. *Beschreibung eines Augen-Spiegels zur Untersuchung der Netzhaut im lebenden auge.* [Description of an eye-mirror for the investigation of the retina in the living eye.] Berlin: A Forstner, 1951.
88. Walker CB. Retinal detachment: technical observations and new devices for treatment with a specially arranged diathermy unit for general ophthalmic service. *Am J Ophthalmol* 1934;17:1.
89. Weve H. Zur Behandlung der Netzhautablösung mittels Diathermie. In: *Abhandlungen aus der Augenheilkunde,* Heft. 14. Berlin: Karger, 1932.

5
Differential Diagnosis

Rhegmatogenous retinal detachment (RRD) must be distinguished from exudative detachment, that is, detachment caused by exudation of fluid from the choroid or retina in the absence of retinal breaks. If the underlying condition can be successfully treated, an exudative detachment will resolve. Rhegmatogenous retinal detachment must also be differentiated from traction retinal detachment, which results from transvitreal traction on the retina, not from a retinal break. Traction detachments may not progress into the macula, but if they do, vitrectomy is the treatment of choice for releasing the traction. RRD can also be confused with entities that resemble it but are not retinal detachments at all. Retinoschisis and choroidal detachment fall into this category. This chapter discusses the features that help the ophthalmologist to make the correct diagnosis.

RHEGMATOGENOUS RETINAL DETACHMENT

If no break can be found, the diagnosis of presumed RRD can be made only after the conditions outlined in this chapter have been excluded. A history of light flashes or floaters followed by progressive visual field loss strongly suggests RRD. It is also possible, however, for patients with malignant melanoma to notice light flashes (8) and for patients with cells in the vitreous from inflammatory conditions to complain of "floaters."

In RRD, the intraocular pressure is usually lower in the affected eye than in the fellow eye. Pigmented cells ("tobacco dust") may be present in the vitreous cavity and in the anterior chamber (see Fig. 1-3). Detachments caused by flap or operculated tears frequently have associated vitreous hemorrhage. The detached retina undulates with eye movements. It is slightly opaque and often has a corrugated appearance. The subretinal fluid (SRF) is clear, and although in most cases it is nonshifting, the examiner must remember that it is shifting in about 5% of cases, especially those with long-standing detachments (15). Irregular folds are common. Fixed folds, equatorial traction, and other signs of proliferative vitreoretinopathy (PVR) are rare in nonRRD.

EXUDATIVE RETINAL DETACHMENT

Exudative detachments are caused by choroidal and retinal conditions that damage the blood–retinal barriers and allow fluid to pass into the subretinal space. Neoplasms and inflammatory diseases are the leading causes of such detachments. A hallmark of these detachments is "shifting fluid": the SRF responds to the force of gravity, detaching the area of the retina in which it accumulates. For example, when the patient is sitting, the inferior retina is detached (Fig. 5-1). When the patient is then placed in the supine position, the fluid moves posteriorly in a matter of seconds or minutes, and the macula is detached.

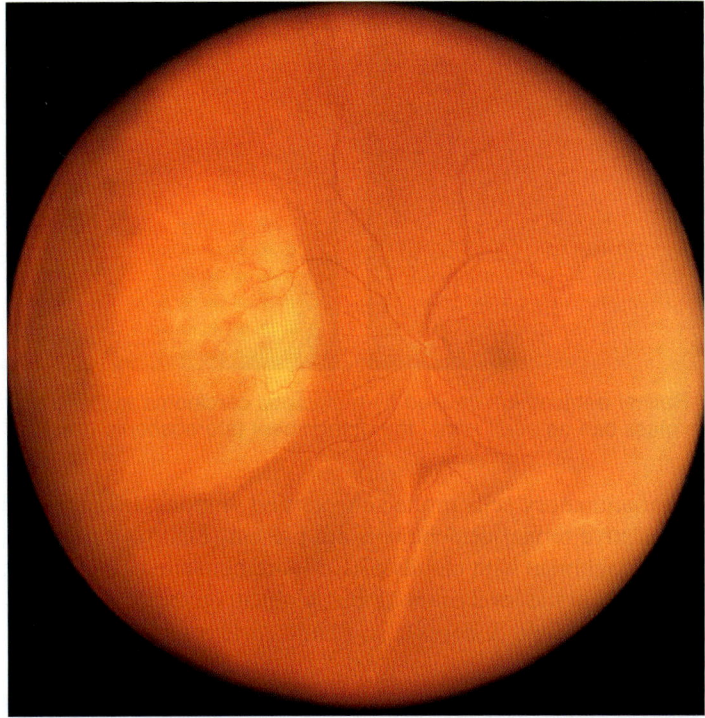

FIGURE 5-1. Retinal detachment caused by choroidal melanoma. The subretinal fluid typically accumulates inferiorly in two bullae.

Another characteristic of exudative detachment is the smoothness of the detached retina (Fig. 5-2), in contrast to the corrugated appearance seen in RRD. Fixed folds are rarely, if ever, seen in exudative detachments. If these folds are seen, even in eyes with neoplasms, the detachment is probably rhegmatogenous (Fig. 5-3). Occasionally, the retina can be elevated enough in exudative detachments to be seen directly behind the lens. This rarely occurs in RRD. Specific causes of exudative detachment are discussed in the following section.

Neoplasms

Melanoma, hemangioma, and metastatic carcinoma of the choroid are the most common neoplastic causes of exudative retinal detachment. In addition to the choroidal mass, which can usually be found by indirect ophthalmoscopy, other features common to exudative retinal detachment, such as shifting fluid, a biomicroscopically clear vitreous, and the absence of a retinal break, are likely to be present.

Inflammatory Diseases

Harada's Disease (Vogt–Koyanagi–Harada Syndrome)

Harada's disease is a bilateral uveitis usually seen in blacks, Asians, and darkly pigmented whites. Systemic manifestations include headache, malaise, tinnitus, and nausea. Meningeal inflammation may cause stiff neck and cerebrospinal fluid pleocytosis. No sexual predilection is present. The patient may have associated papillitis. One usually

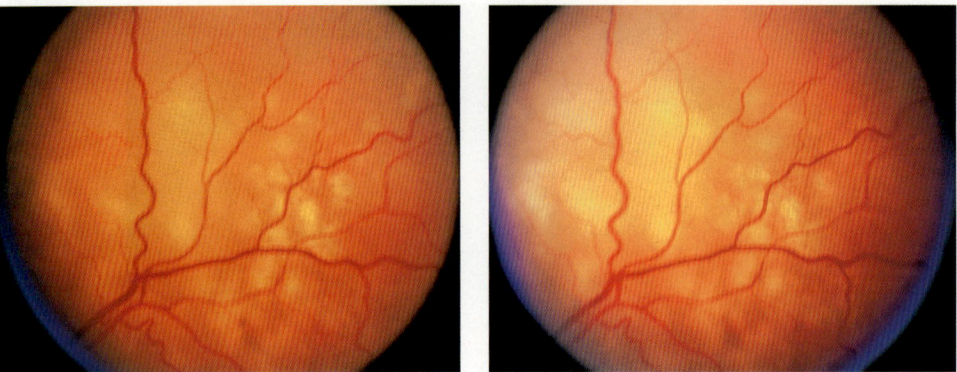

FIGURE 5-2. Retinal detachment caused by metastatic carcinoma to the choroid. The retina is smooth. The mass can be seen under the detachment (stereoscopic view).

sees numerous inflammatory cells in the aqueous and vitreous. In early stages, multiple, dome-shaped exudative retinal detachments are present (Fig. 5-4). Later, they may coalesce into a large detachment with cloudy SRF. Fluorescein angiography reveals multiple, pinpoint leakage spots at the level of the retinal pigment epithelium (RPE) (see Fig. 5-4). Most cases respond well to high doses of systemic corticosteroids.

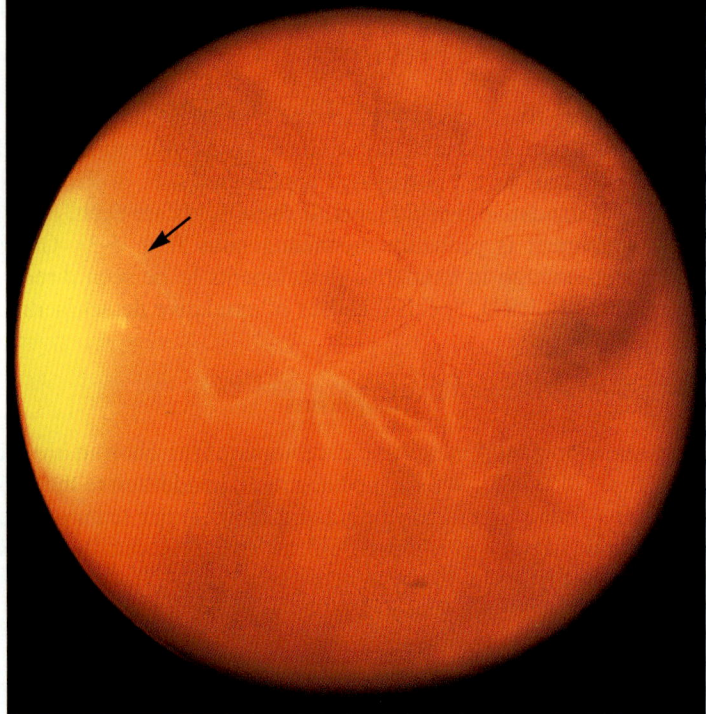

FIGURE 5-3. Rhegmatogenous retinal detachment in an eye with coincidental malignant melanoma (nasal to optic nerve). The rhegmatogenous nature of detachment is shown by the demarcation line *(arrow)* and the fixed fold (inferotemporally). Shifting fluid was not present. The patient elected to have treatment of the melanoma by cobalt plaque. A sclera buckling procedure reattached the retina. (Courtesy of Jerry Shields, M.D., and Sheldon Kaplan, M.D.)

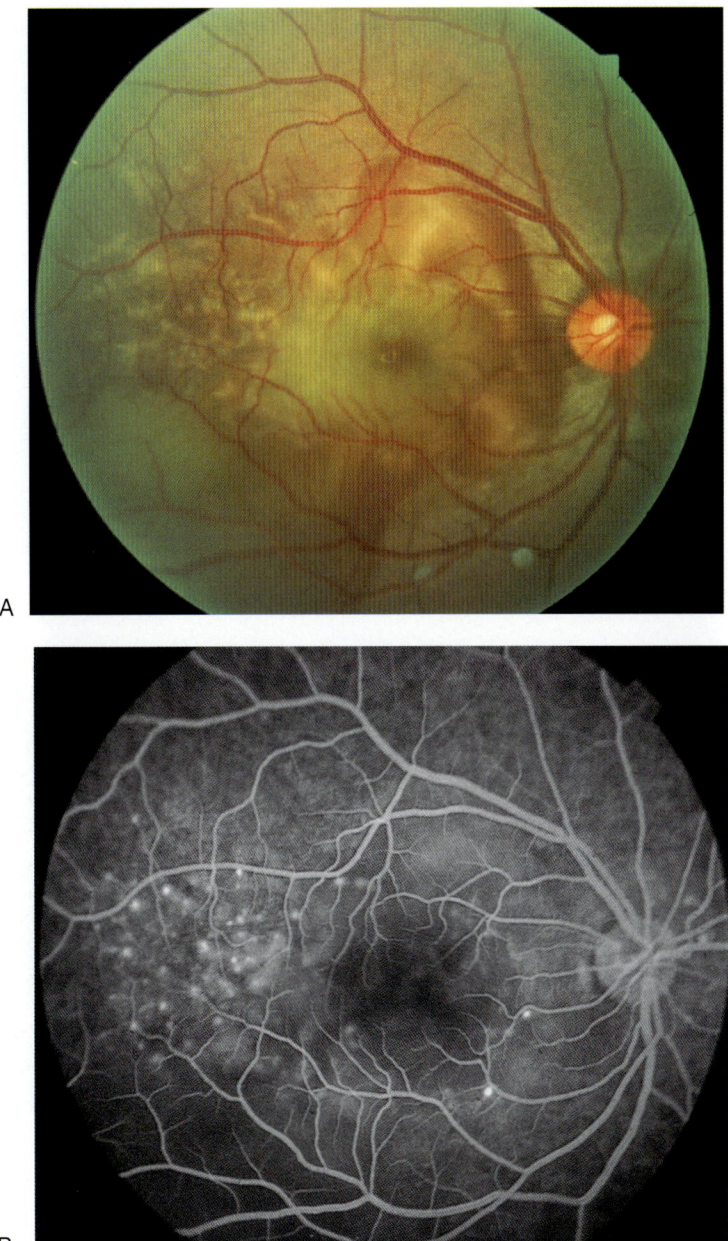

FIGURE 5-4. Harada's disease. **A:** Fundus photograph shows subretinal fluid in the macula and peripapillary area. The corresponding early **B** and late **C** phase fluorescein angiogram photographs demonstrate multiple pinpoint hyperfluorescent dots with leakage of dye into the subretinal space. (From Essentials of Vitreoretinal Disease, Brown, Flynn, Regillo, eds, Thieme Medical Publishers, with permission.)

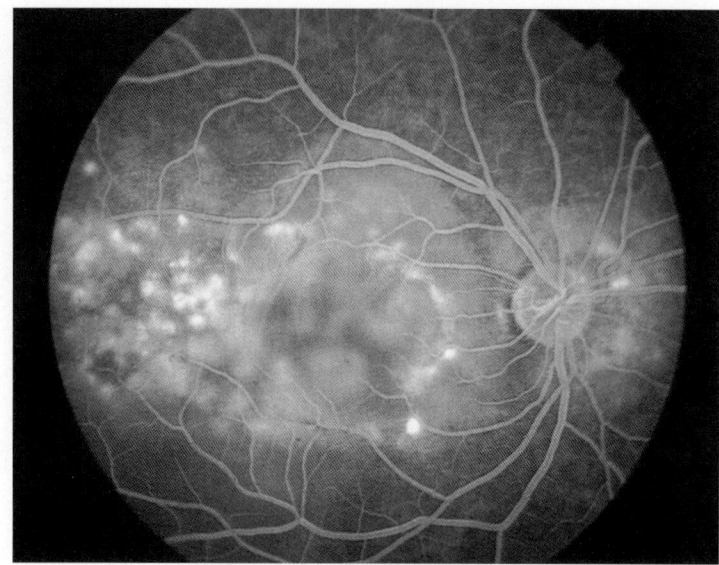

C

FIGURE 5-4. *Continued.*

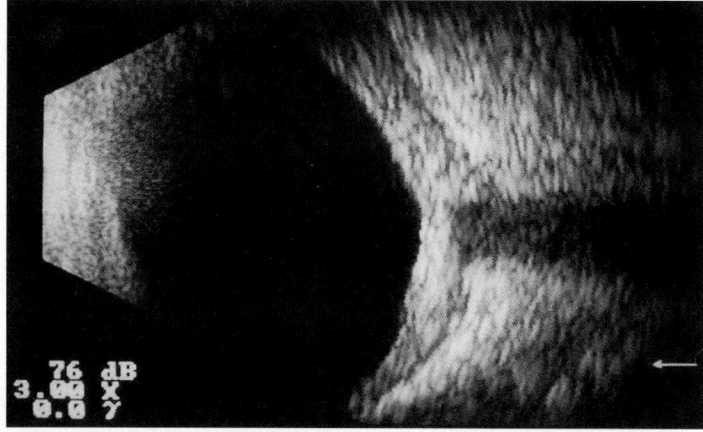

FIGURE 5-5. Posterior scleritis. B-scan ultrasonography shows marked sclerochoroidal thickening. Also visible is a characteristic echolucent zone between the sclera and the orbital tissue corresponding to fluid in the posterior sub-Tenon space.

Posterior Scleritis

Scleral inflammation can cause nonRRD, usually with shifting, cloudy, SRF (2). Women are more commonly afflicted with posterior scleritis than men, and approximately 10% have a collagen-vascular disease. The condition is generally unilateral, with associated anterior scleritis and ocular, brow, or zygoma pain. If the inflammation is intense and localized, it can cause a posterior mass that indents the choroid and RPE. The mass can be found by indirect ophthalmoscopy. Ultrasonography differentiates it from choroidal neoplasms, which it may resemble, by showing a thickened sclera with high internal reflectivity and retrobulbar edema (Fig. 5-5). Corticosteroids or nonsteroidal anti-inflammatory agents usually resolve the inflammation.

Idiopathic Central Serous Chorioretinopathy

For unknown reasons, in idiopathic central serous chorioretinopathy (ICSC), at least one small area of the RPE loses its adhesion to Bruch's membrane, giving rise to RPE detachments. Choroidal fluid then passes through the RPE and accumulates under the sensory retina. In rare cases of ICSC, multiple, large RPE detachments allow passage of sufficient fluid to cause a bullous exudative retinal detachment (3,7,23). Most of these patients have bilateral evidence of ICSC, and some are pregnant, are in renal failure, or are taking systemic corticosteroids (10,17,22). Some have bilateral bullous detachments. Others have a bullous detachment in only one eye, but they have evidence of more typical ICSC in the other eye, with fluid limited to the macula.

ICSC with bullous detachment can be confused with RRD. In an ICSC detachment, one sees shifting fluid, clear vitreous, and no retinal break, findings not characteristic of RRD. In addition, patients with ICSC do not complain of flashes or floaters. They usually notice blurring of central before peripheral vision. Sometimes, significant fibrin exudation is seen adjacent to the RPE detachments. Finally, large RPE detachments in the posterior pole, characteristic of bullous ICSC, can be found by indirect ophthalmoscopy and confirmed by fluorescein angiography. These detachments can sometimes be effectively treated by argon laser photocoagulation.

Uveal Effusion Syndrome

The uveal effusion syndrome is a bilateral condition in which patients with normal-sized eyes have exudative detachment of the peripheral choroid, ciliary body, and retina (9,19). The subretinal fluid typically is seen in the inferior fundus, as it is in other conditions that cause exudative retinal detachment (Fig. 5-6). As in nanophthalmos, these findings are caused by a thickened sclera that hinders uveoscleral outflow. Features that aid in the diagnosis include dilation of episcleral vessels, cells in the vitreous, characteristic leopard-spot RPE changes, and thickening of the choroid on ultrasonography. Resolution of the detachments has been reported after vortex vein decompression (19) and after excision of a lamellar flap of sclera in each quadrant while avoiding the vortex veins (9).

Nanophthalmos

The thickened sclera in these small eyes decreases uveoscleral outflow, often causing an exudative retinal detachment. The correct diagnosis is suggested by the small

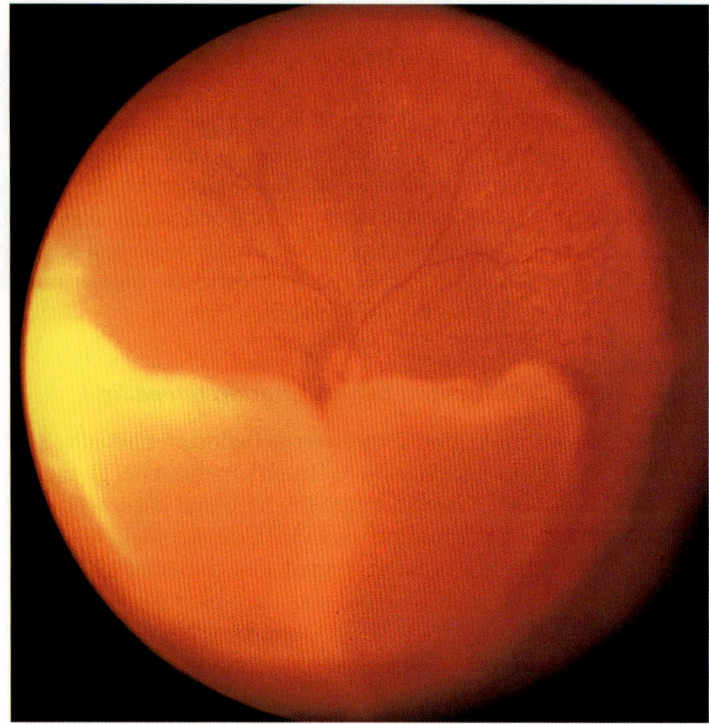

FIGURE 5-6. Exudative retinal detachment in a patient with uveal effusion syndrome. Two large bullae of subretinal fluid are present inferiorly.

cornea, the shallow anterior chamber, the narrow filtration angle, the high lens-to-eye volume ratio, and the absence of retinal breaks. Increased glycosaminoglycans contribute to the abnormal sclera and prevent outflow from the eye (14). The best treatment is decompression of the vortex veins (21) or opening of partial-thickness scleral windows.

Congenital Abnormalities

The morning glory syndrome and choroidal coloboma, both of which are actually rhegmatogenous, are discussed in chapter 3.

TRACTION RETINAL DETACHMENT

Vitreous membranes caused by PVR or penetrating injuries can pull the neurosensory retina away from the RPE, causing a traction retinal detachment. The retina characteristically has a smooth surface and is immobile. The detachment is concave toward the front of the eye and rarely extends to the ora serrata (Fig. 5-7). In most cases, the causative vitreous membrane can be seen ophthalmoscopically or with the three-mirror lens. If the traction can be released by vitrectomy, the detachment usually resolves. In some cases,

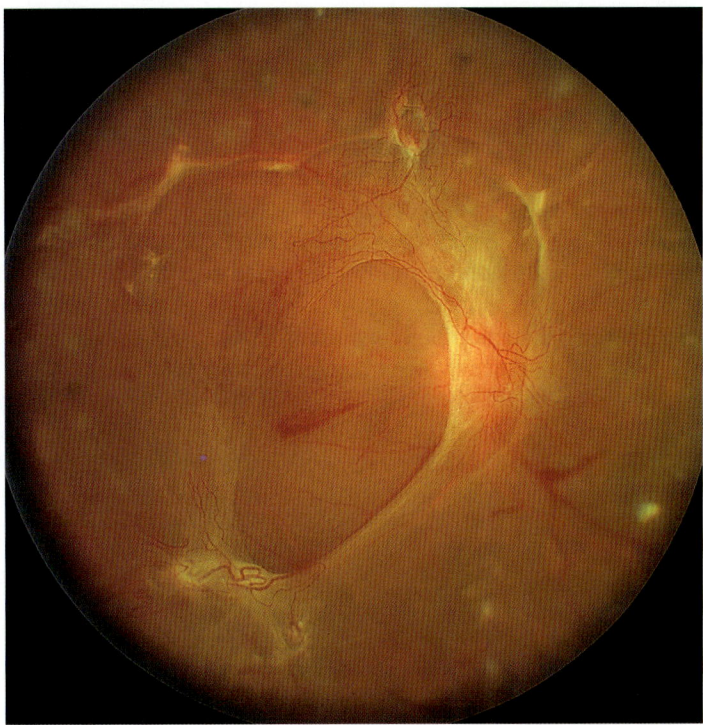

FIGURE 5-7. Traction retinal detachment from proliferative diabetic retinopathy. The detached retina is smooth and is concave toward the pupil.

traction tears the retina and causes an RRD that is convex toward the front of the eye. The retina then becomes more mobile and has the irregular folds and corrugations characteristic of RRD. Treatment consists of a combination of vitrectomy to release the traction and a scleral buckling (SB) procedure to seal the break.

LONG-STANDING RETINAL DETACHMENT

The features of long-standing RRD without PVR are discussed in detail in chapter 2. Because the retina is thin (see Figs. 2-5 and 2-7B) and the causative breaks are usually small, long-standing RRD may be confused with senile retinoschisis. Findings often present in long-standing detachment but not found in retinoschisis are "tobacco dust" (see Fig. 1-3), intraretinal cysts (see Fig. 2-6), white retroretinal dots (see Fig. 2-3), depigmentation or hyperpigmentation of the underlying RPE (see Fig. 2-7), and demarcation lines (see Fig. 2-7).

Long-standing inferior RRD with macular involvement in pseudophakic eyes is occasionally not diagnosed at all; the decreased vision is attributed to pseudophakic cystoid macular edema (CME). The error occurs because the detached retina is thin and relatively transparent and because CME develops in the detached macula. Significant delay in treatment results (16).

RETINOSCHISIS

Clinical Appearance of Uncomplicated Retinoschisis

In degenerative retinoschisis, the retina is split into two layers ("walls") by a viscous substance presumed to be hyaluronic acid (24). The schisis cavity is dome-shaped with a smooth and thin inner wall (Fig. 5-8). Retinoschisis may resemble RRD, but several factors help the ophthalmologist to make the correct diagnosis. First of all, 70% of these patients' eyes are hyperopic, whereas the eyes of patients with RRD are more commonly myopic. Second, in most patients with bullous retinoschisis in one eye, significant retinoschisis is present in the other eye. This is much less likely in eyes with long-standing RRD (1,5). Third, no "tobacco dust" or hemorrhage is present. Fourth, the outer wall of retinoschisis has a pocked or pitted appearance that can be identified with the aid of scleral depression. The retinal vessels are often sheathed. Fifth, prominent cystoid degeneration and "snowflakes" or "frosting" (footplates of Müller cells) (Fig. 5-9) are seen near the ora serrata. Sixth, unless full-thickness retinal detachment is present, the underlying RPE appears normal, and no demarcation line is present. Finally, the absolute scotoma found on visual field testing helps to distinguish retinoschisis from RRD, which causes a relative scotoma.

Retinoschisis–retinal Detachment

In addition to simulating detachment, as discussed previously, degenerative retinoschisis can, in some cases, cause RRD. Breaks in the outer wall (Fig. 5-10), with or without coexistent inner wall holes, can give rise to a detachment that, if progressive, must then be treated

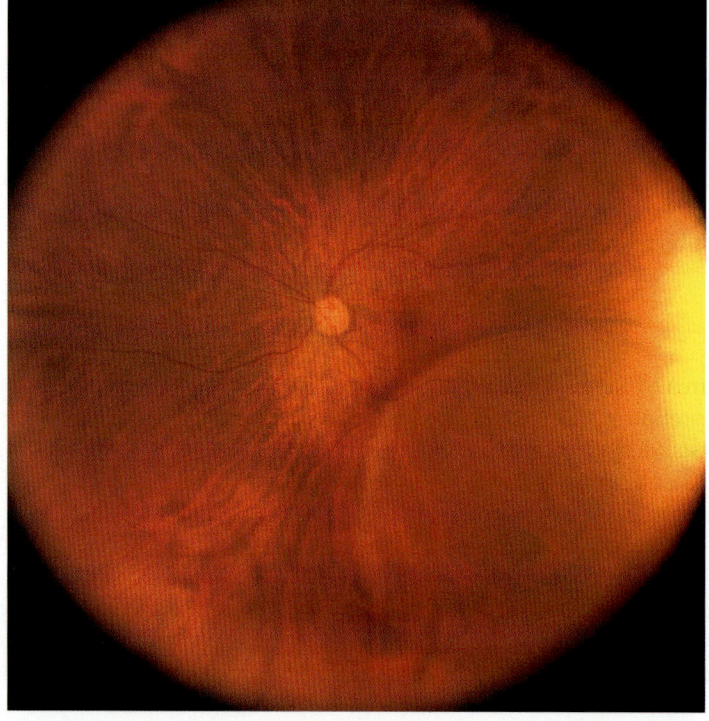

FIGURE 5-8. Degenerative (senile) retinoschisis. Note the dome-shaped smooth inner wall and inferotemporal location. (Courtesy of William H. Annesley, Jr., M.D.)

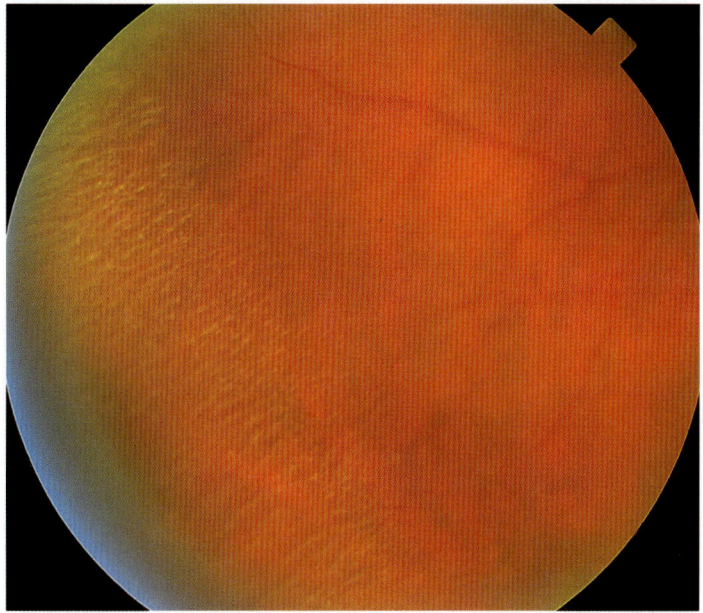

FIGURE 5-9. Snowflake pattern seen near the ora serrata in degenerative retinoschisis.

by the usual procedures (18). When outer wall holes alone are present, retinoschisis–retinal detachments characteristically advance slowly beyond the margins of the schisis cavity. Atrophy of the underlying RPE and demarcation lines are common (5). In some retinoschisis–retinal detachments, the schisis cavity collapses. Then, the combined detached retinal layers resemble a typical RRD (Fig. 5-11). If the examiner has not correctly diagnosed the

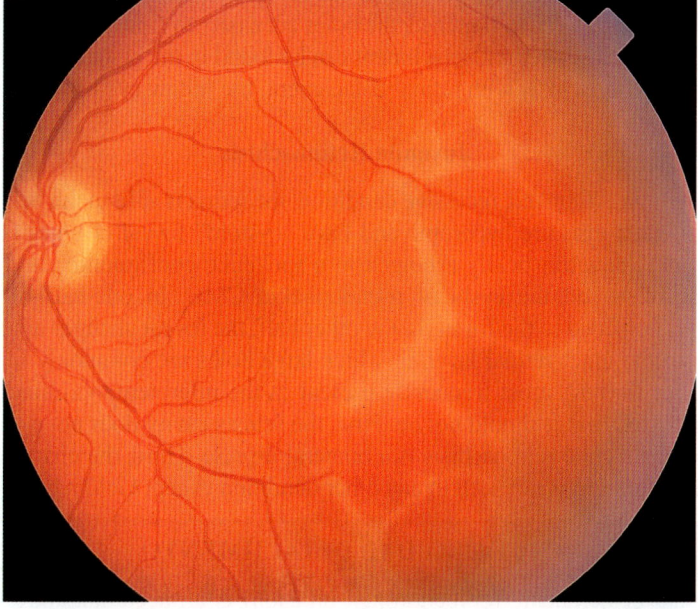

FIGURE 5-10. Outer wall holes in degenerative retinoschisis.

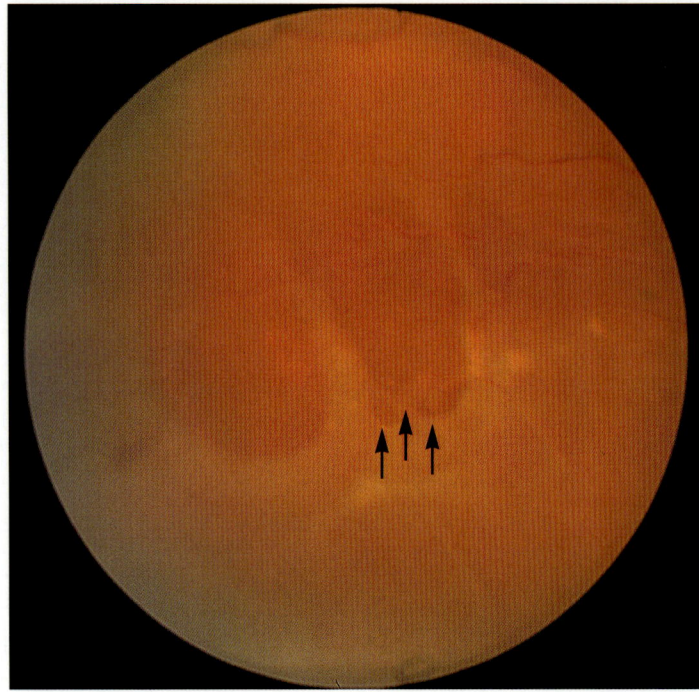

FIGURE 5-11. Two large outer wall holes and three small inner wall holes *(arrows)* in retinoschisis–retinal detachment.

detachment as secondary to retinoschisis, the breaks may not be located. If a retinoschisis–retinal detachment is suspected, the examiner should carefully search posteriorly, where outer wall holes are frequently found. The holes are generally round, with rolled edges (see Fig. 5-11). Occasionally, if holes cannot be found, the surgeon should drain the SRF. When the retina has been flattened, the holes are easier to find. Confirmation of the diagnosis of a retinoschisis–retinal detachment can be found in the patient's other eye; in 95% of patients with retinoschisis with retinal detachment, the fellow eye has retinoschisis (12).

Juvenile Retinoschisis

In this congenital, X-linked, recessive condition, the retina is split in the nerve fiber layer. Almost all affected eyes are hyperopic and have "cystoid" foveal changes (see Fig. 3-8). The "cysts" are characteristically arranged in a spokelike configuration and do not stain with fluorescein, as do the cysts of pseudophakic CME. In one-half of these cases, retinoschisis is confined to the fovea. In the other half, the foveal changes are accompanied by elevation of the inner retinal layer, in which large holes are commonly found (see Fig. 3-9). This latter finding, most frequently present in the inferotemporal quadrant, may be confused with RRD, but it should not be. First, the schisis cavity does not extend to the ora serrata. Second, juvenile retinoschisis is a bilateral disease. Third, the characteristic foveal "cystoid" configuration is not seen in any other condition except Goldmann–Favre disease.

CHOROIDAL DETACHMENT

A "choroidal detachment" (ciliochoroidal effusion) is an accumulation of fluid either within the suprachoroidea and the supraciliaris, the outermost layer of the choroid and the ciliary body, or, rarely, between the choroid and the sclera. Choroidal detachment is usually a sequela of ocular surgery, but it may also accompany ocular inflammatory conditions (6).

Choroidal detachments can be mistaken for RRDs, but they have several distinguishing features. They are orange brown and have a more solid appearance than do RRD because the RPE and choroid are part of the elevated tissue (Fig. 5-12). Hypotony, the elevation of the pars plana, and the absence of a retinal break also help to identify a

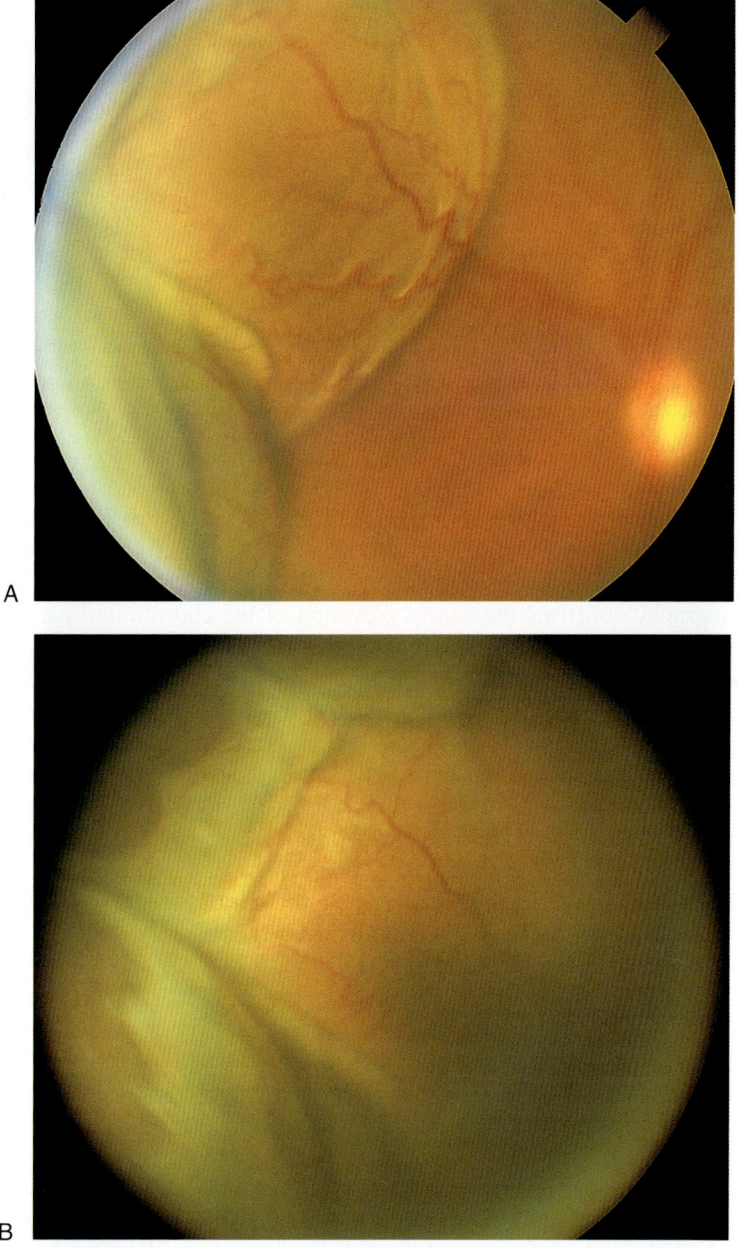

FIGURE 5-12. Choroidal detachment. **A:** Note the "solid" appearance and orange-brown color. **B:** A more anterior view; the pars plana is easily seen.

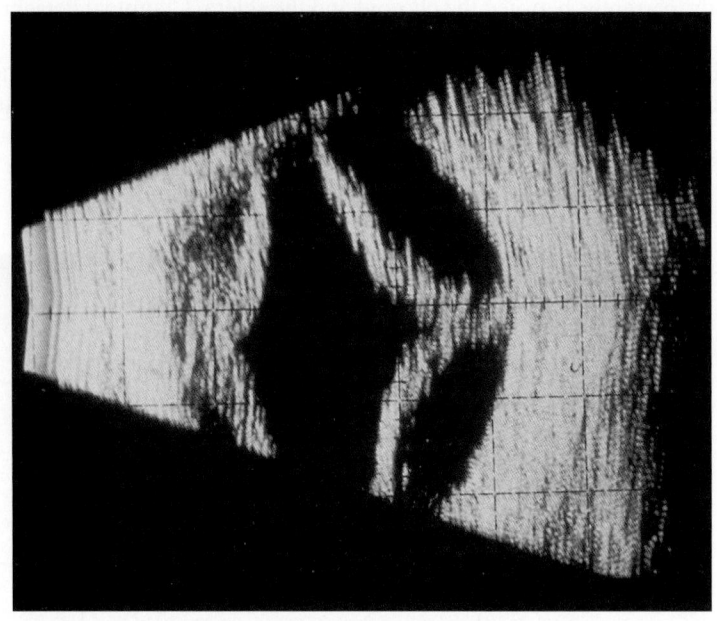

FIGURE 5-12. *Continued.* **C:** B-scan ultrasonography shows the multiple, peripheral, dome-shaped elevations.

choroidal detachment. Initially, a choroidal detachment has a smooth surface, but as it regresses, retinal folds may form. Choroidal detachments may jiggle on eye movements, but they do not undulate like RRDs.

Ultrasonography confirms the serous elevation of the choroid and pars plana, ruling out both neoplasms and retinal detachment (see Fig. 5-12). Choroidal detachments (unless hemorrhagic) transilluminate readily. Choroidal detachment can appear in conjunction with RRD (Fig. 5-13), thus posing an additional diagnostic problem. The coincidence of a brownish choroidal "mass" and a retinal detachment may lead to the mistaken diagnosis of malignant melanoma with associated serous detachment. Certain findings help the examiner to make the correct diagnosis. First, in RRD with choroidal detachments, the eye is usually hypotonous. The retinal detachment is presumed to cause hypotony, which then induces the choroidal detachment. When the ciliary body is detached, aqueous secretion is further decreased, lowering the intraocular pressure still more. Second, the presence of a retinal break and pigmented cells in the aqueous and vitreous helps to identify the retinal detachment as rhegmatogenous. Third, a choroidal detachment associated with RRD transilluminates, whereas a pigmented malignant melanoma does not. Finally, on ultrasonography, a choroidal detachment associated with RRD is acoustically empty, whereas a malignant melanoma is solid.

In some patients with RRD with choroidal detachment and hypotony, the eye becomes inflamed and painful. The anterior chamber depth increases, and concentric folding and posterior bowing of the iris with iridophakodonesis occur. Posterior synechiae may form (11,13,20). The prognosis for retinal reattachment is poor because of the high incidence of PVR. Most authors use topical and periocular corticosteroids to try to reduce the inflammation and the extent of the choroidal detachment before attempting surgical repair. Localizing and treating retinal breaks through the supra-

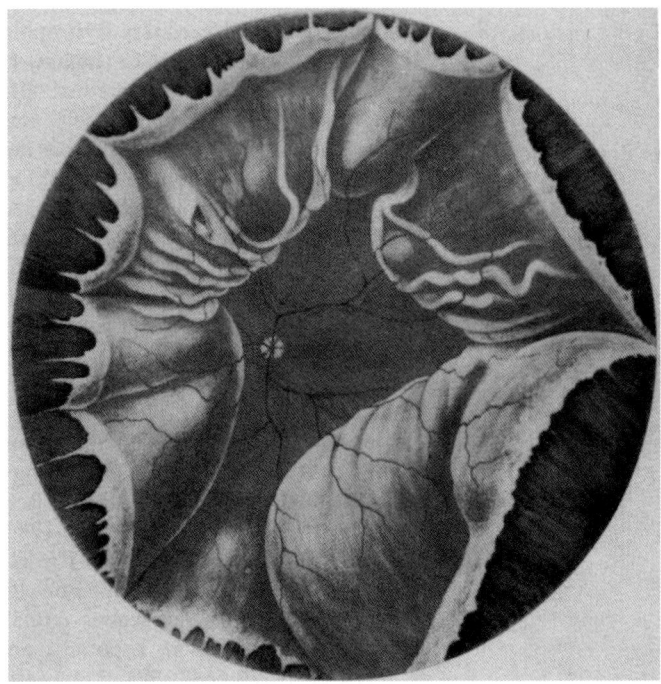

FIGURE 5-13. Combined rhegmatogenous retinal detachment and choroidal detachment. The pars plana is significantly elevated. A superonasal retinal break is present. (Courtesy of C.L. Schepens, M.D., Retina Foundation, Boston).

choroidal fluid is difficult. Therefore, if the fluid is still present, we drain it, place a pars plana infusion cannula, and combine vitrectomy techniques with a SB procedure to repair the detachment.

REFERENCES

1. Ballantyne A, Michaelson I. *Textbook of the Fundus of the Eye.* Baltimore: Williams & Wilkins, 1970.
2. Benson WE. Posterior scleritis. *Surv Ophthalmol* 1988;32:297.
3. Benson WE, Shields JA, Annesley WH Jr, et al. Idiopathic central serous retinopathy with bullous retinal detachment. *Ann Ophthalmol* 1980;12:920.
4. Byer NE. Clinical study of senile retinoschisis. *Arch Ophthalmol* 1968;79:36.
5. Byer NE. Long-term history of senile retinoschisis with implications for management. *Ophthalmology* 1986;93:1127.
6. Finlay A, Fogle J, Green W. Ciliochoroidal effusion. In: *Duane's Clinical Ophthalmology,* edited by Tasman, W, Jaeger, E. Philadelphia: Lippincott–Raven Publishers, 1986:1.
7. Gass JDM. Bullous retinal detachment: an unusual manifestation of idiopathic central serous choroidopathy. *Am J Ophthalmol* 1973;75:810.
8. Gass JDM. Problems in the differential diagnosis of choroidal nevi and malignant melanomas. *Am J Ophthalmol* 1977;83:299.
9. Gass JDM, Jallow S. Idiopathic serous detachment of the choroid, ciliary body, and retina (uveal effusion syndrome). *Ophthalmology* 1982;89:1018.
10. Gass JDM, Little H. Bilateral bullous exudative retinal detachment complicating idiopathic central serous chorioretinopathy during systemic corticosteroid therapy. *Ophthalmology* 1995;102:737.
11. Gottlieb F. Combined choroidal and retinal detachment. *Arch Ophthalmol* 1972;88:481.
12. Hagler WS, Woldoff HS. Retinal detachment in relation to senile retinoschisis. *Trans Am Acad Ophthalmol Otolaryngol* 1973;77:99.
13. Jarrett WHD. Rhegmatogenous retinal detachment complicated by severe intraocular inflammation, hypotony, and choroidal detachment. *Trans Am Ophthalmol Soc* 1981;79:664.

14. Kawamura M, Tajima S, Azuma N, et al. Immunohistochemical studies of glycosaminoglycans in nanophthalmic sclera. *Graefes Arch Clin Exp Ophthalmol* 1996;234:19.
15. Kirkby GR, Chignell AH. Shifting subretinal fluid in rhegmatogenous retinal detachment. *Br J Ophthalmol* 1985;69:654.
16. Lakhanpal V, Schocket SS. Pseudophakic and aphakic retinal detachment mimicking cystoid macular edema. *Ophthalmology* 1987;94:785.
17. Polak BC, Baarsma GS, Snyers B. Diffuse retinal pigment epitheliopathy complicating systemic corticosteroid treatment. *Br J Ophthalmol* 1995;79:922.
18. Regillo C, Custis P. Surgical management of retinoschisis. *Curr Opin Ophthalmol* 1997;8:80.
19. Schepens CL, Brockhurst RJ. Uveal effusion. 1. Clinical picture. *Arch Ophthalmol* 1963;70:189.
20. Seelenfreund MH, Kraushar MF, Schepens CL, et al. Choroidal detachment associated with primary retinal detachment. *Arch Ophthalmol* 1974;91:254.
21. Singh OS, Simmons RJ, Brockhurst RJ. Nanophthalmos: a perspective on identification and therapy. *Ophthalmology* 1982;89:1006.
22. Sunness JS, Haller JA, Fine SL. Central serous chorioretinopathy and pregnancy. *Arch Ophthalmol* 1993;111:360.
23. Tsukahara I, Uyama M. Central serous retinopathy with bullous retinal detachment. *Graefes Arch Clin Exp Ophthalmol* 1978;206:169.
24. Yanoff M, Fine B. In: *Ocular Pathology*. Hagerstown: Harper & Row, 1975:416.

6

Fundus Examination and Preoperative Management

INDIRECT OPHTHALMOSCOPY

If one could have only one instrument for the evaluation and management of retinal detachment, it would be the Schepens binocular indirect ophthalmoscope.

Principles and Advantages

In indirect ophthalmoscopy, light from the patient's fundus is focused by a lens into an intermediate image, which is viewed by the observer (Fig. 6-1). The observed image is upside down and inverted (Fig. 6-2). The headpiece of the binocular indirect ophthalmoscope is constructed so the light of a high-intensity electric bulb is focused onto a mirror that reflects the light into the patient's eye and onto the retina (Fig. 6-3). Because the mirror is mounted above the view box, the beam of light entering the patient's eye (illumination beam) is separated from the light rays viewed by the examiner (observation beams) (see Fig. 6-3). This arrangement prevents the corneal light reflex of the illumination beam from interfering with viewing (see Fig. 6-3). Stereoscopic vision is provided by the view box, which contains prisms that optically "narrow" the examiner's pupillary distance; otherwise, the light rays exiting from the patient's pupil could not reach both the examiner's pupils (Fig. 6-4).

The indirect ophthalmoscope offers several advantages over other techniques in the evaluation of retinal detachment (9,11,17–20). The strong illumination provided by the headlamp and the light-gathering capability of the hand lens enable the examiner to see through hazy media. When combined with scleral depression, it provides the best view of the peripheral retina. Finally, this instrument makes a wide area of the retina visible at one time, thereby helping to ensure that no abnormalities are missed (Fig. 6-5).

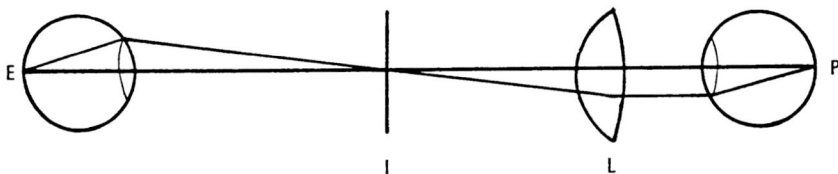

FIGURE 6-1. Indirect ophthalmoscopy. *(A)* Rays from a point in the patient's fundus *(P)* are focused by a lens *(L)* into an intermediate image *(I)*, which is viewed by the examiner *(E)*.

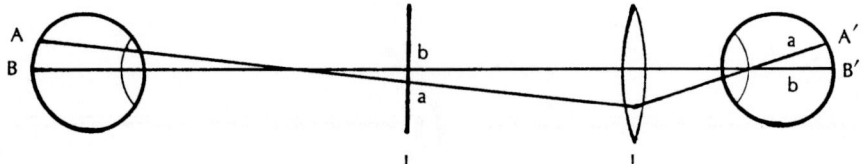

FIGURE 6-2. The relative position of rays of light *a* and *b* from points *A* and *B* in the patient's fundus is reversed at the intermediate image *(I)*, so *a* strikes the examiner's superior retina at *A'*. Because the examiner's inferior visual field is "seen" by the superior retina, *A* appears to be inferior to *B*.

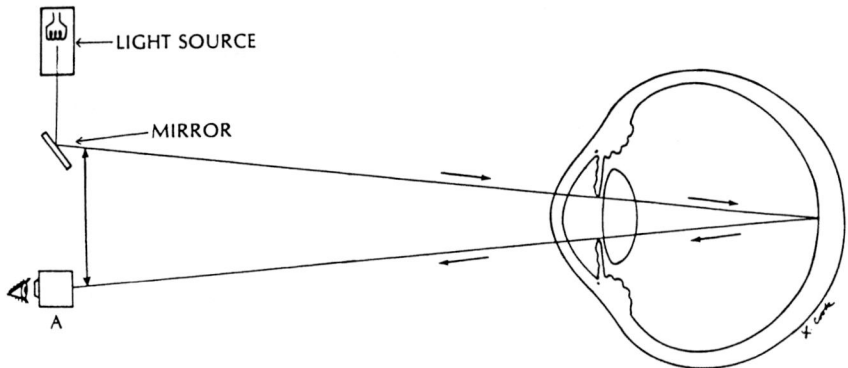

FIGURE 6-3. The path of light rays entering the eye (illumination beam) is separated from those leaving it (observation beam), minimizing corneal light reflexes.

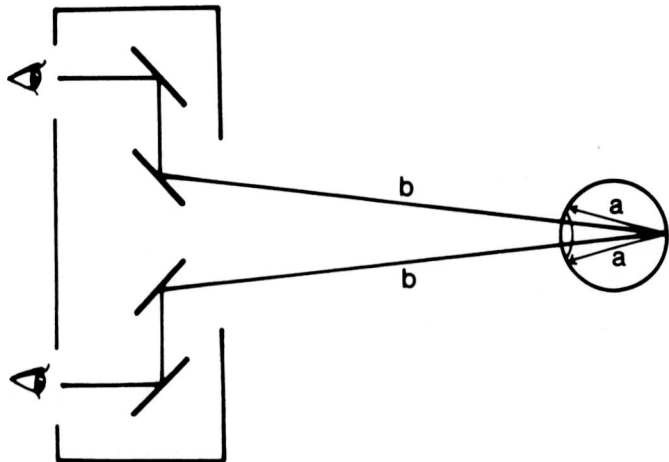

FIGURE 6-4. Prisms in the view box of the binocular indirect ophthalmoscope "narrow" the examiner's pupillary distance. Therefore, from points in the patient's fundus, an observation beam *(b)* can reach each of the examiner's eyes. Without the view box, binocular vision would be impossible because light rays *(a)*, aimed at each of the examiner's eyes, could not exit through the pupil.

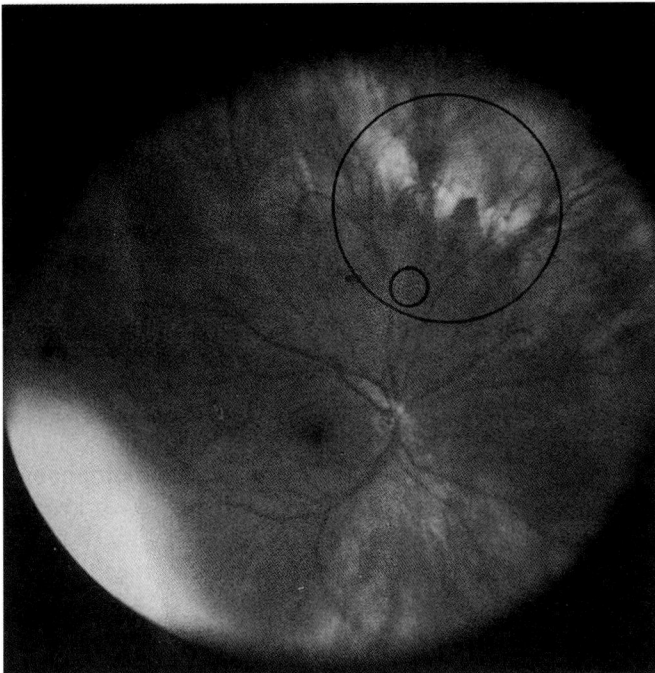

FIGURE 6-5. The *large circle* indicates the area of the fundus that can be seen at one time with the indirect ophthalmoscope and the large 20-diopter lens. The *small circle* indicates the area that can be seen with the direct ophthalmoscope. Clearly, detection of the long-standing retinal detachment with demarcation line is easier with the indirect ophthalmoscope.

Technique

Several aspheric lenses are available. The 14-diopter lens has the highest magnification of the commonly used lenses (3.6×), but it is difficult to use because of its long focal length (7 cm). The 30-diopter lens (f = 3.3 cm) is often preferred by beginners because it is easy to use, especially in patients with small pupils, but it does not provide adequate magnification (1.5×) for finding small breaks. We prefer the 20-diopter lens (f = 5 cm), which is easy to use and provides a magnification of 2.3×. (18) Any lens should be held with the more convex surface toward the examiner (see Fig. 6-1). It is slightly tilted to move the two light reflexes (one from each surface of the lens) away from the examiner's viewing axis (Fig. 6-6). To minimize the corneal light reflex, the mirror should be adjusted so the illumination beam is in the top of the field of view of the eyepieces. For small pupils, the light must be directed still higher (Fig. 6-7), or, alternatively, a smaller light beam can be used.

The patient should be reclining comfortably, and the pupil should be dilated widely. Initially, the transformer rheostat should be set at a low voltage. Higher light intensities can be tried later, if the patient becomes less sensitive to light. Bilateral cycloplegia and topical anesthesia reduce photophobia and enhance cooperation. The superior periphery should be examined first: the periphery because it is less sensitive to light than is the posterior pole, and the superior periphery because photophobic patients have less pain on upgaze. When patients attempt to close their eyes, thus inducing Bell's phenomenon, examination of the inferior retina is difficult, if not impossible. To counteract this tendency,

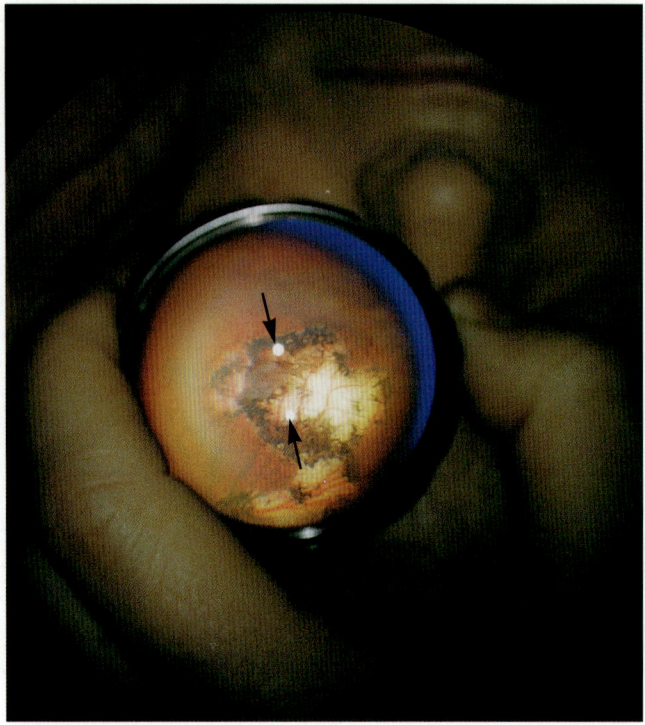

FIGURE 6-6. Proper use of the hand lens. The lens is tilted to separate the light reflexes *(arrows)* on its surfaces.

the examiner must constantly encourage the patient to keep both eyes open. Sometimes, a fixation target such as the patient's thumb or a mark on the ceiling is helpful.

Beginners frequently make the error of standing too close to the patient (Figs. 6-8 and 6-9). It is much easier for the examiner to obtain a clear fundus image if his or her arm is extended. This is especially important if the pupil is small.

The examiner's head should be positioned to look directly into the quadrant examined. To examine the nasal periphery, the examiner should stand on the same side as the eye being examined (Figs. 6-10 and 6-11); for the temporal periphery, the examiner should stand on the opposite side (Figs. 6-12 and 6-13). The hand lens is shifted from the right

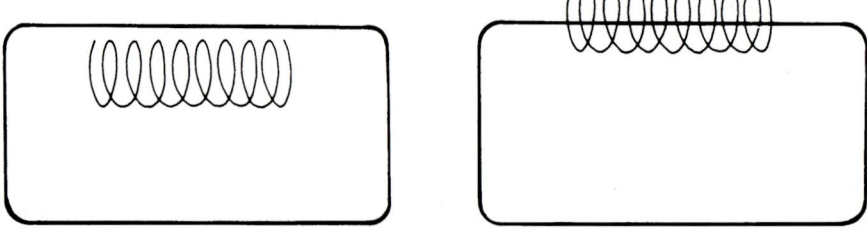

FIGURE 6-7. For viewing through adequately dilated pupils *(left)*, the reflected light (filament) should be at the top of the examiner's field of vision *(enclosed area)*. For viewing through small pupils *(right)*, the mirror is positioned so only a small strip of light is seen at the top of the field of vision.

CHAPTER 6/FUNDUS EXAMINATION AND PREOPERATIVE MANAGEMENT   79

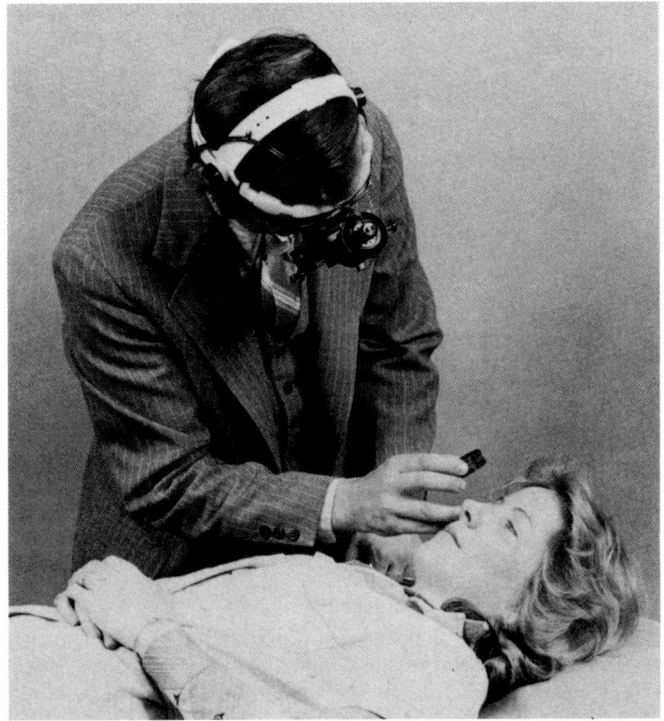

FIGURE 6-8. Examiner standing too close to the patient.

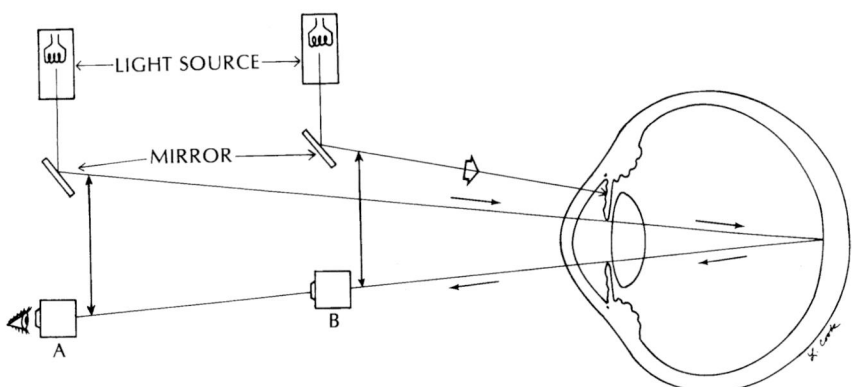

FIGURE 6-9. The distance between the illumination beam and the observation beams is fixed *(double-headed arrows)*. When the examiner stands at position A, the illumination beam can enter the patient's pupil and the observation beams can exit. At position B, the illumination beams *(open arrow)* cannot enter the eye. If the examiner lowered his or her head, the eye would be illuminated, but the observation beams could not exit.

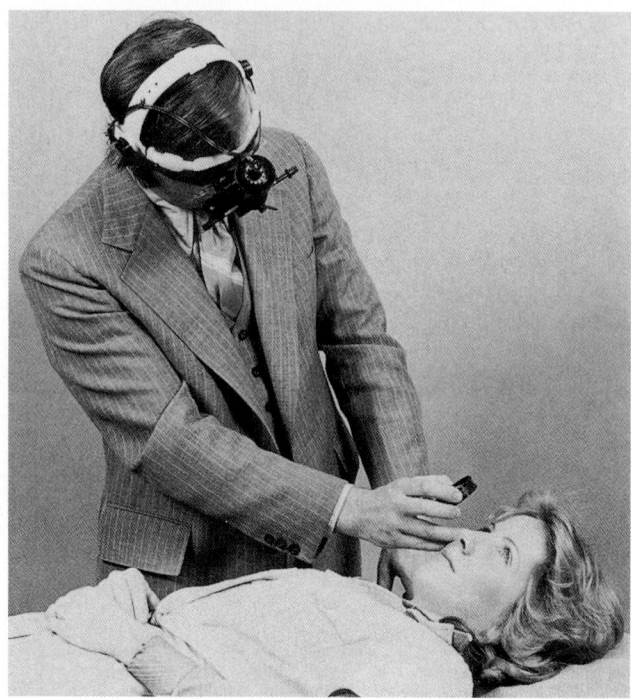

FIGURE 6-10. Examination of the superonasal periphery, right eye. The patient keeps both eyes open and looks up and to the left. The examiner's arm is extended. The examiner stands on the patient's right, holds the lens in the right hand and steadies it by resting his or her finger on the patient's face.

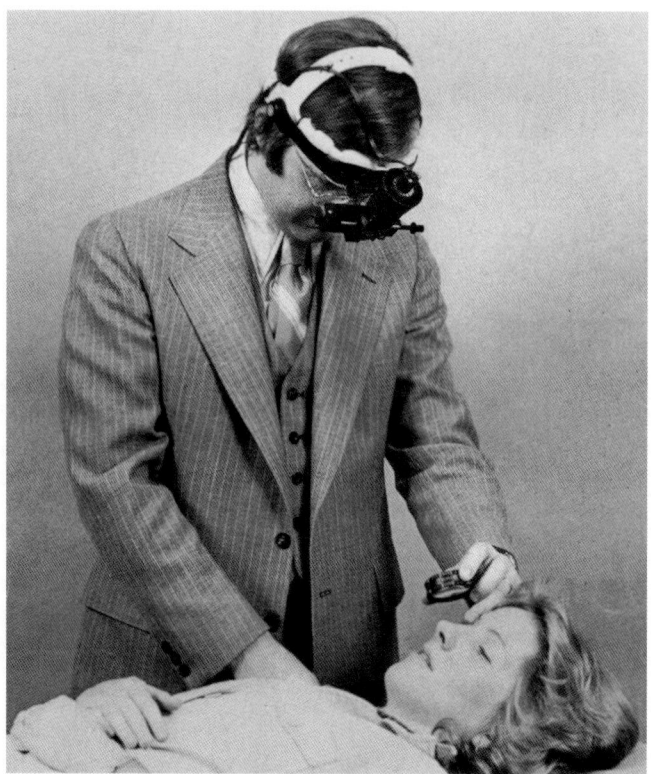

FIGURE 6-11. Examination of the inferonasal periphery, right eye. The patient looks down and to the left. The examiner remains on the patient's right but holds the lens in the left hand.

CHAPTER 6/FUNDUS EXAMINATION AND PREOPERATIVE MANAGEMENT   81

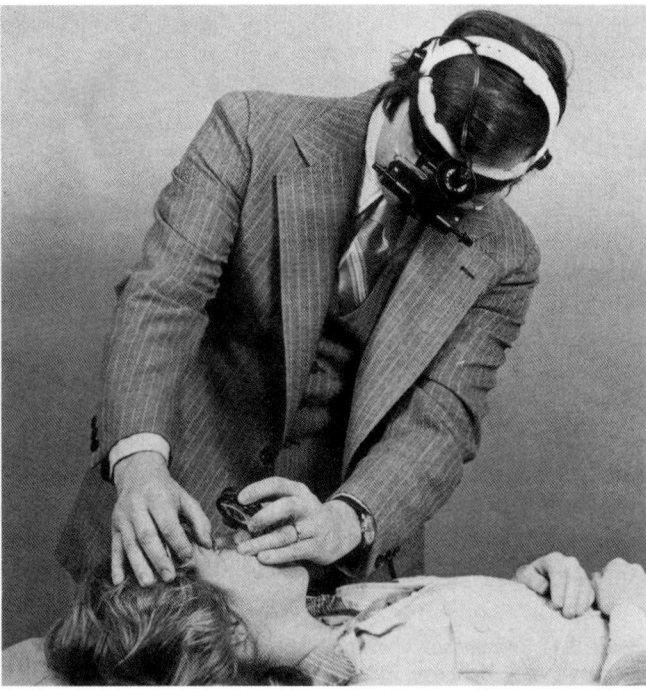

FIGURE 6-12. Examination of the superotemporal periphery, right eye. The examiner has moved to the patient's left side. The lens is held in the left hand. The patient looks up and to the right. The patient's face is rolled to the left so the nose is not an obstacle.

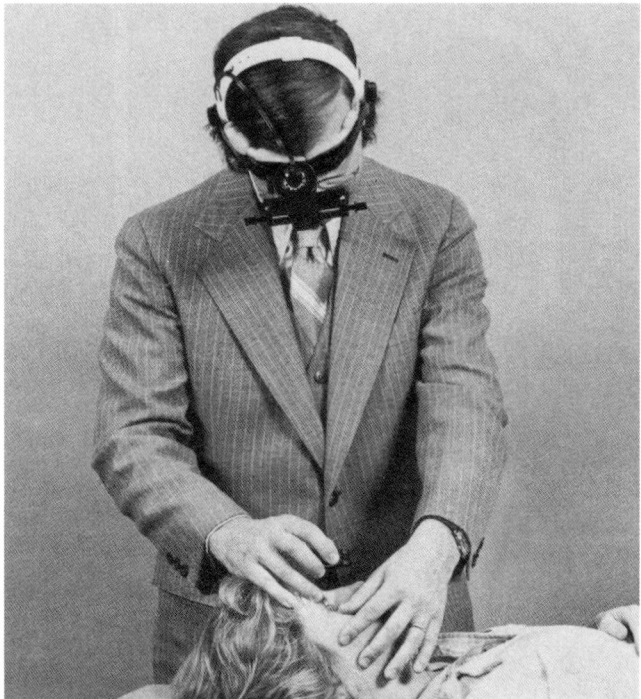

FIGURE 6-13. Examination of the inferotemporal periphery, right eye. The examiner remains on the patient's left but has shifted the lens to the right hand.

hand to the left as necessary to avoid clumsy maneuvering, especially during scleral depression. The patient's nose becomes less of an obstacle to viewing the temporal periphery when the patient rolls his or her head toward the examiner while looking temporally.

The pupillary aperture appears elliptical to the examiner when the peripheral retina is viewed. This makes stereoscopic viewing more difficult and decreases the amount of light that can enter the eye. The examiner must increase the voltage of the light source and tilt his or her head slightly so part of the illumination beam can enter the eye and one of the observation beams can exit (Figs. 6-14 and 6-15). This achieves only a monocular view.

When a patient has a small pupil, it is easier for the examiner to focus on the retina if the pupil is viewed while the examiner holds the lens at a distance further than the focal length of the eye and the lens is then slowly moved toward the pupil.

Fundus Drawing

Two ways exist to correct for the inverted image of the indirect ophthalmoscope. The first is to observe the retina, then mentally correct for the inverted image, drawing the findings as they are, not as they are seen. The second is to invert the drawing pad and then to draw the findings as they are seen. When the drawing (Fig. 6-16) is finished, the findings will be correctly positioned.

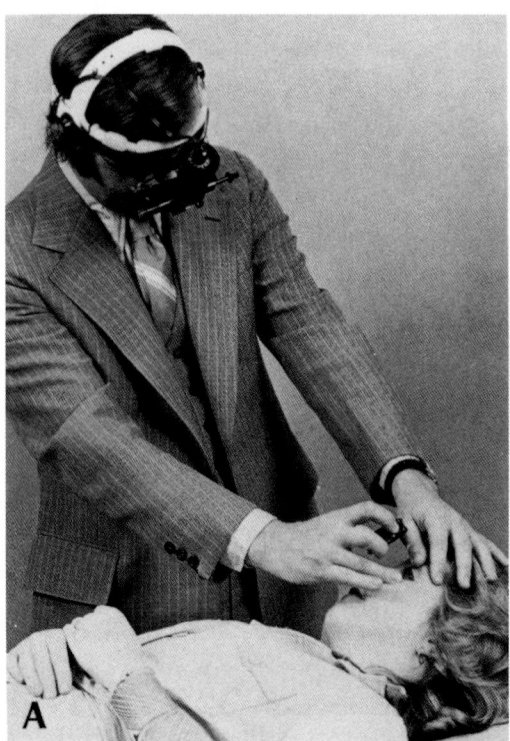 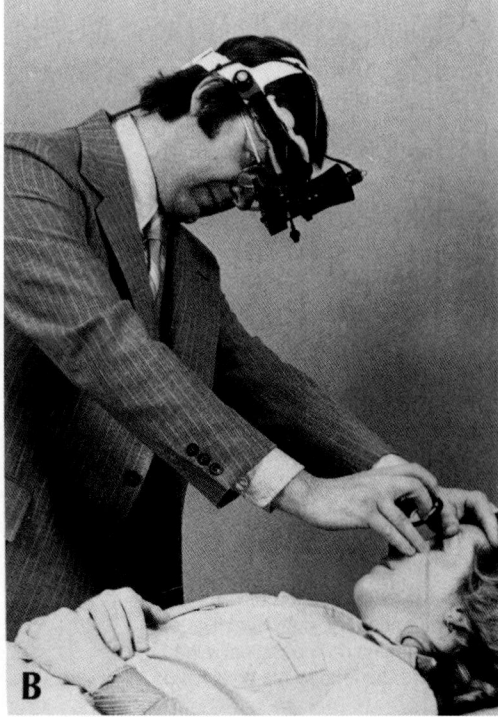

FIGURE 6-14. A: Examiner's head is incorrectly positioned for examination of the temporal periphery. **B:** Examiner's head is properly tilted so the eye is well illuminated and a monocular image can be seen.

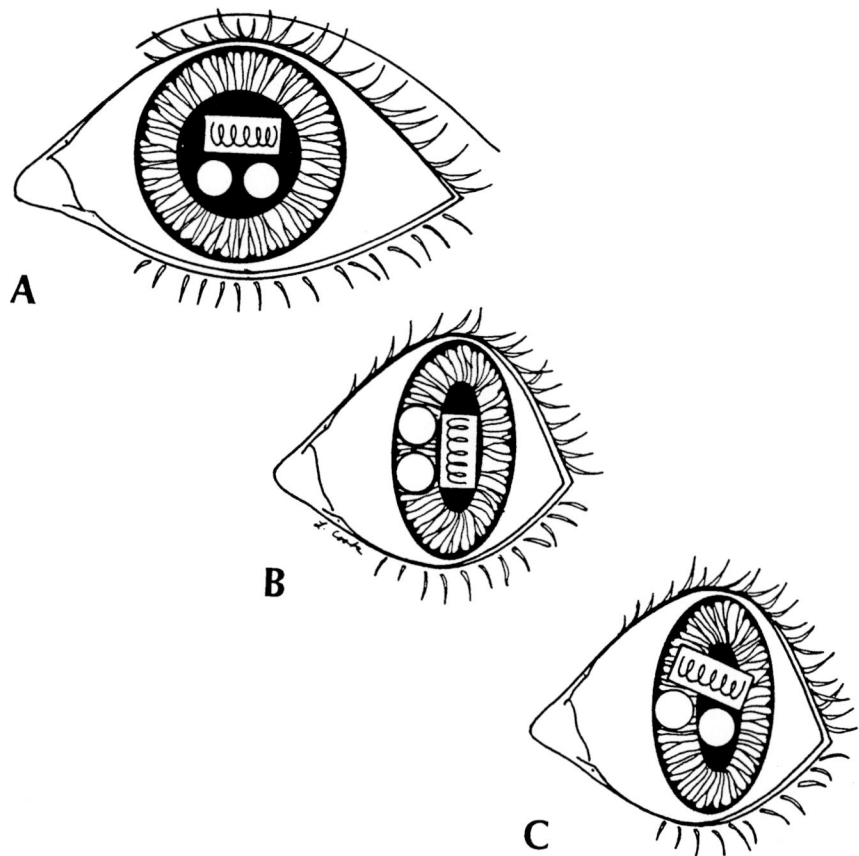

FIGURE 6-15. A: Viewing the posterior pole through a large pupil. The illumination beam (filament) enters through the top, leaving ample room for the observation beams (*white circles*) below. Binocular vision is provided. **B:** The pupillary aperture becomes elliptical when the examiner tries to see the far periphery. If the examiner does not tilt his or her head, the illumination beam can enter the eye, but the observation beams cannot emerge. **C:** The examiner must tilt his or her head so part of the illumination beam can enter the eye. Often, only a monocular view of the fundus is possible, because only one of the observation beams can emerge from the eye.

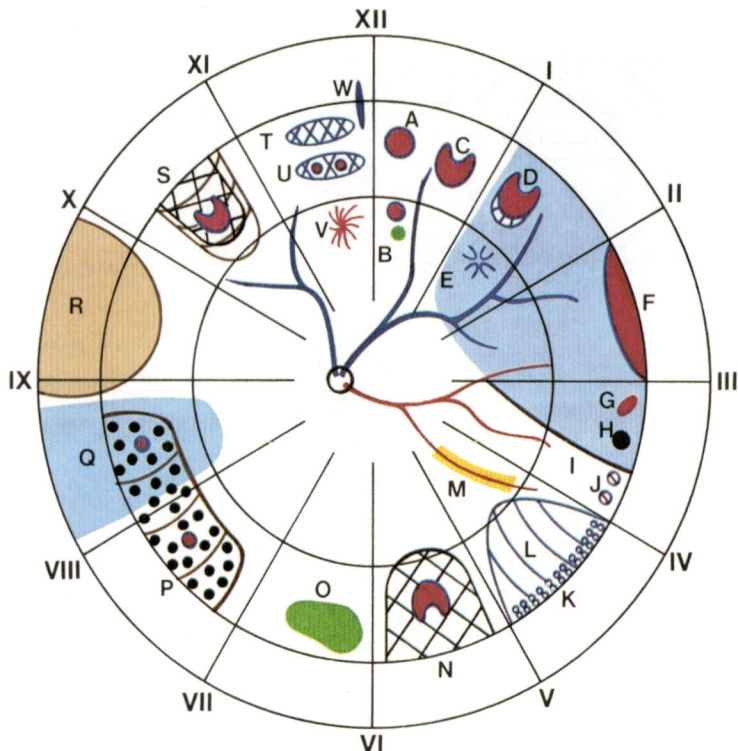

FIGURE 6-16. Schematic drawing of retinal findings. Arteries and intraretinal or subretinal hemorrhages are red. Veins are blue. Red outlined by blue indicates retinal breaks. Attached retina is white. Detached retina is blue. Intraretinal and subretinal exudates are yellow. Chorioretinal scarring (pigment epithelial proliferation) is black. Any choroidal mass or indentation is brown. (Clearly, a label is required to distinguish a choroidal detachment from a malignant melanoma.) Anything in the vitreous (e.g., hemorrhage, foreign body) is green. Here, too, a label is often required *(A)* round hole; *(B)* operculated tear; *(C)* flap tear; *(D)* flap tear with posteriorly rolled edge; *(E)* fixed fold; *(F)* retinal dialysis (disinsertion); *(G)* retinal hemorrhage; *(H)* intraretinal pigmentation; *(I)* demarcation line; *(J)* cobblestones; *(K)* peripheral cystoid degeneration; *(L)* senile retinoschisis; *(M)* exudate along a retinal artery; *(N)* flap tear surrounded by cryotherapy scarring; *(O)* vitreous opacity; *(P)* two round holes on a circumferential scleral buckle surrounded by diathermy scars; superiorly, the retina has redetached; *(Q)* detachment of nonpigmented epithelium of the pars plana; *(R)* choroidal mass; *(S)* flap tear surrounded by cryotherapy scarring on a radial scleral buckle; *(T)* lattice degeneration; *(U)* lattice degeneration with atrophic round holes; *(V)* vortex vein ampulla; *(W)* meridional fold.

To examine the fundus completely, one may start at the optic nerve and follow each of the retinal vessels to the periphery, or a scanning technique can be used. Keeping one's eyes and the hand lens aligned, the examiner swings his or her gaze along the periphery (Fig. 6-17). This serves two purposes. First, the entire retina is examined. In cases of retinal detachment, holes can be recognized when a sudden change in the brightness of the subretinal layers is noted. A hole is perceived as a discontinuity in the nearly uniform translucency of the detached retina (Fig. 6-18); when the observer's gaze is moving, the discontinuity becomes easier to see because of the contrast between the detached retina and the now visible layers underneath (Fig. 6-19). Slightly wiggling the lens from side to

CHAPTER 6/FUNDUS EXAMINATION AND PREOPERATIVE MANAGEMENT   85

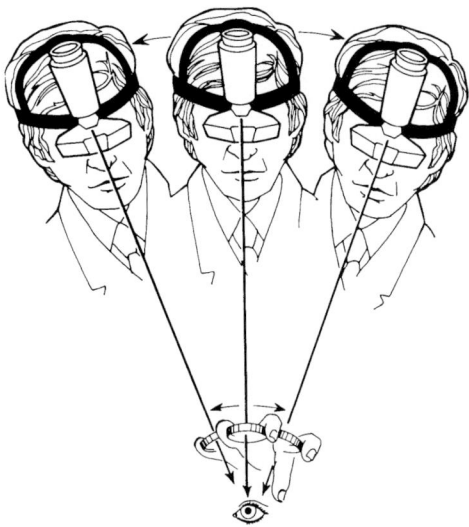

FIGURE 6-17. Scanning technique for examining the retina. The examiner keeps his or her eyes and lens aligned while viewing the retina.

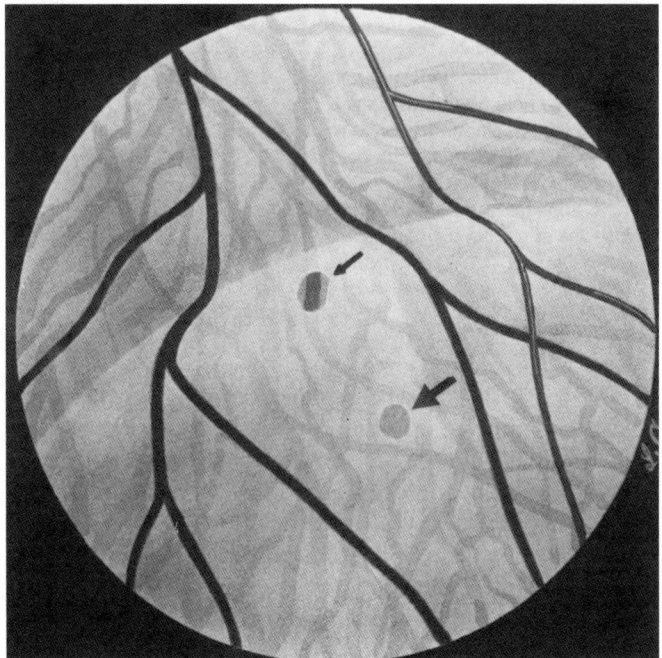

FIGURE 6-18. Retinal breaks are perceived as discontinuities in the detached retina. One hole *(small arrow)* appears as a dark spot because a choroidal vessel underlies it. The other *(large arrow)* is more difficult to see because of lack of contrast between the retina and the subretinal layers.

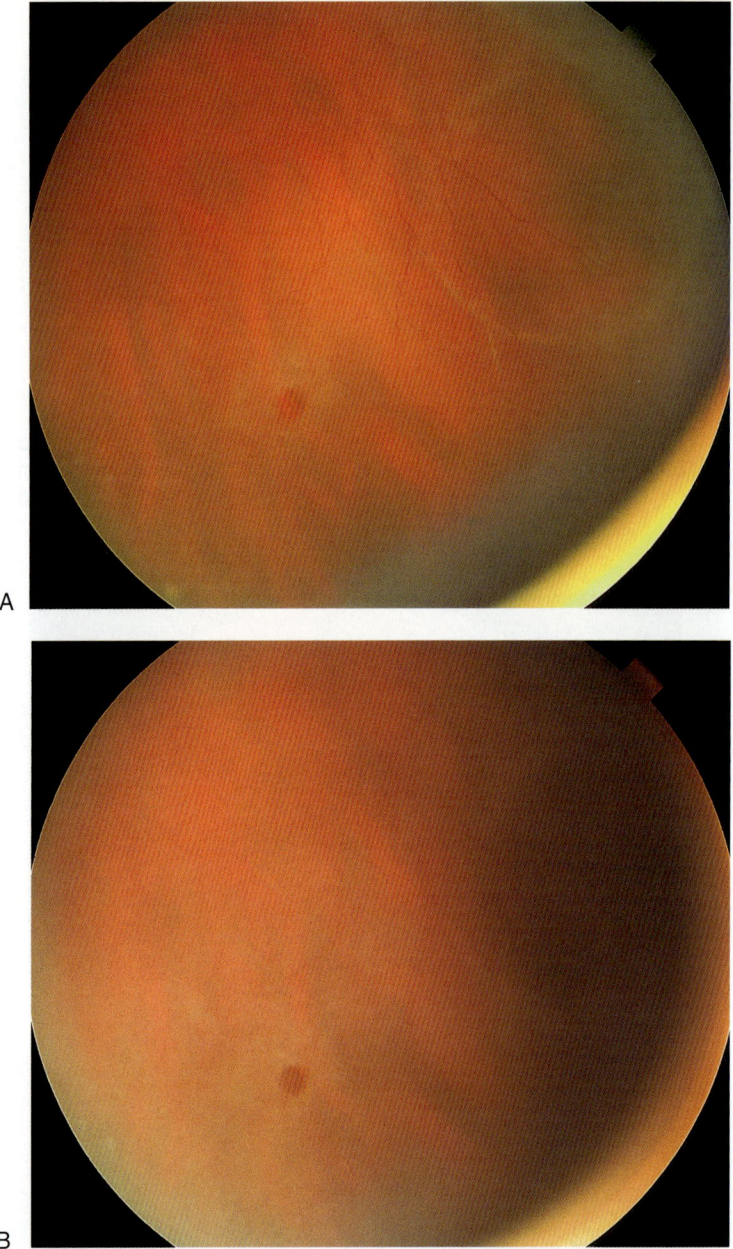

FIGURE 6-19. Long-standing retinal detachment with a small atrophic hole and a macrocyst. The retina is thin. Under the detachment is an area of pigmentation between choroidal blood vessels. **A:** The hole appears to be a dark spot because the choroidal pigmentation is seen through it. **B:** Viewed from a different angle, the hole appears lighter.

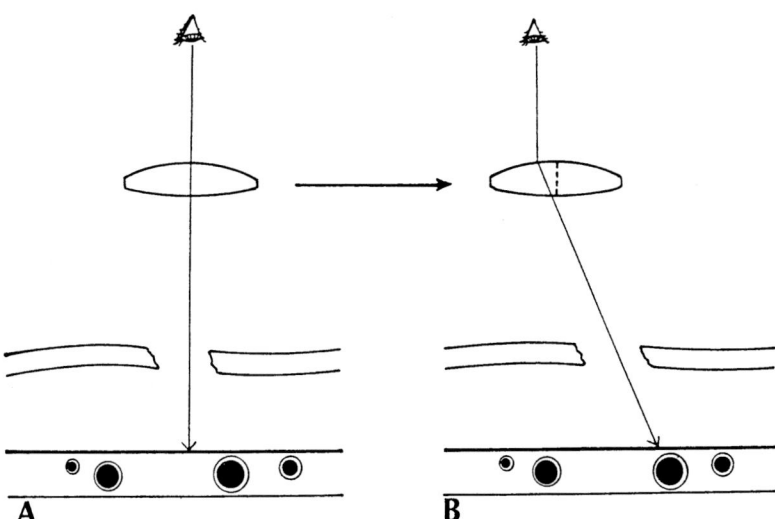

FIGURE 6-20. Use of the prism effect of the lens to find retinal breaks. **A:** The break is initially difficult to find because of little contrast between the detached retina and the background. **B:** As the lens moves, the retina appears to move with it. A choroidal vessel is suddenly seen more clearly, identifying the break.

side produces a prism effect that also helps to reveal discontinuities in the retina (Fig. 6-20).

No matter what the patient's complaint, the fellow eye must be carefully examined. For example, in patients with retinal detachment, the examiner must look for retinal breaks or other abnormalities that may require prophylactic treatment (3).

Scleral Depression

In patients with retinal detachment or posterior vitreous detachment (PVD), after the retina has been thoroughly scanned, the peripheral retina should be examined with scleral depression to detect small holes, especially those near the ora serrata. In some patients, this region cannot be seen at all without indentation. Beginners should not attempt scleral depression until they are adept at viewing the retina anterior to the equator without it. Otherwise, the scleral depression will afford little or no information and the patient will have suffered needlessly. Effective scleral depression can be achieved by the original thimble-type depressor designed by Schepens, the longer pencil-like depressor, a cotton-tipped applicator, and even a large paper clip.

Scleral depression helps in four ways to detect small breaks. First, it increases the contrast between the intact retina and the break. The indented choroid retinal pigment epithelium (RPE) is darker than the unindented choroid RPE and darker still than the intact retina, features that enable the examiner to locate the break, which appears as a dark spot (Figs. 6-21 and 6-22). Second, the decreased retinal translucency that results from scleral depression may increase the contrast between the hole and the retina, thus allowing the hole to be seen. The retina appears less translucent because it is seen at a more acute angle (Fig. 6-23). Moreover, the increased angle may aid the examiner to see the posterior edge of a break. Third, the flaps of tiny breaks at the posterior vitreous base can sometimes be seen as the sclera is indented (Fig. 6-24). Fourth, in patients with small

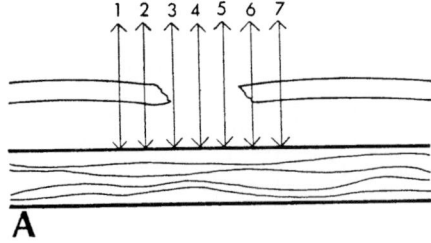

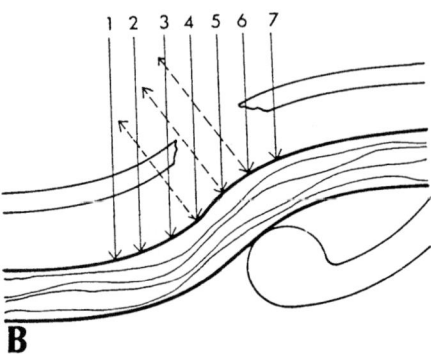

FIGURE 6-21. Scleral depression changes the brightness of the subretinal layers. **A:** Without indentation, light rays 3, 4, and 5 are reflected directly back to the examiner. **B:** With indentation, some light rays are reflected away from the examiner, so the indented area appears darker.

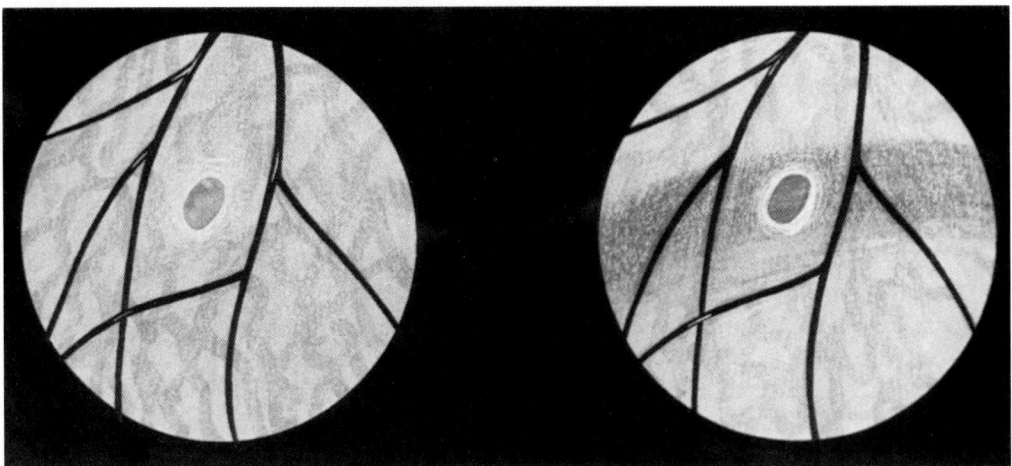

FIGURE 6-22. The use of scleral depression to find retinal breaks. *Left*, the retinal hole can barely be seen because of little contrast between the retina and the underlying choroid. *Right*, scleral depression darkens the underlying choroid. The hole is seen as a dark spot.

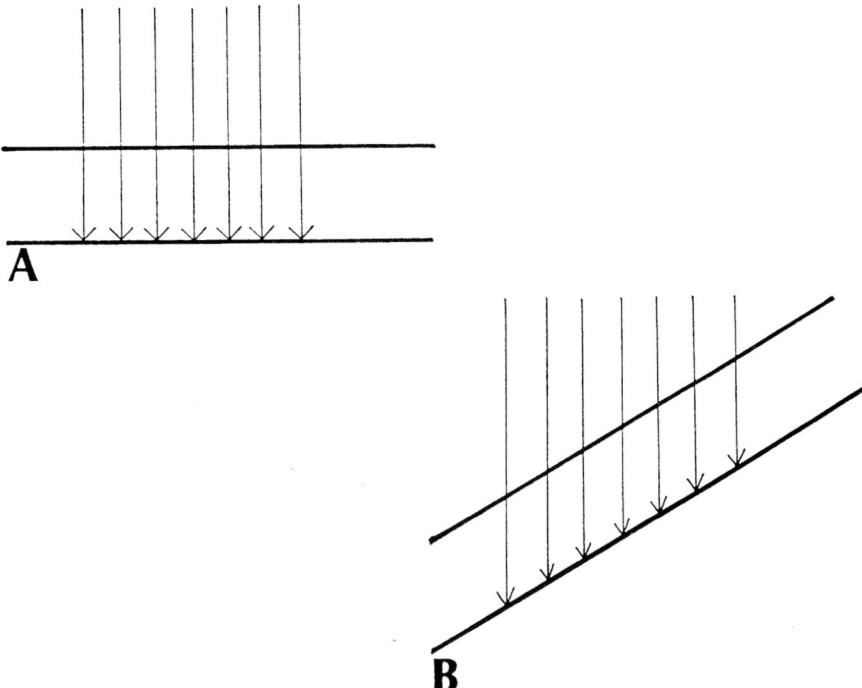

FIGURE 6-23. A: Without scleral depression, light rays have a short path through the retina. **B:** Retina tilted by scleral depression. The light rays must travel a longer path through the retina, which therefore appears less translucent.

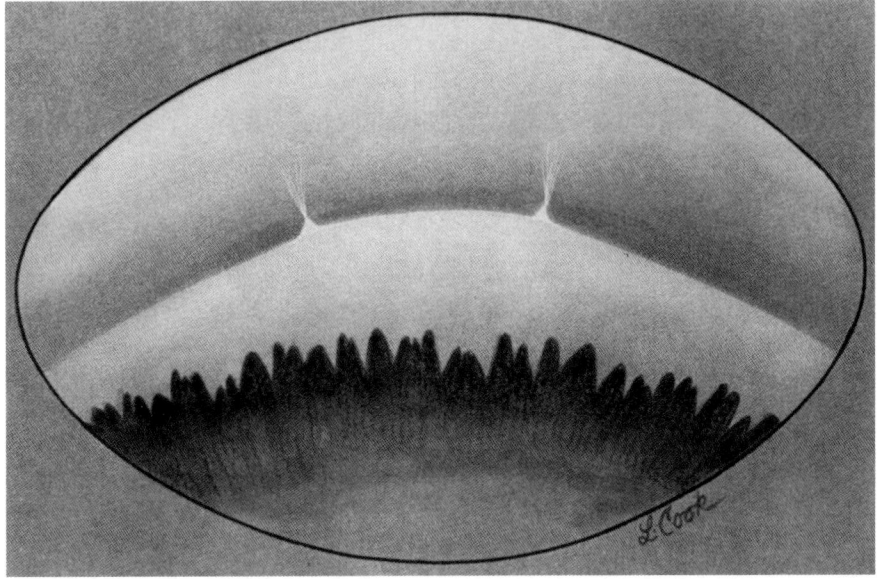

FIGURE 6-24. Indirect ophthalmoscopic view of tiny flap tears with vitreous traction, demonstrated by scleral depression at the posterior vitreous base.

pupils, depression can bring the peripheral retina into view. In all cases, constant movement of the scleral depressor maximizes the chances of finding a small break.

Scleral depression may cause pain. It raises the intraocular pressure and is therefore especially painful in eyes with a high initial pressure. Glaucoma patients must be examined gently. In addition, the examination stretches and compresses the eyelids and may thereby cause discomfort. To minimize this complication, scleral depression should be started superiorly because the upper eyelid is looser and more flexible than the lower.

The patient looks down, and the examiner places the depressor near the lid margin or in the lid crease, following the eyelid up as the patient looks up. Beginners should hold the depressor vertically so the indentation can be found easily with the indirect ophthalmoscope. The examiner merely follows the shaft of the depressor down into the eye. If the indentation is not seen, the examiner should scan the fundus, moving his or her head from side to side. Holding the depressor vertically also simplifies the problem of orienting one's movements in the inverted upside-down field of the indirect ophthalmoscope (Fig. 6-25). Anteroposterior movements are easily made. For examining more posteriorly, the observer simply moves the depressor toward the optic nerve. Circumferential movements are more difficult, but they become automatic with practice. The beginner simply has to remember that the depressor should be moved opposite the direction suggested by the view of the retina.

If the superior ora serrata is to be viewed, the patient should look as far superiorly as possible (Fig. 6-26). Beginners will see the ora serrata most easily in highly myopic eyes. If areas of the superior retina posterior to the equator are to be examined, the patient must look slightly inferiorly (Fig. 6-27).

Scleral depression is most difficult at the 9:00 and 3:00 positions because the eyelid is shorter here and because the canthal ligaments resist the posterior movement of the depressor. Direct scleral depression at the canthus is painful. Moreover, the depressor may slip off the eyelid and may strike the patient's eye. The following techniques help to avoid these problems. First, the depressor is placed on the superior eyelid, above the horizontal axis. It is then rotated downward toward the canthus, carrying the eyelid down with it. The lid becomes more slack when the patient, his or her head rolled away from the ex-

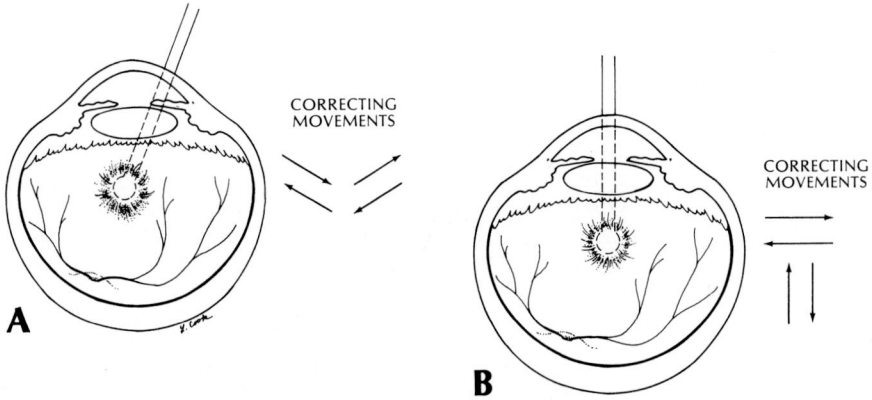

FIGURE 6-25. A: Incorrect technique for scleral depression. Making diagonal correcting movements is difficult because of the upside-down and backward image of the indirect ophthalmoscope. **B:** Correct technique for scleral depression. The depressor is held vertically, so horizontal and vertical correcting movements can be made easily.

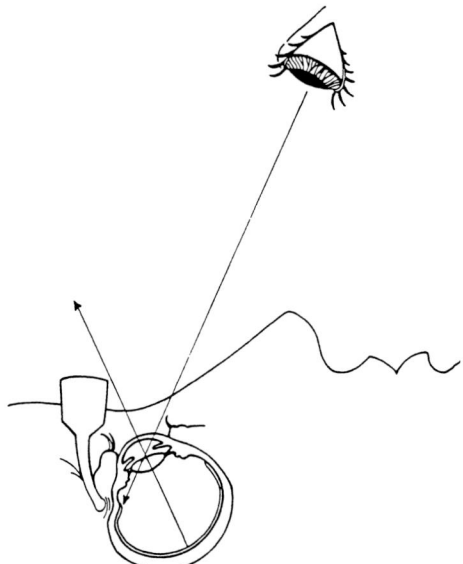

FIGURE 6-26. The ora serrata can be seen best when the patient looks as far superiorly as possible.

aminer, is not looking into an extreme position of gaze (Fig. 6-28). Second, a cotton-tipped applicator, being blunter and softer than a metal depressor, may be better tolerated. Finally, if the foregoing techniques are unsuccessful, one can easily depress the conjunctiva directly after topical anesthesia has been administered (Fig. 6-29).

Scleral depression should be avoided in patients who have had recent intraocular surgery. Instead, the examiner should wait until the patient is in the operating room, when the wound can be inspected and, if needed, reinforced. Depression should also be avoided in eyes with an acute traumatic hyphema or with a suspected scleral rupture.

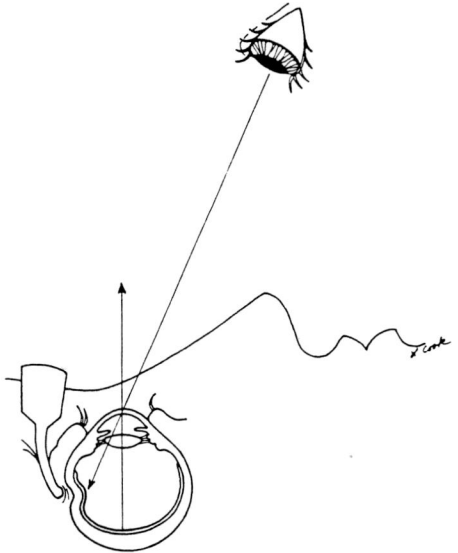

FIGURE 6-27. To view the midperiphery, the examiner should have the patient look slightly inferiorly.

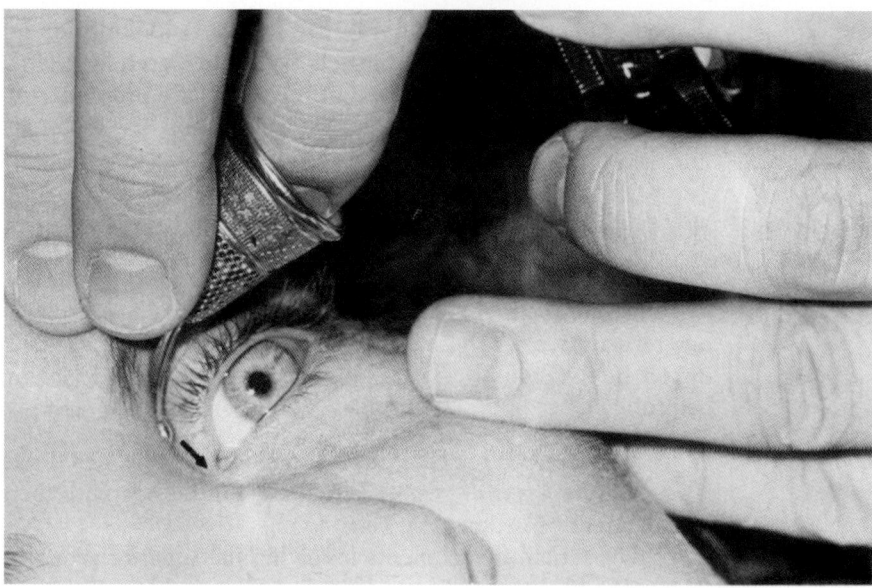

FIGURE 6-28. Scleral depression of the nasal periphery. The patient's head is rolled away from the examiner. The patient looks straight ahead, keeping the eyelid slack. The scleral depressor is placed on the superior eyelid above the horizontal axis. It is then rotated downward toward the canthus *(arrow)*, carrying the eyelid with it.

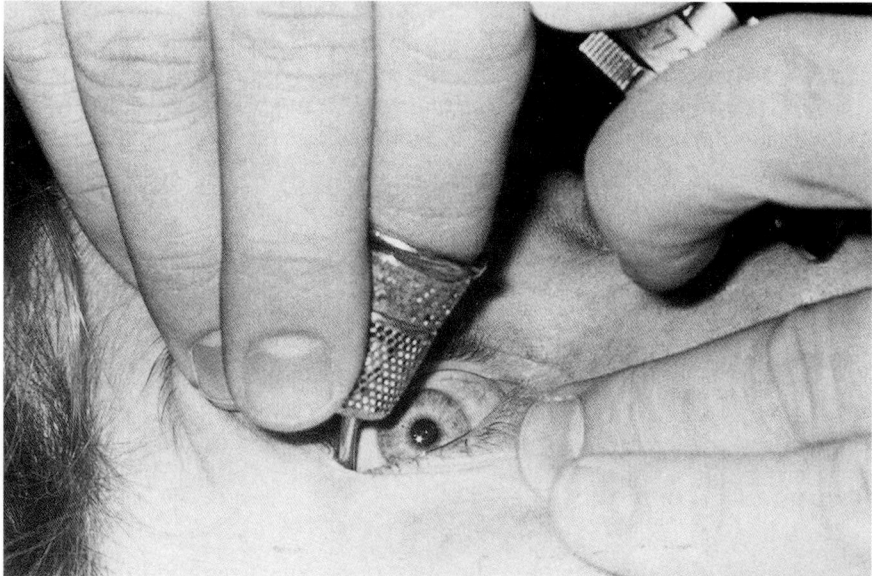

FIGURE 6-29. Examination of the temporal periphery. If the eyelid is not slack enough to allow depression, the scleral depressor can be placed on the anesthetized conjunctiva.

BIOMICROSCOPY

Goldmann Three-mirror Contact Lens

The Goldmann three-mirror lens is used when high magnification is required. It is most useful in patients in whom it is difficult to find breaks with indirect ophthalmoscopy and in patients in whom it is difficult to determine whether a retinal break is full or partial thickness. Although nearly all breaks can be found with indirect ophthalmoscopy and scleral depression, in some cases, tiny breaks may be found with the Goldmann three-mirror lens.

Wide-field Contact Lenses

Visualization of the peripheral retina may be difficult in pseudophakic eyes because of opacification of the posterior capsule or shrinkage of the anterior capsular opening. The first step is to make a wide posterior capsulotomy with the neodymium: yttrium aluminum garnet laser. If this fails, the Mainster and Volk wide-field contact lenses combined with ocular rotation, lens tilting, and scleral depression are helpful in visualizing the retina anterior to the equator (14).

Handheld Lenses

The Volk aspheric lenses are positive lenses that permit magnified, indirect ophthalmoscopy of the retina. They are especially helpful when looking for breaks from the posterior pole to the midperiphery. In eyes with small pupils, the 90-diopter aspheric lens is best. When more magnification is required, 60- and 78-diopter lenses are available.

FINDING THE RETINAL BREAKS

The configuration of the retinal detachment suggests the location of at least one retinal break (13). The basic principle is that gravity helps subretinal fluid (SRF) to dissect inferiorly and retards superior dissection. The following hints may be helpful:

1. For superior retinal detachments crossing the 12:00 meridian, a break is within $1\frac{1}{2}$ hours of 12:00 on the side with the greater inferior extent of detachment (Fig. 6-30).
2. For retinal detachments involving the superior retina but not crossing the 12:00 meridian, a break is within $1\frac{1}{2}$ hours of the most superior edge of the detachment (Fig. 6-31).
3. A focal spot of pigment may help to locate a break because such a spot sometimes appears in the flap of a tiny horseshoe tear (see Fig. 6-31).
4. For inferior detachments higher on one side, a break is located on that side (Fig. 6-32).
5. For inferior detachments with equal upward extent on both sides, a break is usually found near 6:00 (Fig. 6-33).
6. Inferior breaks usually do not cause highly bullous retinal detachments. Therefore, when large bullae are seen inferiorly, the surgeon must look carefully for a superior retinal break (15).
7. When no breaks are found in an inferior retinal detachment, a superior break may be leaking fluid down a shallow peripheral trough (Fig. 6-34). Locating these breaks is sometimes facilitated by having the patient's head tilted far backward, allowing the fluid to shift up toward the break (Fig. 6-35).

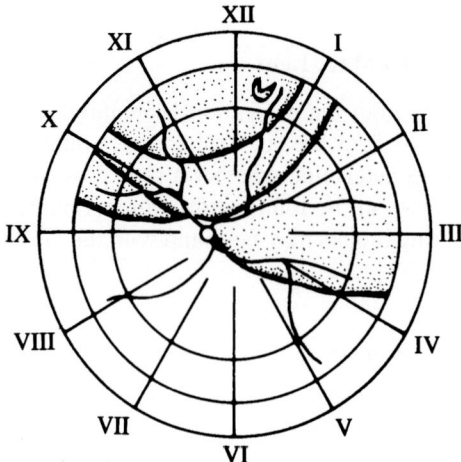

FIGURE 6-30. A superior retinal detachment that crosses the 12:00 meridian. A break is found near the 12:00 position on the side with the greater inferior extent of detachment, in this case the temporal side.

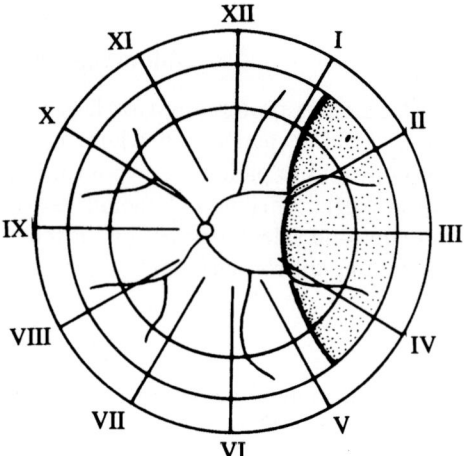

FIGURE 6-31. A superior retinal detachment that does not cross the 12:00 meridian. A break is found within 1½ hours of its most superior margin. A focal pigmented spot alerts the examiner to the location of the break, which can only be seen with scleral depression.

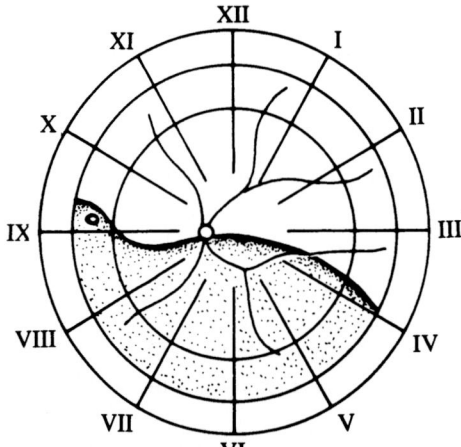

FIGURE 6-32. An inferior detachment that is higher on the nasal side. A break is located on that side (at the 8:45 position).

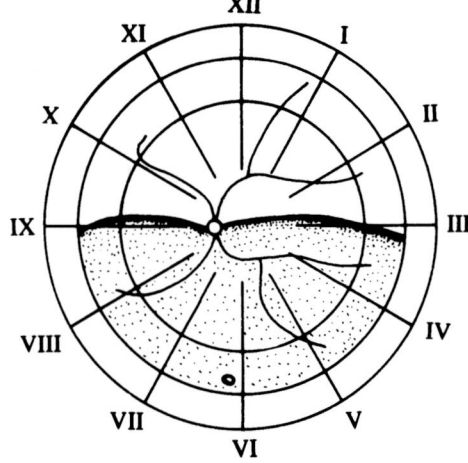

FIGURE 6-33. An inferior detachment with equal superior extent on both sides. A break is found near the 6:00 position.

CHAPTER 6/FUNDUS EXAMINATION AND PREOPERATIVE MANAGEMENT 95

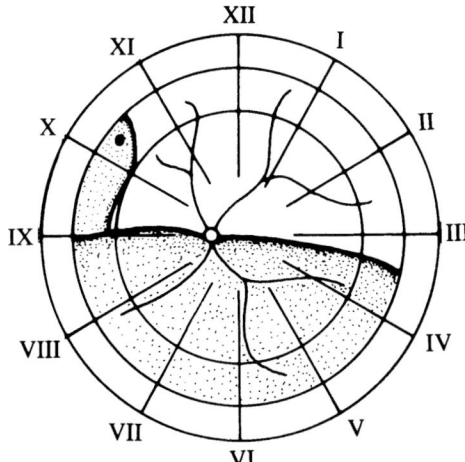

FIGURE 6-34. When no inferior break is found in an inferior retinal detachment, the examiner should look for a superior break that is leaking fluid along a shallow peripheral trough.

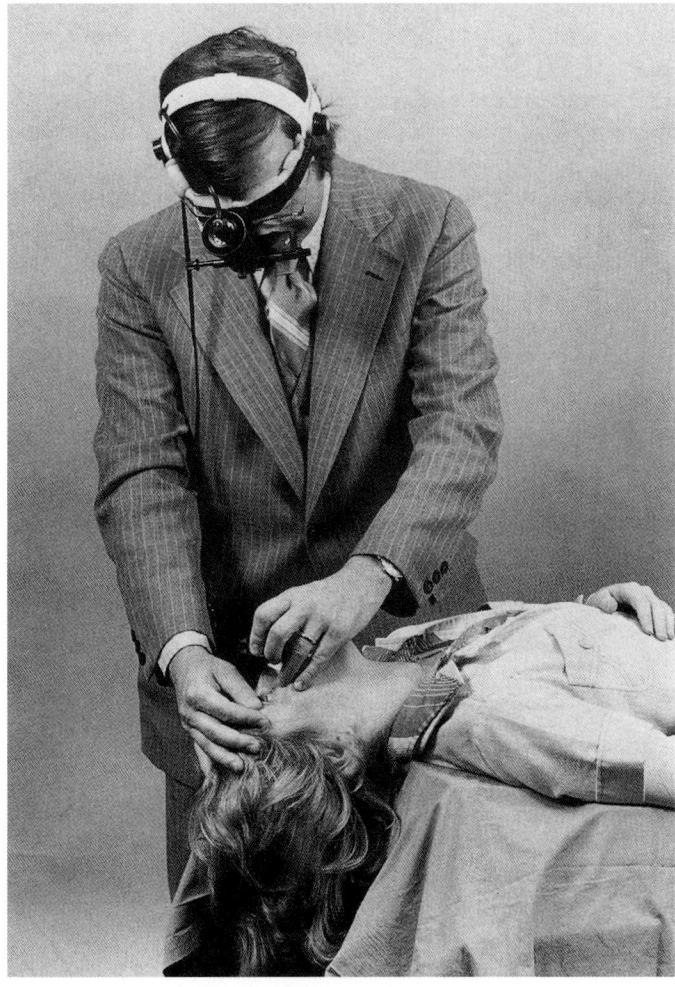

FIGURE 6-35. Patient's neck is hyperextended to allow fluid to shift superiorly.

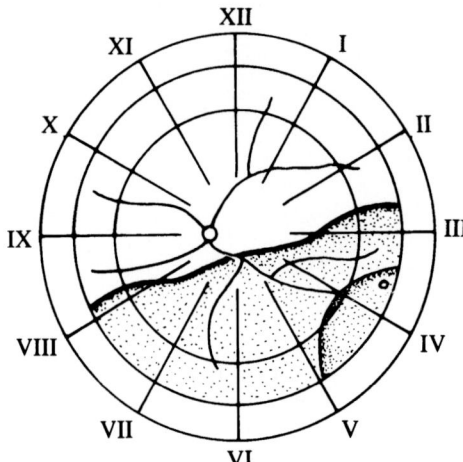

FIGURE 6-36. A demarcation line (from the 3:30 to the 5:00 position) has failed to contain a retinal detachment. A break must be present between the demarcation line and the ora serrata.

8. If a demarcation line is present in a superior quadrant, a hole must exist between the line and the ora serrata (Fig. 6-36). This is usually also true for demarcation lines in inferior quadrants, but occasionally, fluid trickling down from a superior break may cause an inferior demarcation line in the absence of a superior one.
9. Until proven otherwise, one should suspect that a break is present at the end of meridional folds, especially in aphakic retinal detachments.
10. In pseudophakic retinal detachments, the surgeon should carefully examine the posterior border of the vitreous base for tiny flap tears (see Fig. 6-24).
11. In high myopes with a posterior staphyloma, a break may be found anywhere in the posterior pole, not necessarily in the fovea.
12. In high myopes, a peripheral break may allow the accumulation of fluid in a posterior staphyloma, even though a connection between the break and staphyloma is not apparent.

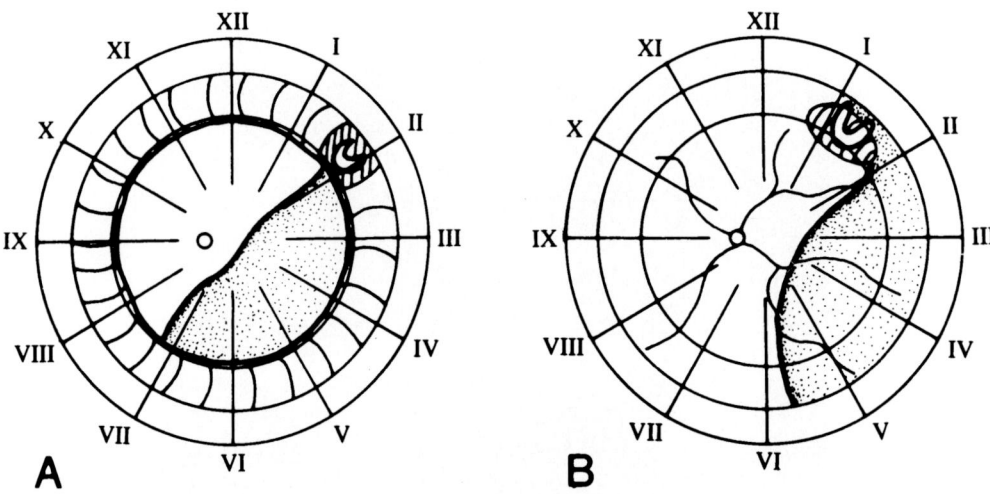

FIGURE 6-37. Redetached retina. **A:** The encircling scleral buckle *(parallel curved lines)* was not placed far enough posteriorly to seal the horseshoe tear. **B:** The segmental circumferential buckle was not placed far enough anteriorly.

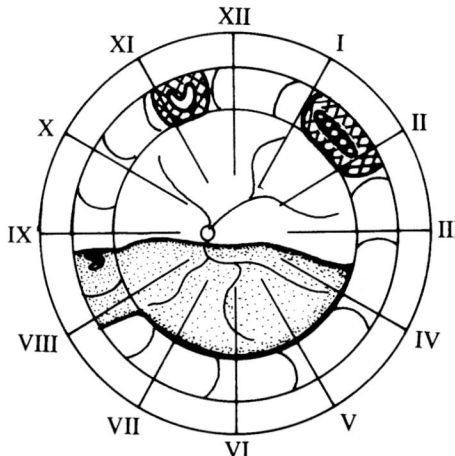

FIGURE 6-38. Redetached retina. A break is often found where the subretinal fluid crosses over the scleral buckle (from the 8:00 to the 9:00 position).

13. In redetachments, the surgeon should first see whether the original break or breaks have reopened (Fig. 6-37). If not, a break may be found in the most superior area where SRF crosses over the scleral buckle (Fig. 6-38). If no SRF crosses over the buckle, the break is probably posterior to it (Fig. 6-39).
14. When a break is not easily located, the patient should be examined while he or she is seated. The slight shift of the fluid may facilitate the detection of breaks.
15. In 3% of patients with retinal detachment, no definite break is ever found (5).
16. When a bullous retinal detachment is present, a break previously hidden by retinal folds sometimes appears after the SRF has been drained during the surgical procedure.

The foregoing discussion in no way implies that the remainder of the retina need not be examined after a break has been found in the expected location. Fifty percent of retinal detachments have more than one break (17). If any retinal break is not closed, the operation is likely to fail.

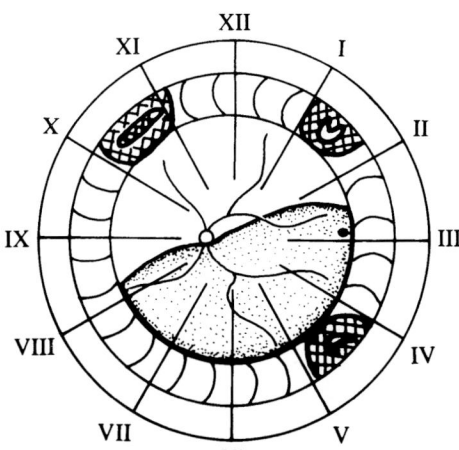

FIGURE 6-39. Redetached retina. No fluid crosses over the scleral buckle. A break is found posterior to the buckle (3:00 position).

PREOPERATIVE MANAGEMENT

Medical Evaluation

A careful medical evaluation is important, especially in cases of complicated retinal detachment in which the procedure may last 2 or more hours and is to be done with the patient under general anesthesia. Allergies must be identified. The anesthesiologist must be alerted if the patient has glaucoma and is being treated with anticholinesterase drugs, such as phospholine iodine. Because these drugs lower blood pseudocholinesterase, succinylcholine should not be used in conjunction with general anesthesia, or the patient will have prolonged respiratory paralysis.

Prevention of Infection

Even in the absence of clinical infection, some surgeons routinely treat patients preoperatively with prophylactic antibiotics. Patients' eyelashes are trimmed so they do not contaminate the operative field and so postoperative secretions can be more readily wiped away.

Binocular Patching

Binocular patching and bed rest, in almost all cases, prevent the spread of the retinal detachment. Moreover, significant quantities of SRF may be absorbed, especially in superior bullous retinal detachments (1,2,10,12). The fluid is not as readily absorbed in aphakic and inferior retinal detachments (10). The decreased elevation of the detachment facilitates the localization of breaks and sometimes allows a nondrainage procedure to be performed.

Informed Consent

The ophthalmologist must document in the chart what he or she tells patients because they are likely to forget unpleasant details. A prospective study found that only 23% of patients retained knowledge of surgical risks (16).

Pupillary Dilatation

Maximal cycloplegia and mydriasis are obtained if, beginning 1 hour before the surgical procedure, three applications of cyclopentolate 1% and phenylephrine 2.5% are given at 15-minute intervals. If the pupil will not dilate enough to allow peripheral retinal examination, iris hooks can be used at the start of the procedure (see Fig. 7-26). If a dense cataract prevents satisfactory examination, we combine cataract extraction, vitrectomy, and scleral buckling (SB) at the same sitting.

Timing of Surgery

In many cases, even if the macula is threatened, it will not detach if the operation is scheduled on the following day, especially if the patient is bilaterally patched. Further, emergency late-night surgery for retinal detachment does not give better visual results than surgical procedures done the next day (8). However, because detachment of the macula may lead to permanent visual loss, when the detachment is close to the center of the macula, repair is usually performed on the day the patient presents with this condition. If the macula has been detached for less than a day, the surgical procedure is nearly always done within a day, because prompt retinal reattachment can often restore much of the central vision. If the macula has been detached for 2 to 7 days, waiting a day or two does not make a difference in visual results, but the operation should be done within a few days. If the macula has been detached for more than a week, the timing of the surgical repair is still less critical (4,6,7).

REFERENCES

1. Algvere P, Rosengren B. Active immobilization of the eye in the treatment of retinal detachment. *Mod Probl Ophthalmol* 1977;18:286.
2. Algvere P, Rosengren B. Immobilization of the eye: evaluation of a new method in retinal detachment surgery. *Acta Ophthalmol* 1977;55:303.
3. Benson WE. Prophylactic therapy of retinal breaks. *Surv Ophthalmol* 1977;22:41.
4. Burton T. Recovery of visual acuity after retinal detachment surgery. *Trans Am Ophthalmol Soc* 1982;80:475.
5. Griffith RD, Ryan EA, Hilton GF. Primary retinal detachments without apparent breaks. *Am J Ophthalmol* 1976;81:420.
6. Grupposo S. Visual results after scleral buckling with silicone implant. *Arch Ophthalmol* 1975;93:327.
7. Gundry MF, Davies EW. Recovery of visual acuity after retinal detachment surgery. *Am J Ophthalmol* 1974;77:310.
8. Hartz AJ, Burton TC, Gottlieb MS, et al. Outcome and cost analysis of scheduled versus emergency scleral buckling surgery. *Ophthalmology* 1992;99:1358.
9. Havener WH, Gloeckner S. *Atlas of Diagnostic Techniques and Treatment of Retinal Detachment.* St Louis: CV Mosby, 1967.
10. Hofmann H, Hanselmayer H. Frequency and extent of spontaneous flattening of retinal detachments by patient immobilization. *Klin Monatsbl Augenheilkd* 1973;12:178.
11. Hovland KR, Elzeneiny IH, Schepens CL. Clinical evaluation of the small pupil binocular indirect ophthalmoscope. *Arch Ophthalmol* 1969;82:466.
12. Lean JS, Mahmood M, Manna R, et al. Effect of preoperative posture and binocular occlusion on retinal detachment. *Br J Ophthalmol* 1980;64:94.
13. Lincoff H, Gieser R. Finding the retinal hole. *Arch Ophthalmol* 1971;85:565.
14. Lincoff H, Kreissig I. Finding the retinal hole in the pseudophakic eye with detachment. *Am J Ophthalmol* 1994;117:442.
15. Lyall M. Retinal holes. *Arch Ophthalmol* 1972;88:228.
16. Priluck IA, Robertson DM, Buettner H. What patients recall of the preoperative discussion after retinal detachment surgery. *Am J Ophthalmol* 1979;87:620.
17. Rosenthal ML, Fradin S. The technique of binocular indirect ophthalmoscopy. *Highlights Ophthalmol* 1967;9:179.
18. Rubin ML. The optics of indirect ophthalmoscopy. *Surv Ophthalmol* 1964;9:449.
19. Schepens CL. A new ophthalmoscope demonstration. *Trans Am Acad Ophthalmol Otolaryngol* 1947;51:298.
20. Schepens CL. Progress in detachment surgery. *Trans Am Acad Ophthalmol Otolaryngol* 1951;55:606.

7
Scleral Buckling Procedure

As with all methods available to repair a detached retina, the goal is to reapproximate the edges of the retinal break to the underlying retinal pigment epithelium (RPE). Closure of the break eliminates the access of liquid vitreous to the subretinal space, thereby allowing the RPE and choroid to pump out the subretinal fluid (SRF), reattaching the retina. With scleral buckling (SB), this is accomplished by sewing on an inert substance to the sclera and indenting it (Fig. 7-1). Cryotherapy is used with SB to make a permanent chorioretinal scar around the break, ensuring long-lasting closure and preventing late reattachment. The basic steps of the surgical technique are detailed in this chapter.

ANESTHESIA

Scleral buckling can be performed with the patient under either local or general anesthesia. Local anesthesia is provided by a retrobulbar or peribulbar block combined with a facial block and intravenous sedation (3,41,72). It has several potential advantages over general anesthesia: the total operating room time is decreased, bleeding is less, recovery from anesthesia is faster (allowing the patient to return home sooner), and perioperative mortality may be slightly decreased, especially when the patient has multiple systemic medical problems (41). A standard retrobulbar or peribulbar injection through the inferior eyelid, however, may not entirely eliminate pain or uncomfortable pressure sensation when extensive retracting or pulling on extraocular muscles is required and when encircling or large buckling elements are used. In anticipation of this possibility, some surgeons augment the anesthesia with a supratrochlear block preoperatively. Alternatively, a posterior, sub-Tenon's infiltration of the anesthetic agent using a blunt cannula can be performed, or the degree of intravenous sedation can be increased during the operation (55,70).

Rare, but potentially serious, complications of local anesthesia include perforation of the globe, retrobulbar hemorrhage, and injection into the optic nerve. Risk factors for globe perforation include axial myopia (e.g., axial lengths of 26 mm or more), the presence of a posterior or inferior staphyloma, a history of previous SB procedures, and the use of multiple injections (22,62). Injections into the optic nerve can result in optic neuropathy, compression and occlusion of the central retinal artery or vein, and infusion of the anesthetic into the subarachnoid space, which can have life-threatening sequelae such as seizures and central nervous system depression with respiratory arrest (1,44,74,82).

Compared with uncomplicated anterior segment operations, the surgical times required for SB procedures tend to be less predictable and are generally much longer. When local anesthesia is used, the patient may become restless or may have discomfort elsewhere from having to lie still during such a long procedure. These issues, coupled with the occasionally incomplete ocular pain relief that accompanies local anesthesia as described earlier, prompt many surgeons to prefer general anesthesia for most scleral buckle procedures.

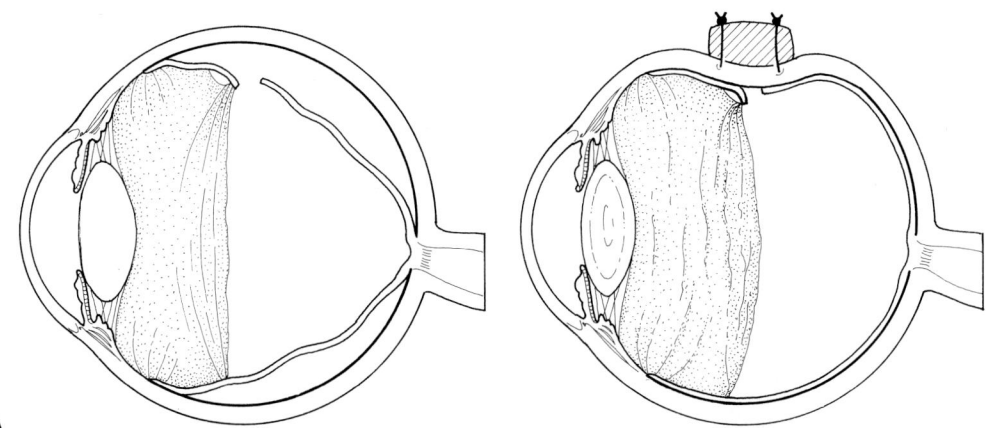

FIGURE 7-1. A: Principle of scleral buckling. Retinal detachment is caused by a flap-like retinal tear (The vitreous gel at the posterior base region can be seen holding the break open.) **B:** The eye wall under the tear is indented, relieving the vitreoretinal traction and effectively eliminating the access of liquid vitreous to the subretinal space. The subretinal fluid resorbs and the retina reattaches.

PREOPERATIVE PREPARATION

Shortly before the procedure begins, the pupil is dilated with a combination of short- and long-acting topical mydriatic agents such as phenylephrine, tropicamide, and cyclopentolate. In the operating room, after local or general anesthesia is administered, the skin around the eye is cleansed in the usual fashion for ocular surgery. A 5% to 10% povidone–iodine solution (Betadine) is instilled at that time to minimize the risk of postoperative infection further. The operative field is then covered with sterile drapes, and the globe is exposed with an eyelid speculum. Some surgeons trim the patient's eyelashes before preparing and draping. However, the adhesive drapes made specifically for eye surgery are usually sufficient to keep the lashes off the surgical field.

INCISION

The conjunctiva and Tenon's capsule are opened by performing a peritomy. In initial operations, the peritomy can be made either at the limbus or 4 mm posterior to it. The limbal peritomy has several advantages. It is opened and closed faster, requires less suture material for closure, covers the site of surgery with an intact layer of tissue, causes less bleeding, does not shorten the fornices, is less likely to cause symblepharon, and causes less postoperative adhesion of Tenon's capsule to the sclera, thereby facilitating reoperation (46).

The limbal conjunctiva and Tenon's capsule are tented up with toothed forceps and are incised down to the sclera with blunt scissors (Fig. 7-2). Tenon's capsule is separated from the perilimbal sclera by blunt dissection, so the incision can be made as close to the limbus as possible for 360 degrees (Fig. 7-3). When a single radial sponge (see later) is to be placed, a 180-degree incision usually suffices. Two relaxing incisions (Fig. 7-4), 180 degrees apart, serve to avoid tearing the conjunctiva. Additional blunt dissection between Tenon's capsule and the sclera is performed posteriorly (Fig. 7-5), so the rectus muscles can be hooked and bridled. A 4-0 black silk suture is passed under the muscle and is tied. Before proceeding further, the surgeon must look for areas of thin sclera. Otherwise, perforation of the globe may occur during localization. In the rare cases in which adequate

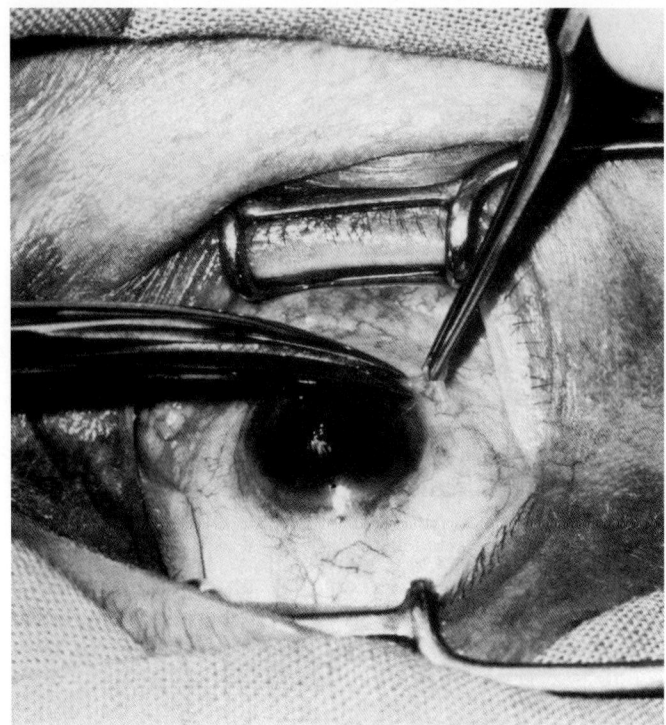

FIGURE 7-2. Limbal peritomy. The conjunctiva and Tenon's capsule are tented up with toothed forceps and are incised with blunt scissors.

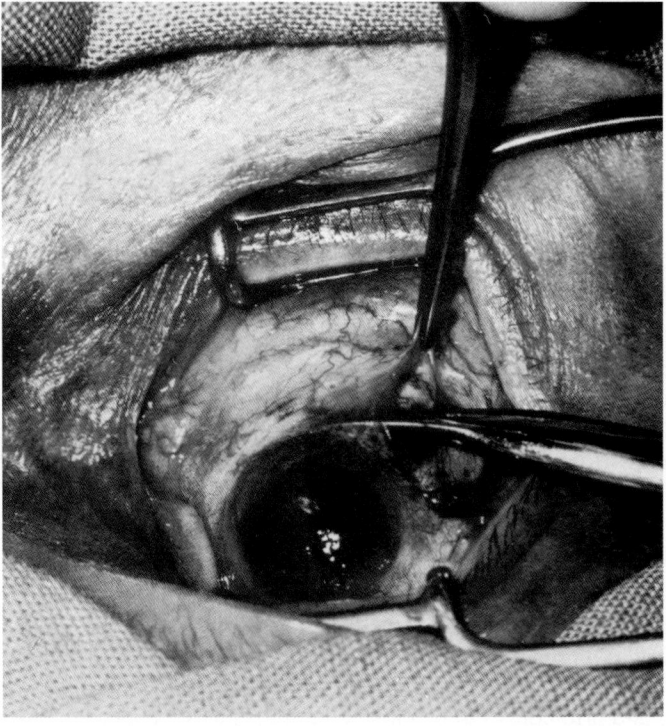

FIGURE 7-3. Tenon's capsule is undermined by blunt dissection so the incision can be as close to the limbus as possible.

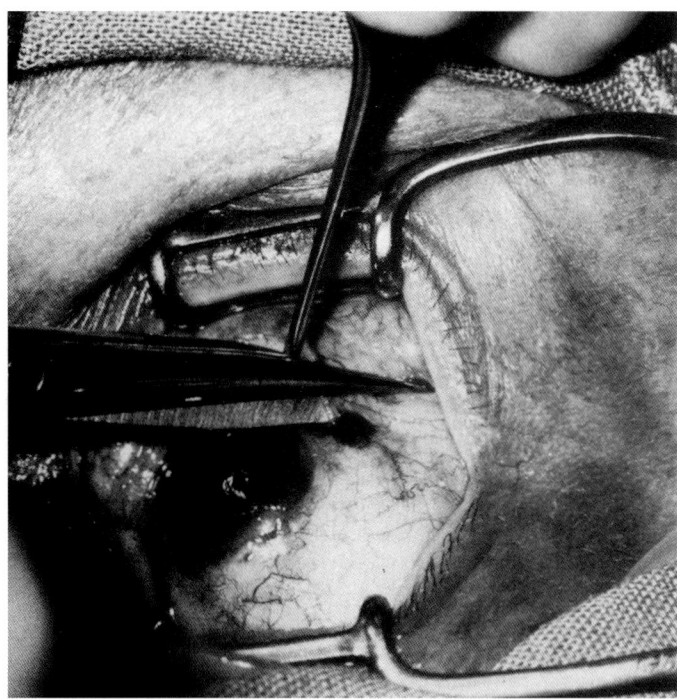

FIGURE 7-4. Radial relaxing incisions of the conjunctival peritomy are made to prevent tearing later in the procedure.

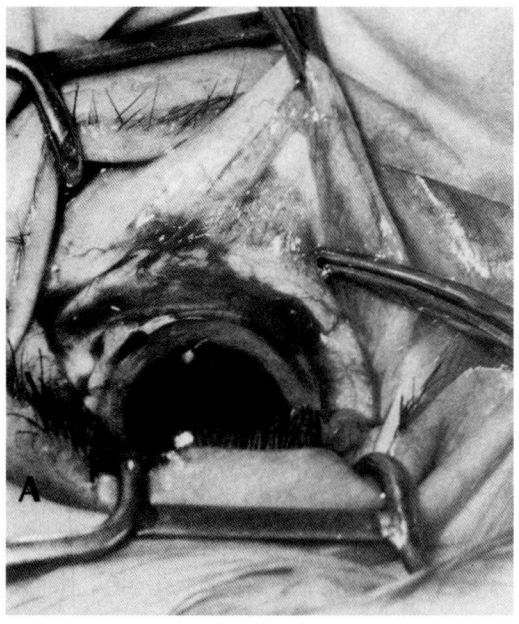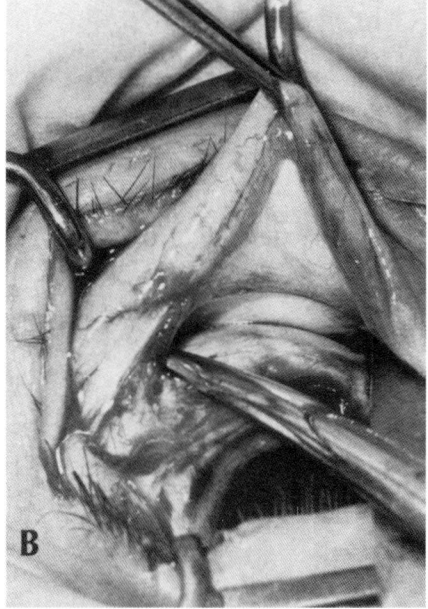

FIGURE 7-5. Posteriorly, Tenon's capsule is loosely adherent to the sclera, and blunt dissection easily separates it from the sclera. **A:** The closed tips of curved scissors are placed on the sclera in the middle of the quadrant and then are moved posteriorly. **B:** The blades are then opened behind the rectus insertions, spreading the dissection laterally. (When removing the scissors, the tips should be closed again to avoid striking the rectus insertion sites.)

exposure cannot be obtained, a lateral canthotomy is performed, and one or more muscles are disinserted. A traction suture is placed into the stump of the tendon.

LOCALIZATION

To place the buckling element correctly, the surgeon must localize all breaks that the buckle is to cover (i.e., the sclera underlying them must be marked). We localize with a blunt-tipped diathermy electrode and use the indirect ophthalmoscope for visualization. The intensity of the diathermy should be tested first on anterior sclera to ensure an adequate but not excessive scleral coagulation. The assistant steadies the eye by holding two bridle sutures while the surgeon, using a cotton-tipped applicator for scleral depression, locates the meridian of the break. The diathermy electrode is then introduced into this meridian. Keeping the wrist cocked to ensure that only the tip of the instrument indents the sclera, the surgeon makes a few brief applications of diathermy on the sclera underlying the retinal break. The eye is then rolled forward, and additional diathermy is applied to make a well-visualized, permanent mark (Fig. 7-6).

Instead of diathermy, various blunt indenting instruments can be used to localize and mark the position of the breaks. A temporary dehydration spot is created when focal pressure is applied to the sclera by the instrument. A permanent mark is then made with a surgical pen. This is the preferred technique when either a staphyloma or thin sclera is present in the region of the retinal break. In this situation, a diathermy electrode is more likely to penetrate the globe, and its use should be avoided.

For small breaks, the posterior edge alone is localized; for large flap tears, the posterior edge and both anterior horns; for lattice degeneration with holes, both ends of the degeneration; for dialyses, the ends of the dialysis as well as the point in the center of the

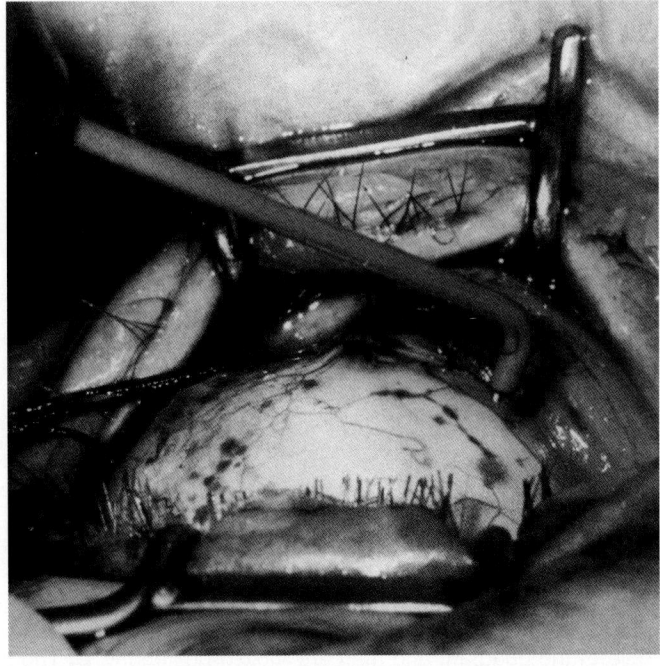

FIGURE 7-6. The diathermy coagulation is reinforced to make an easily visible, permanent mark.

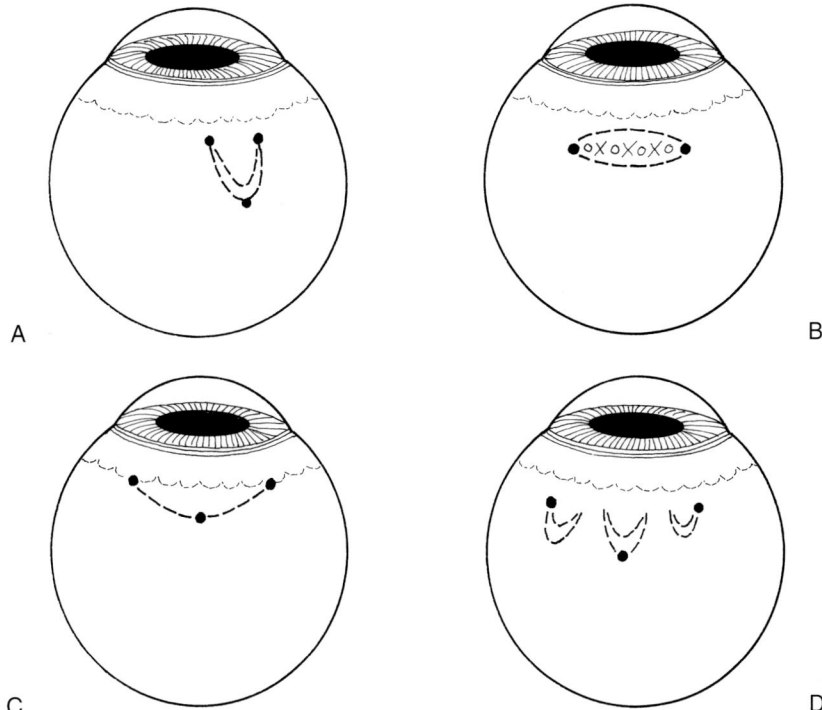

FIGURE 7-7. Localization technique for various types of retinal tears: single flap tear **(A)**, holes or tears in lattice degeneration **(B)**, large retinal dialysis **(C)**, and cluster of tears **(D)**. (The *broken line* represents the ora serrata.)

dialysis where the surgeon estimates that the retina will fall. Anterior and posterior localization of long tears is important, because many tears are not radial (Fig. 7-7).

In highly bullous detachments, parallax can lead the surgeon to localize more posteriorly than the actual position of the break (Fig. 7-8). This error can be minimized by first localizing the least elevated part of the break, generally its anterior border. This then

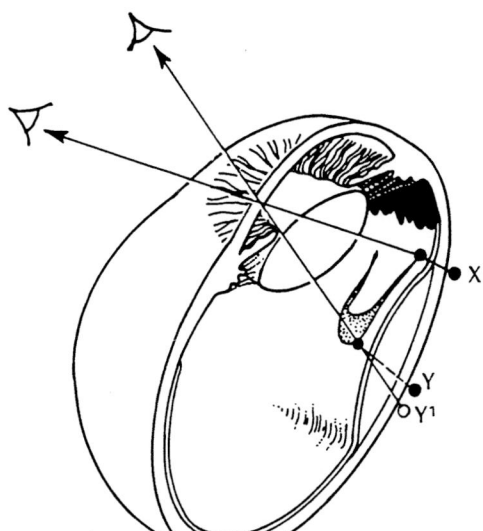

FIGURE 7-8. Because of parallax, the apex of the break appears to be more posteriorly located (Y^1) than it really is. If the retina were flat, the apex would be at Y, not at Y^1.

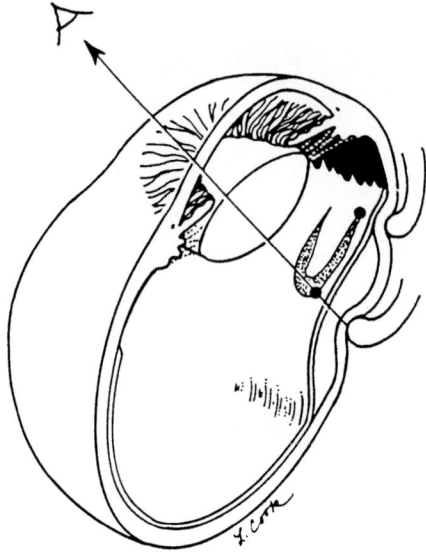

FIGURE 7-9. Errors induced by parallax can be minimized if the less elevated anterior horn is localized first. Then the localizing instrument, functioning as a scleral depressor, is slid posteriorly under indirect ophthalmoscopic control until the surgeon determines that the apex has been reached. The sclera is then marked at this point.

serves as a reference point as the diathermy electrode is gently slid posteriorly under indirect ophthalmoscopic control until the posterior border of the break has been judged to be reached (Fig. 7-9). Sometimes, focal hyperpigmented hyperplasia of the RPE, which can be seen through the retinal break, indicates the origin of the retinal break. In rare cases, accurate localization of the breaks can be achieved only after the retina has been flattened by a combination of drainage of the SRF and an injection of saline into the vitreous cavity. Finally, after the known breaks have been localized, the surgeon must fully reinspect the retina for any that may have been missed. If the preoperative examination has been difficult, this final check is all the more important.

RETINOPEXY

A firm adhesion between the retina and either the RPE or Bruch's membrane is required to seal the retinal breaks adequately and to achieve long-lasting retinal reattachment. Currently, cryotherapy is the most frequently used modality with SB to induce this adhesion.

Cryotherapy

Freezing focally destroys the choriocapillaris, RPE, and outer retinal layers. The formation of a firm chorioretinal scar results over the ensuing weeks (52). An adequate adhesion may sometimes result from cryotherapy of the surrounding RPE alone, that is, without visible freezing effects to the overlying detached retina around the break. However, experimental evidence indicates that such treatment results in a relationship between the sensory retina and the RPE similar to the relatively weak adhesion found in eyes without detachment (48,52). A histologically strong adhesion results when the RPE and the sensory retina are both frozen during treatment, because tight junctions are later seen between Müller cells and the RPE or Bruch's membrane (48,52). The surgeon should avoid freezing RPE that will not come into contact with the retina when it is attached. Freezing within the break does not increase the strength of the adhesion. Such freezing only releases more pigment into the vitreous and the SRF and may contribute to proliferative vitreoretinopathy (PVR; see later) (14).

The pressure of the cryoprobe on the sclera forces fluid from the eye. As the eye softens, high indentation by the probe is possible. Therefore, breaks in attached retina should be frozen first, and breaks in highly detached retina should be frozen last. As the assistant steadies the patient's eye with the rectus muscle bridle sutures, the surgeon, viewing with the indirect ophthalmoscope, surrounds the tears with 2 to 3 mm of retinal freezing to ensure adequate adhesion. The surgeon's wrist must be kept cocked outward so only the tip of the cryoprobe indents the eye. Beginners tend to indent the eye with the shaft of the probe, mistaking this indentation for the indentation of the probe's tip. When treatment is then applied, the freezing tip of the probe can cause severe damage posterior to the area of visualization. Most cryoprobes have a small knob 180 degrees away from the freezing tip to aid the surgeon in orienting the probe. The freezing portion of the tip must be pressed squarely against the globe.

When the retina is frozen, it turns white. This retinal opaqueness aids in differentiating small retinal breaks from small patches of thin retina. Normal and thin retina both turn white when frozen. Full-thickness retinal breaks appear dark in contrast to the adjacent frozen retina. Even after thawing, the sensory retina remains slightly more opaque than adjacent retina. This opacification helps the surgeon to verify that the treatment applications have been contiguous. Scleral depression makes this change easier to see.

After the first application, the surgeon keeps the probe in place until the iceball has thawed; then, watching retinal landmarks, the surgeon gently moves the probe just enough to place the next contiguous lesion. An alternative method of treatment allows the surgeon to check the accuracy of the localization marks. Under direct visualization, the probe is frozen to the mark on the sclera. The eye is then rolled backward to verify the treatment with the indirect ophthalmoscope. Retinal freezing is observed surrounding the break if the localization mark is correct (Fig. 7-10).

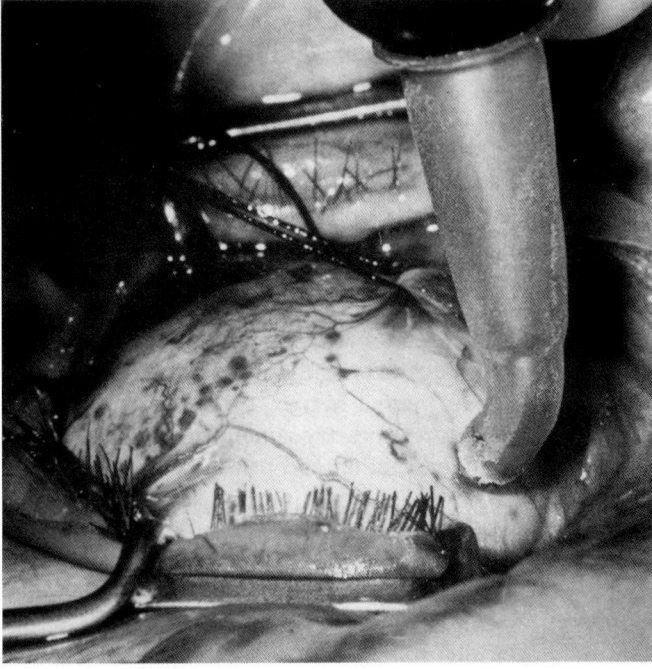

FIGURE 7-10. Checking the accuracy of localization. The cryoprobe tip is frozen to the localization mark. The eye is then rolled backward for indirect ophthalmoscopy. The surgeon should be able to confirm proper placement of the treatment by observing freezing of the retina surrounding the break.

The firmer the indentation, the faster the rate of freezing because choroidal flow, which acts as an insulator, is stopped. Excessive indentation can close the central retinal artery. After a few consecutive applications, the surgeon must relax the pressure on the eye to permit ocular circulation. If a break is highly elevated, the surgeon should not indent excessively, especially if the eye has recently undergone intraocular surgery or has a scleral staphyloma. When these conditions are present, the SRF should be drained before cryotherapy.

Laser Photocoagulation

Traditionally, laser was not an option with SB procedures because the available delivery systems such as endolaser probes and laser indirect ophthalmoscopes allowed for adequate laser update to occur only once the retina was attached. For this reason, these modalities have been mainly used in the setting of a detached retina approached with vitrectomy, applied after the retina is flattened during the operation with internal tamponading agents such as air, perfluorocarbon liquid (PFCL), or silicone oil (see chapter 9, Alternative Techniques). However, a transcleral diode laser probe has been developed that permits laser retinopexy around a tear in detached retina and therefore may be used as a substitute for cryotherapy in SB (37,54). Although favorable results have been reported, the experience with this technique to date is limited, and the full spectrum of potential risks and benefits compared with those of established methods has not yet been analyzed.

SCLERAL BUCKLING

Indenting the sclera and choroid toward the retinal breaks ("scleral buckling") promotes settling of the detached retina. With good intraoperative apposition of the layers in the region of the break, the SRF completely, and often quickly, resorbs postoperatively. Scleral buckling permanently relieves vitreoretinal traction, which, if unrelieved, can reopen a retinal break despite otherwise adequate cryotherapy or diathermy treatment. Scleral buckling can also favorably counteract the adverse features of early PVR. For example, when placing the buckle under a fixed fold, the force from the fold pulls the retina toward the RPE instead of away from it, thereby facilitating retinal reattachment in this setting (58).

Explant Material

The element that is sutured to the surface of the sclera to indent it is referred to as an explant. Explants may be radial (perpendicular to the ora serrata) or circumferential (parallel to the ora serrata). The latter may be segmental or encircling. All permanent explant material currently used is made of silicone (66). Two basic varieties are used: silicone sponge and solid silicone (Fig. 7-11). Available sponges are 80 mm long and are either round (3, 4, and 5 mm in diameter), elliptical (7.5 × 5.5 mm), oval (5 and 7.5 mm), or rectangular (12 × 4 mm). Solid silicone is available in various sizes and shapes.

Suture Technique

Explants are held in place by mattress sutures of 5-0 monofilament nylon, 4-0 or 5-0 Dacron, or 4-0 or 5-0 Supramyd. Thinner sutures tend to erode out of the sclera. Colored sutures are easier to locate in reoperations than white ones.

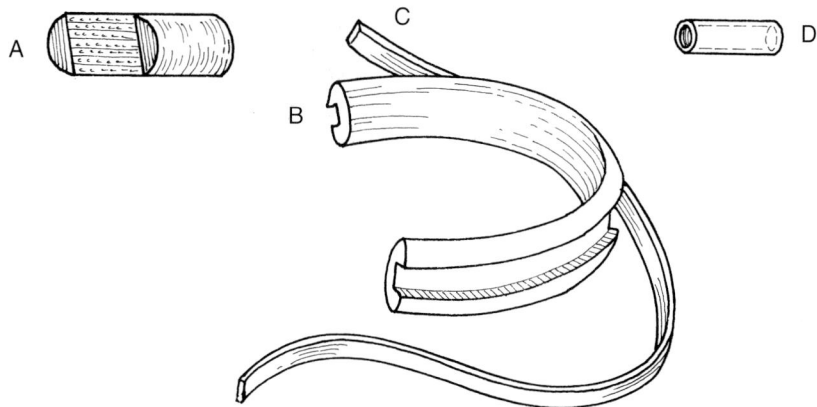

FIGURE 7-11. Scleral buckle elements: silicone sponge **(A)**; grooved, solid silicone tire **(B)**; silicone encircling band **(C)**; and silicone (Watzke) sleeve **(D)**.

The assistant provides exposure and steadies the globe with the bridle sutures adjacent to the break. Tenon's capsule is held back with a Schepens retractor. The surgeon further immobilizes the globe by grasping the tendon of a rectus muscle with toothed forceps (Fig. 7-12). Stabilizing the globe is easier if the suture needle moves away from, rather than toward, the tendon grasped. Therefore, to secure a radial explant, for example, it is best to use a double-armed suture and to pass each needle in an anterior-

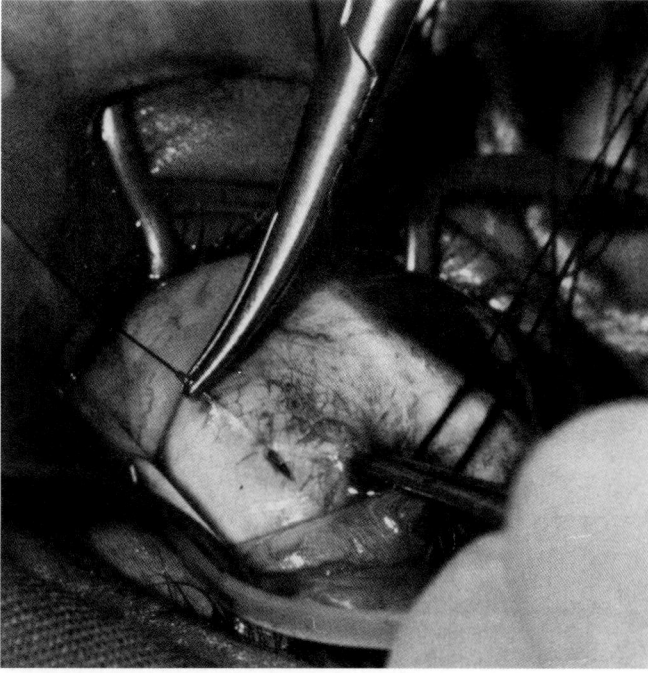

FIGURE 7-12. Placement of a scleral suture for a circumferential buckle. The assistant provides exposure and stability by means of two bridle sutures and a retractor. The surgeon further steadies the eye by grasping a rectus muscle tendon with toothed forceps.

to-posterior direction (Fig. 7-13). An added benefit of this approach is that the suture is tied posteriorly, where Tenon's capsule is thicker; therefore, late erosion of the suture knot is less likely.

Placement of deep scleral sutures in a hypotonous eye without accidental perforation of the choroid is difficult. If the eye is soft, the assistant should increase the pressure to a nearly normal level by gentle indentation. If the break is located under a rectus muscle, the assistant can aid in the placement of sutures by retracting the muscle with a muscle hook. Alternatively, the muscle can be temporarily disinserted. Finally, a circumferential explant can be used instead of a radial one because the sutures can then be placed to either side of the muscle.

Scleral bites should be both deep and long, so the suture will not erode out of the sclera postoperatively. A spatula needle must be used. Its tip is introduced slowly into the sclera (Fig. 7-14A). When the proper depth has been reached, the needle is carefully pushed along between scleral lamellae (see Fig. 7-14B). Proper depth can be verified by gently lifting the needle while keeping it parallel to the sclera (see Fig. 7-14C). The needle must not be allowed to lose its depth (see Fig. 7-14D) because it is difficult and dangerous to regain depth once it has been lost. When the bite has been completed, the surgeon should push the needle through to its hub and should remove it following the curve of the needle. If the spatula needle is twisted during this maneuver, the sharp edge may cut through the choroid and cause bleeding. It may also cut into the overlying sclera and weaken it.

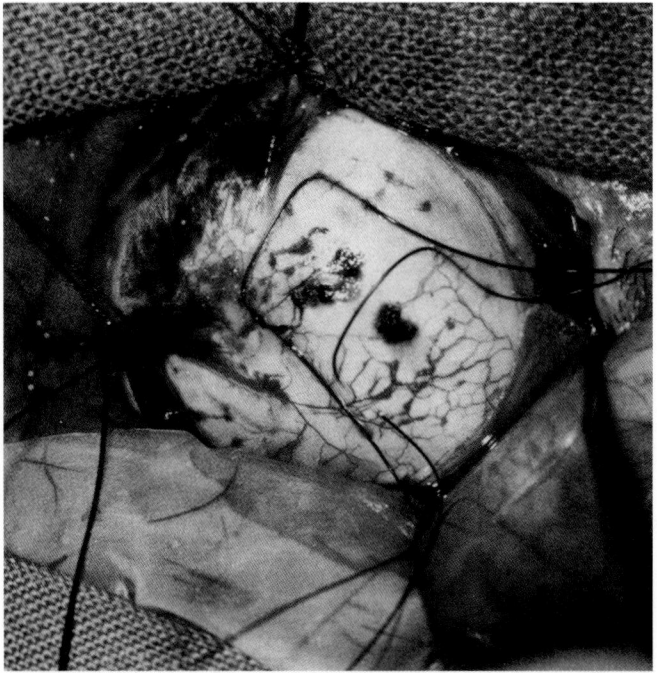

FIGURE 7-13. Double-armed sutures placed anterior to posterior in preparation for a radial buckle. The anterior horns and apex of the flap tear have been localized with diathermy. (For purposes of illustration, the diathermy marks have been darkened with methylene blue.)

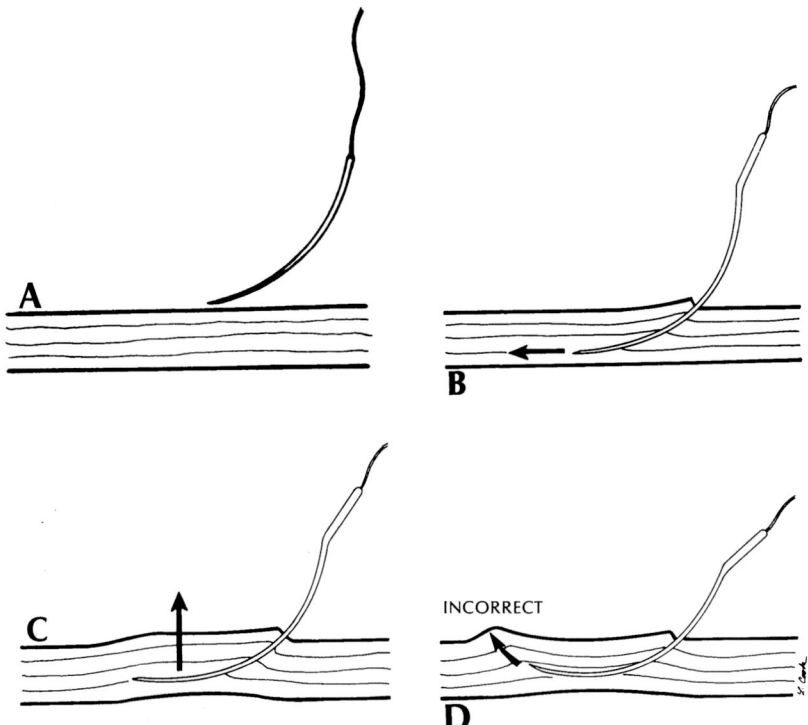

FIGURE 7-14. Placement of a scleral suture. The proper needle orientation of approach **(A)** and needle depth **(B)** are obtained. The needle is then guided between the scleral lamellae, parallel to the surface *(arrow)*. **C:** While advancing through the scleral lamellae, the proper depth can be verified by gently lifting the needle from time to time. **D:** Premature loss of depth will occur if the needle begins to point upward.

Radial Explants

Radial explants are preferred over circumferential explants for closing wide horseshoe tears because they cause much less fishmouthing of the posterior edge (see later) (50,61). They are also recommended for the treatment of extremely posterior breaks because it is easier to place radially rather than circumferentially oriented sutures far back on the sclera.

Silicone sponges are usually used for radial explants. The explant should extend 1 to 2 mm beyond the margins of the break. A 5-mm sponge adequately closes a break 3 mm wide. A 7.5-mm sponge closes breaks 5 to 6 mm wide. Larger breaks require two sponges placed side by side or a 12-mm sponge trimmed to the required size. Cutting a sponge in half lengthwise reduces its bulk without decreasing the width of the explant (Fig. 7-15). Adequate indentation can still be obtained.

The arms of the suture are placed 2 to 3 mm farther apart than the width of the sponge; for example, for a 5-mm width sponge, the sutures are placed 7 mm apart; for a 7.5-mm width sponge, 9 to 10 mm apart. One suture suffices for a small break. For larger breaks, two are needed (see Fig. 7-13). To prevent the fishmouth phenomenon, the surgeon should begin the posterior bite at the level of the apex of the tear and carry it 3 mm posteriorly. The anterior suture starts 2 mm anterior to the horns of the tear.

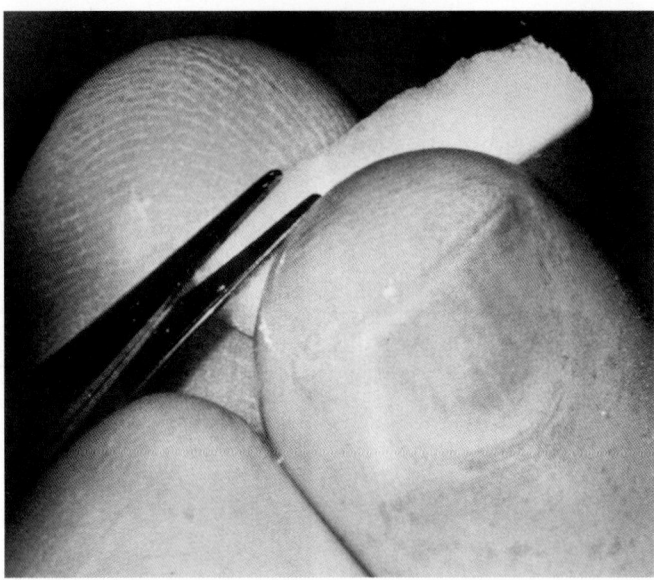

FIGURE 7-15. The sponge can be cut in half lengthwise to reduce its bulk.

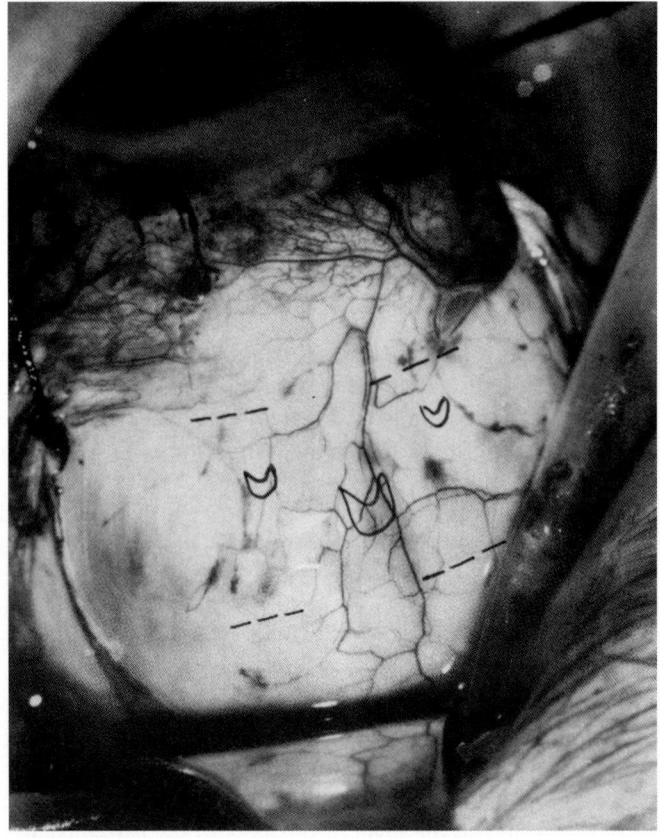

FIGURE 7-16. Three retinal breaks at different levels. A circumferential explant is required. *Broken lines* indicate the proper location of the mattress sutures.

Circumferential Explants

A circumferential explant is indicated for wide retinal breaks (80 to 90 degrees) such as a dialysis, for multiple breaks at different distances from the ora serrata (Fig. 7-16), and for detachments in which no break is found. Circumferential explants can be either sponge or solid silicone. The width of the explant depends on the anteroposterior length, not width, of the break.

The sutures are asymmetrically placed so the break will lie on the crest or anterior slope of the buckle (see Fig. 7-16). The posterior bite of the mattress suture usually must be made 3 to 4 mm posterior to the localizing mark of the apex of the tear. To buckle the anterior horns of flap tears, the anterior bite must be 1.5 mm anterior to their localizing marks. Then the distance between the sutures is measured, and an explant 2 mm less in width is selected.

If the surgeon uses an explant that is too small, it may shift anteriorly or posteriorly, uncovering part of the break and leading to failure of the operation. If no break has been found, the explant must buckle the posterior vitreous base and must extend the length of the detachment. If the explant encounters a rectus muscle, the explant must be placed under, not over, the muscle.

ENCIRCLING

Traction along the entire vitreous base region can be reduced permanently by a silicone band or sponge that encircles and constricts the eye (Table 7-1). Encircling is indicated when one sees evidence of early PVR, such as fixed folds, retinal tears with posteriorly rolled edges, or equatorial traction folds (Fig. 7-17). It is often used in the treatment of aphakic or pseudophakic retinal detachments because of their relatively high risk of developing PVR and of having missed or new breaks postoperatively. Some surgeons also advocate the use of encircling in patients with high myopia, especially when one sees extensive lattice degeneration or retinal breaks outside the area of detachment. It is also used to treat detachments in which no breaks have been found.

When using an encircling element, care must be taken not to pull the band too tight because this may result in postoperative chronic or severe pain, intrusion of the band, or anterior segment necrosis (20,83). In most cases, an indentation of 1 mm suffices to release vitreous traction, but a higher amount of indentation (e.g., 2 to 3 mm) is recommended in patients with PVR. If the scleral indentation is obtained by tightening the encircling element, the axial length of the globe is increased. On the other hand, if the surgeon desires some scleral shortening to counteract PVR, the indentation should be made by placing two mattress sutures in each quadrant, so the sclera can be wrapped around the explant (38).

Maximal reduction of vitreoretinal traction can be achieved only if the encircling band constricts the posterior vitreous base region. In the presence of strong vitreous traction, this area can be located by an equatorial fold or by a row of small flap tears. Otherwise,

TABLE 7-1. *Common indications for encircling*

Early proliferative vitreoretinopathy (PVR)
Aphakia or pseudophakia
High myopia
Extensive lattice degeneration
No retinal breaks found

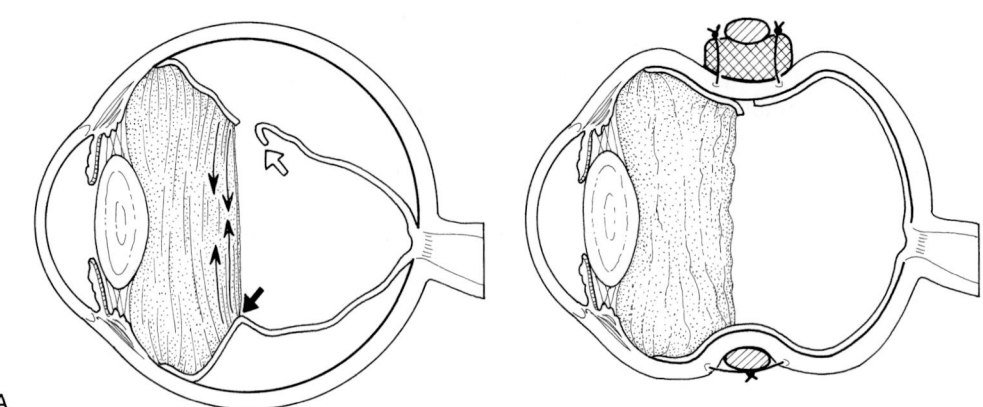

FIGURE 7-17. A: Retinal detachment with signs of early proliferative vitreoretinopathy: an equatorial retinal fold *(closed arrow)*, a posteriorly rolled edge of the retinal break *(open arrow)*, and strong transvitreal traction *(large arrows)*. An encircling procedure is indicated. **B:** The radial sponge adequately closes the break, and an encircling band provides support of the entire vitreous base region, relieving the vitreoretinal traction elsewhere.

the surgeon should place the encircling band 2 to 3 mm from the ora serrata, where the posterior vitreous base is generally located. The band can be anchored to the sclera by mattress sutures (Fig. 7-18) or by belt loops (Fig. 7-19). Anchoring mattress sutures are often preferred over belt loops because repositioning intraoperatively is more readily accomplished with sutures.

Small breaks (1 mm in diameter) can be closed by a 2-mm wide silicone band. The breaks must lie on the crest and anterior slope of the band. Therefore, the anterior bite of the scleral suture is placed at the level of the localization mark. When additional width is required to close a large break, a radial explant can be placed under the encircling band.

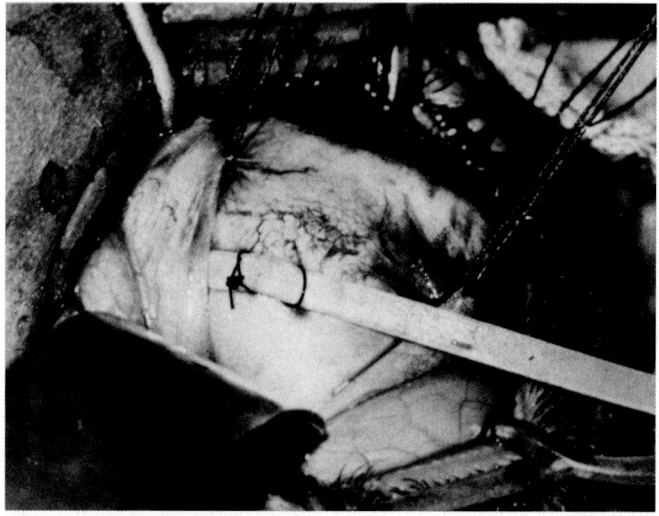

FIGURE 7-18. Silicone encircling band anchored to the sclera by a mattress suture. The sutures are tied and cut before drainage of subretinal fluid.

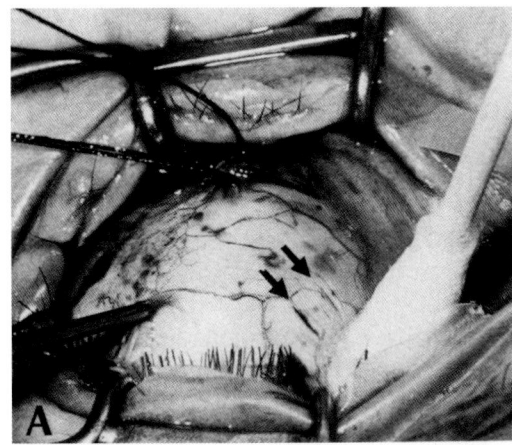
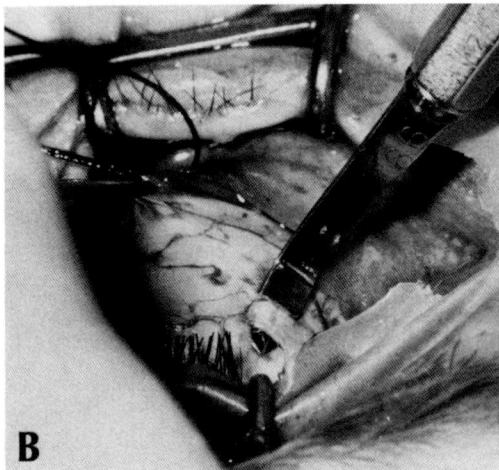
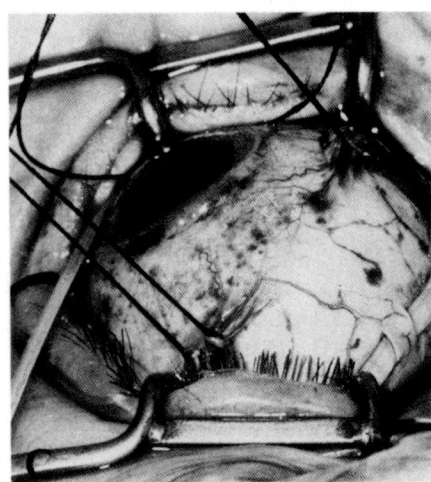

FIGURE 7-19. Encircling band anchored with belt loops. **A:** Two 3-mm grooves *(arrows)* are made 2.5 mm apart. **B:** A no. 66 Beaver or equivalent blade makes a small tunnel between the grooves. **C:** The encircling band is then placed through the tunnel.

For multiple breaks at different levels, a segmental circumferential explant can be combined with an encircling band. Alternatively, the eye can be encircled with a wide, 4-mm band or with a 5- or 7.5-mm sponge.

If the encircling procedure has been elected to treat a detachment in which no holes have been found, cryotherapy should be applied to the vitreous base over the length of the detached retina.

SCLERAL BUCKLING WITHOUT THERMAL ADHESION

In 1975, Zauberman and Rosell postulated that thermal adhesion is not necessary if vitreous traction can be successfully counteracted by a SB procedure (84). This concept was tested by several groups. The consensus was that, in the immediate postoperative period, cryotherapy played no role in the rate of reattachment (4,18,25). However, with long-term follow-up, eyes in patients who had undergone cryotherapy had a lower rate of redetachment than eyes in patients who had not (4,18). Some retinas redetached because the original break reopened as buckle height decreased (18) or simply because fluid seeped through the untreated break (4). These retinas could be reattached by photocoagulation. The high incidence of PVR (10% to 34%) in eyes not treated by cryotherapy contradicts the hypothesis that cryotherapy promotes PVR.

DRAINAGE OF SUBRETINAL FLUID

Indications for Drainage

External drainage of SRF during a SB procedure only should be performed when judged to be necessary for surgical success because it is an invasive step that can result in serious complications (Table 7-2) (80,81). When the retinal break cannot be closed at surgery, and it is apparent that vitreous traction (as in PVR or diabetic traction detachment) will prevent postoperative settling of the retina, the SRF should be drained. Extremely bullous detachments, particularly if inferior in location, may not settle well postoperatively without drainage, and they should also be drained. Finally, drainage of the SRF may be indicated in cases of retinal detachment with large tears, because such detachments similarly do not settle well and because space may be required for supplemental, internal tamponade with an intravitreal gas bubble.

Other situations in which to consider draining SRF include detachment in eyes with poor retinal circulation, staphylomatous sclera, or recent intraocular surgery because the indentation of the scleral buckle can cause a rise in intraocular pressure that could close the central retinal artery or rupture the globe. Drainage of the fluid softens the eye and allows it to accommodate the indentation without a precipitous rise in pressure. Because of poor outflow facility, drainage should also be considered in eyes with advanced glaucoma; without it, they may sustain optic nerve damage before the intraocular pressure has returned to normal. Eyes with high myopia, senile choroidopathy, or long-standing retinal detachment tend to absorb fluid poorly and are often treated with a drainage procedure (64). Last, many surgeons use drainage when no retinal breaks are found intraoperatively and during buckle revisions (i.e., retinal detachment reoperations.)

Lincoff and others (16,47,49,51,60,67) believe that most other cases can be managed without drainage of SRF, and in a prospective, randomized study, Hilton found no statistical difference between the rate of reattachment in drainage and nondrainage cases (39). Nevertheless, many retinal surgeons choose drainage in a high percentage of their cases. The reason for this is that other surgeons found that nondrainage procedures have a slightly lower initial rate of reattachment and a concomitantly higher rate of reoperation (17,49). Common causes of failure in nondrainage procedures are inadequate indentation, inaccurate placement of the scleral buckle, vitreous traction, meridional folds, and fishmouthing. Although the reoperation is usually successful (17,47,49), it has its own complications. First, should drainage be required, the inflammation caused by the initial operation increases the likelihood of choroidal bleeding from the drainage perforation. Second, postoperative explant infection and extrusion are more common after reopera-

TABLE 7-2. Possible indications for draining subretinal fluid

Early proliferative vitreoretinopathy (PVR) or significant vitreoretinal traction
Extremely bullous retinal detachments
Extremely large retinal tears
Inferior retinal detachments
Chronic retinal detachments
Recent intraocular surgery
Staphylomatous sclera
Advanced glaucoma
No retinal breaks found
Reoperations (scleral buckle revisions)

TABLE 7-3. *Major intraoperative complications of draining subretinal fluid*

Choroidal bleeding
Suprachoroidal hemorrhage
Subretinal hemorrhage
Retinal perforation
Retinal incarceration
Vitreous incarceration or loss

tion than after initial operations (27). In addition, the patient again faces the danger of anesthesia and the psychic trauma of surgery, as well as the potential for additional hospitalization. Finally, some patients refuse the reoperation.

Complications

When the procedure is performed properly, major complications related to the drainage maneuver are rare (39,43,80,81). In a large series by Wilkinson and Bradford (81), the planned drainage of SRF appeared possibly associated with anatomic failure in only 2 of 556 cases (0.4%). However, even without causing retinal redetachment, the complications of draining can still be a source of permanent visual acuity loss.

The four major complications of the drainage perforation are choroidal bleeding, retinal incarceration, loss of formed vitreous, and retinal perforation (Table 7-3) (81). The draining needle may lacerate a large-caliber choroidal vessel and may lead to suprachoroidal, subretinal, or vitreous hemorrhage. High myopes, elderly patients, and patients with Ehlers–Danlos syndrome are particularly prone to this complication. If blood accumulates under the fovea, the eye may not regain good visual acuity (Fig. 7-20). Both reti-

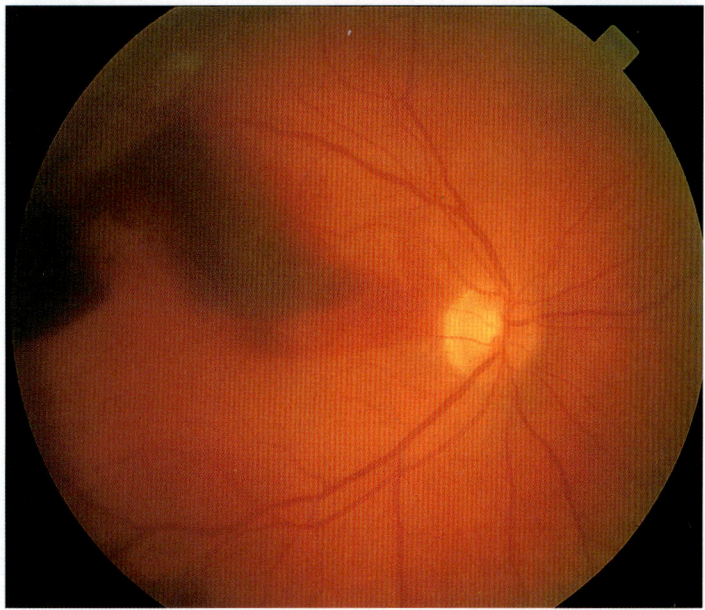

FIGURE 7-20. Large subretinal hemorrhage from the drainage site. The visual acuity was counting fingers.

nal incarceration and loss of formed vitreous can cause macular pucker or retinal folds, which may keep adjacent breaks open (Fig. 7-21). Vitreous loss in this setting also appears to be associated with a high incidence of PVR. Retinal perforation by the drainage instrument usually does not cause postoperative visual loss, but it does require treatment and buckling of the iatrogenic hole.

Technique

Because few large choroidal blood vessels are present just above or below the medial or lateral rectus muscle (Fig. 7-22) and under the superior or inferior rectus muscles, these are prime drainage sites. The chances of hemorrhage are further minimized if the choroid is perforated anteriorly. It is best to drain through sclera in the area that will be buckled because, should the retina be perforated or incarcerated at the drainage site, the repair will not entail placing additional sutures in a soft eye. Drainage under a large bulla of SRF allows a good quantity of fluid to drain before the retina settles over the drainage site and closes it. Adequate SRF under the drainage site is also important to avoid retinal perforation by the drainage needle. Two final considerations in selecting a drainage site are (a) that possible hemorrhage from a nasal perforation is less likely to reach the fovea than is one from a temporal site and (b) that the stiff retina of a fixed fold rarely incarcerates.

Once the drainage site has been selected, transillumination can be used to locate large choroidal blood vessels (Fig. 7-23) (28). This procedure is especially helpful if the drainage site is located posteriorly. The surgeon must be careful in the occasional patient

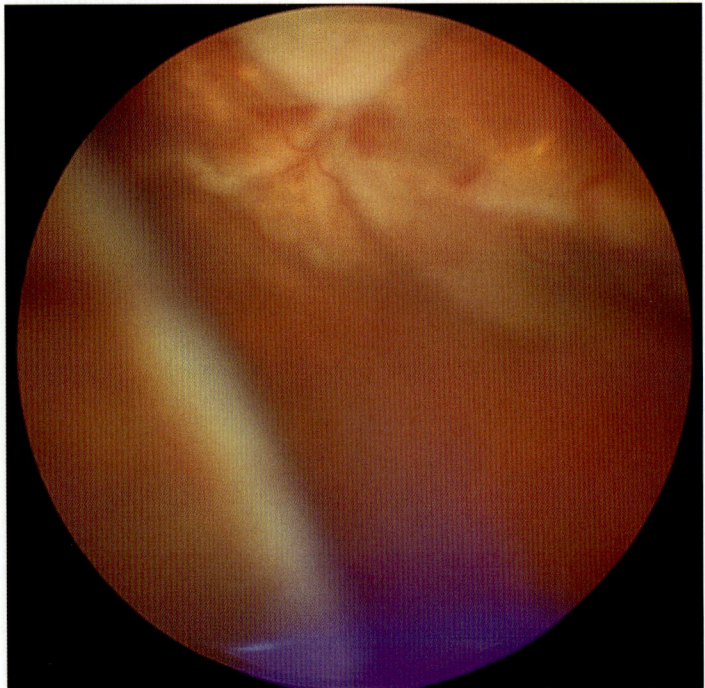

FIGURE 7-21. Incarceration of the retina into a drainage site. The resultant retinal folds can keep adjacent breaks open.

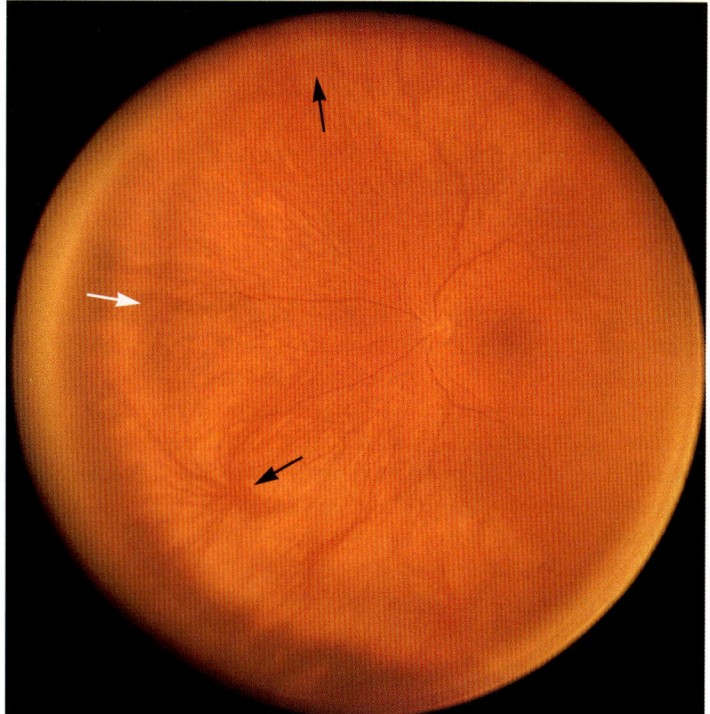

FIGURE 7-22. Vortex vein ampullae *(black arrows)* and large choroidal veins are rarely found just above or below the horizontal meridian, which is marked by the long ciliary nerve *(white arrow)*.

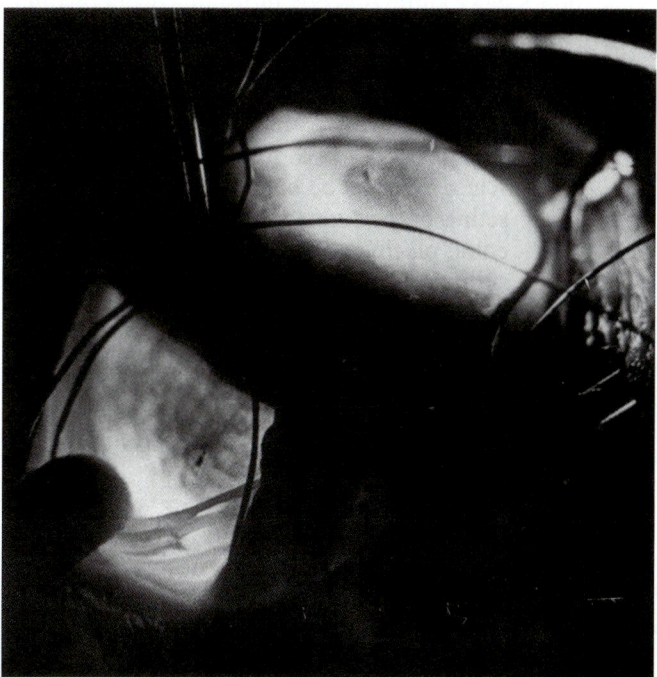

FIGURE 7-23. Transillumination of the globe verifies that no large choroidal vessels cross the drainage site.

with rhegmatogenous retinal detachment (RRD) with shifting fluid. The fluid may move away from the selected drainage site, and the retina may be perforated accidentally. Tilting the operating table toward the drainage site helps to keep SRF over it.

External drainage of SRF is typically performed in a two-step fashion: creation of a full-thickness scleral incision (sclerotomy) followed by perforation of the choroid (choroidotomy) to reach the subretinal space. A one-step approach using a 25-gauge needle has also been described, but it requires ophthalmoscopic guidance and is more cumbersome (11,15). The sclerotomy can be either a simple, radial scleral cutdown or an incision in the bed of a small, triangular scleral flap (Fig. 7-24A). Regardless of the style of the scleral incision, the best drainage is obtained if ultimately no scleral fibers overlie the choroid at the drainage site. A longer cutdown provides better exposure and allows for safe removal of these deep scleral fibers. The thicker the sclera, the longer the cutdown necessary. The scleral flap or cutdown is closed by a preplaced absorbable suture if an explant will be covering the drainage site; if not, it should be closed by a preplaced nonabsorbable suture. (Some surgeons do not believe that any suture closure is necessary if the drain site is covered by the explant.) To reduce the possibility of hemorrhage, the blunt conical electrode is used to treat the exposed choroid with several applications of low-intensity diathermy (see Fig. 7-24A).

The eye must be normotensive for drainage. If the intraocular pressure is too high, it must be lowered by acetazolamide, mannitol, or anterior chamber paracentesis. Otherwise, when the choroid is perforated, sudden decompression can cause choroidal hemorrhage or rapid evacuation of the SRF, followed by retinal or vitreous incarceration. If the intraocular pressure is too low, the assistant should indent the eye with a cotton-tipped applicator to restore the pressure to nearly normal. The choroid is then perforated with the diathermy needle electrode (see Fig. 7-24B), a 27-gauge hypodermic needle, a tapered suture needle, or a Ziegler knife. A gentle thrust to a depth of 1 mm is sufficient to perforate the choroid.

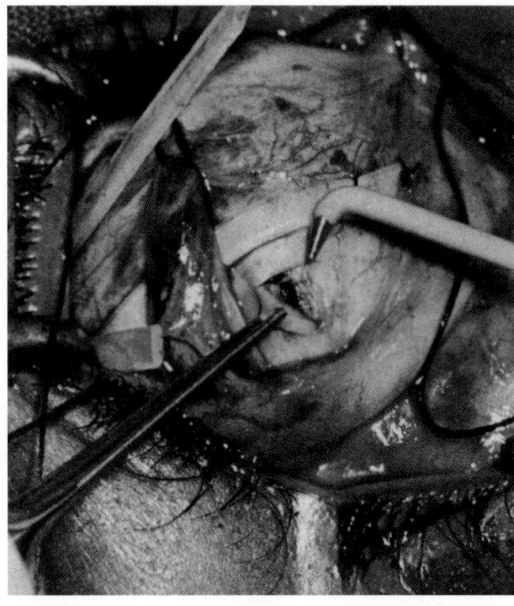

FIGURE 7-24. A: External drainage of subretinal fluid. The choroid is exposed in the bed of a small, triangular scleral flap and is treated with multiple applications of low-intensity diathermy using the blunt conical electrode.

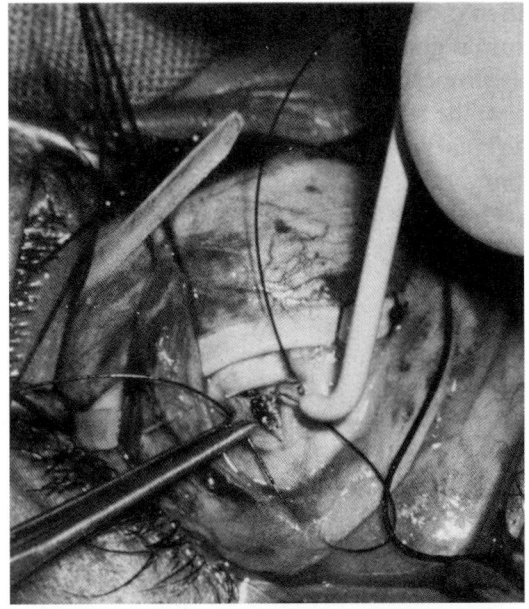

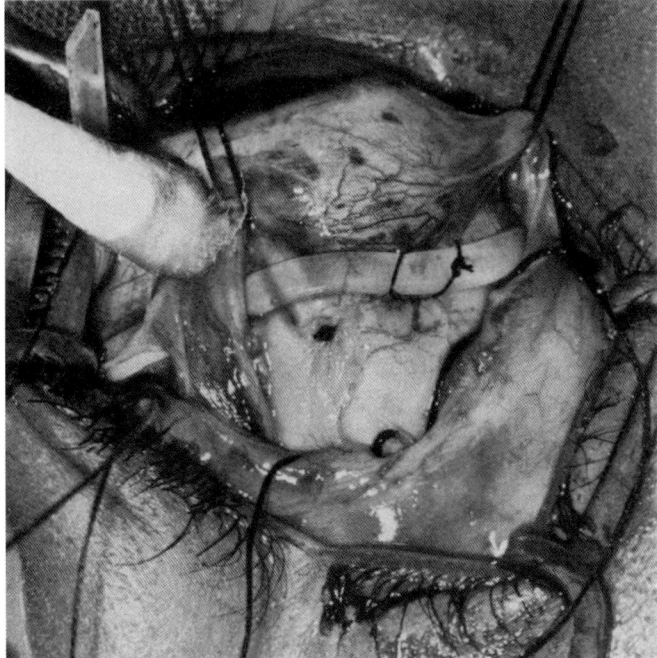

FIGURE 7-24. *Continued.* **B:** Perforation of the choroid with the needle electrode. The needle enters the eye tangentially to reduce the possibility of retinal perforation. A suture is preplaced for closing the scleral flap after drainage, particularly if the drain site is not located in an area to be directly buckled. During drainage, the surgeon pulls outward on the flap to prevent retinal incarceration. **C:** The scleral flap is closed immediately after drainage.

Alternatively, high-intensity argon laser photocoagulation directed to the bed of the full-thickness sclerotomy with a laser endoprobe can be used to drain the SRF (9). External laser choroidotomy has been shown to be at least as safe and effective as needle choroidotomy and may be the preferred method to use in draining shallow retinal detachments or when diathermy is not available (5,43). With this technique, the end of the probe is positioned about 1 mm from the choroid, and single applications are administered to the bare choroid at increasing power until draining begins. The recommended starting laser settings are 0.2 seconds duration and 1.0 W power. It is particularly important with this technique that no residual scleral fibers be present at the base of the scleral incision.

Regardless of the method used to enter the subretinal space, when the SRF begins to drain, gentle indentation of the globe opposite the drainage site helps to shift fluid toward it. Excessive pressure on the eye to force SRF out of the eye may cause retinal incarceration and must be avoided. Traction on the edge of the scleral flap with small forceps helps to hold the sclera and choroid away from the retina, thereby reducing the chances of incarceration (see Fig. 7-24B).

When little or no SRF remains, small hemorrhage or pigment granules usually will appear at the drainage site. At this time, the fundus must be inspected to see whether SRF is present over the drainage site. If so, gentle lateral traction on the scleral flaps may allow further drainage. Occasionally, another choroidal perforation is required. It is rarely necessary to drain until all the SRF is gone or even until the break is flat on the buckle, as long as the buckle is properly placed and of adequate height. When enough fluid has been drained, the suture over the drainage site is tied immediately (see Fig. 7-24C). This prevents retinal incarceration, which could otherwise result from a sudden elevation in intraocular pressure owing to manipulation of the globe. If the perforation site is in a lamellar dissection bed, the scleral flap suture closest to it is immediately closed for the same reason.

INTRAVITREAL INJECTIONS

An injection of fluid, air, or gas into the vitreous cavity through the pars plana will need to be performed to repressurize the eye if severe hypotony persists after draining SRF and securing the buckling elements in place. If the retinal breaks are adequately supported by the buckle indentation effect, sterile balanced saline solution suffices. However, if the break remains elevated significantly off the buckle at this time and the break is located in the superior 240 degrees, then gas is preferred because it serves the dual purpose of immediate globe repressurization and postoperative break closure (internal tamponade).

A persistently elevated detachment with hypotony after copious drainage can be encountered when draining is attempted near large tears. In such cases, liquid vitreous can pass through the tear and out of the eye through the drainage site. The eye becomes soft, but the amount of fluid under the retina remains the same. When this situation is recognized, the surgeon should close the drainage site, tie the scleral buckle in place, and then inject air or, preferably, gas through the pars plana to augment closure of the break (Fig. 7-25).

The specific characteristics of the gases currently available for this purpose and technique used to administer them are discussed in detail in chapter 8, Pneumatic Retinopexy. In general, just enough gas is injected directly into the vitreous cavity to restore the intraocular pressure to the normal range. If too much gas is injected, the excessive rise in

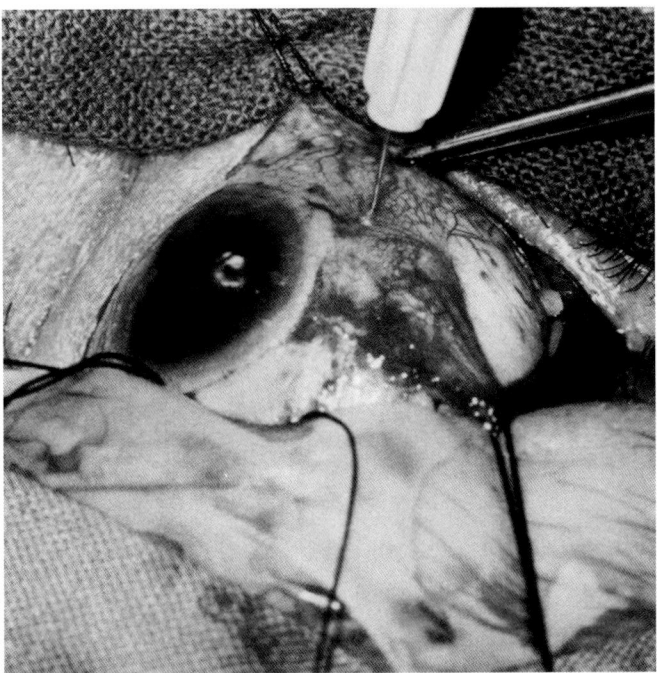

FIGURE 7-25. Gas injection for globe repressurization and supplemental, internal tamponade of the retinal break. The injection is delivered through the pars plana 4 mm from the limbus, using a 30-gauge needle. Note the direction of the needle toward the middle of the vitreous cavity, avoiding both the lens and any highly detached retina.

intraocular pressure may occlude the central retinal artery, incarcerate the retina in a drainage site, rupture the globe through a weakened area, or tear out scleral sutures. If the procedure is properly performed, complications from the injection itself are rare (see chapter 8, Pneumatic Retinopexy).

If the patient is under general anesthesia and nitrous oxide is being used, the surgeon must monitor the intraocular pressure closely and should avoid injection of a large volume of any gas. Nitrous oxide rapidly diffuses into the injected gas bubble and may cause a precipitous elevation of the intraocular pressure (71). Investigators have suggested that the nitrous oxide should be turned off 15 minutes before injection of the gas to avoid this complication (73).

INTRAOPERATIVE PROBLEMS

Retrobulbar Hemorrhage

If, after retrobulbar or peribulbar anesthesia, the eye becomes rock hard owing to an expanding hemorrhage in the closed orbital space, the surgeon must act immediately to prevent a retinal artery occlusion. The orbit must be decompressed by rapidly performing a lateral canthotomy and possibly also a 360-degree peritomy. This is a rare complication of local anesthesia, whether using a retrobulbar or a peribulbar approach.

Small Pupil

Until recently, if the pupil did not dilate well preoperatively, sector iridectomy, laser pupilloplasty, or cumbersome suture pupillary stretching techniques were the only alternatives for obtaining a larger pupillary aperture. Now, flexible iris hooks are available that allow for effective and relatively easy and reversible pupillary stretching (Fig. 7-26). Four small, evenly spaced paracentesis tracks at the limbus are all that is needed, and this maneuver can performed at the beginning of the procedure.

Corneal Opacification

Corneal transparency may be decreased by contact with the solutions used for sterile preparation of the operative field. Excessive scleral depression during localization or treatment may cause epithelial edema. This is the result of transient but large increases in intraocular pressure that can occur during these maneuvers (29). A clearer view of the fundus can be obtained if the cloudy corneal epithelium is removed with a rounded blade. The epithelium usually heals postoperatively in 1 to 2 days, but healing may take longer in diabetic patients.

Posterior Exposure

Placement of sutures for posteriorly located breaks is sometimes difficult. Adequate exposure is usually provided by a lateral canthotomy. If this does not suffice, disinsertion of a rectus muscle may be necessary. A traction suture placed through the stump of the muscle enables the surgeon to manipulate the eye to obtain the desired exposure. Extremely posterior retinal breaks are often best managed by vitrectomy techniques (see chapter 9, Alternative Techniques).

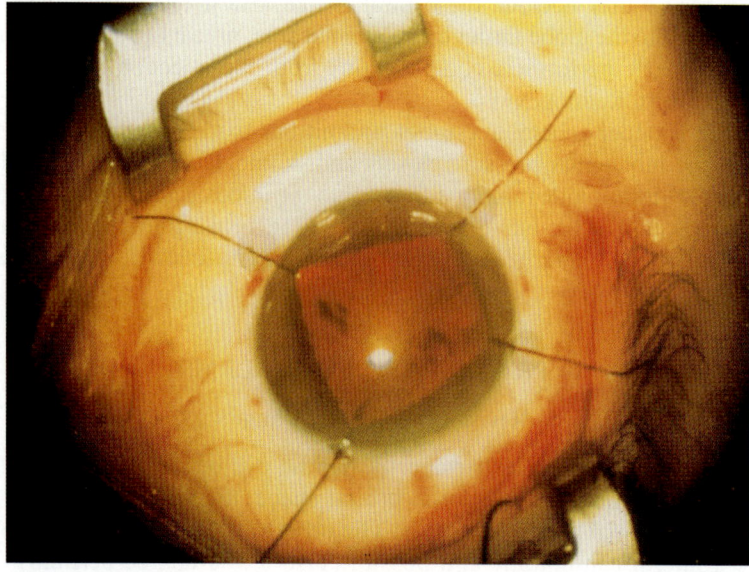

FIGURE 7-26. Iris retractors to augment pupillary dilation (Courtesy of Grieshaber, Inc., Kennesaw, Georgia.)

Staphyloma

Placing sutures into thin sclera is dangerous because the choroid may accidentally be perforated. Moreover, the sutures may pull out postoperatively. The scleral sutures should be placed in adjacent thicker sclera or in the insertion of a rectus muscle. Because the mattress suture is then wider than actually required, one must use a larger explant than is needed to close the break (Fig. 7-27). Shallow bites can be reinforced with cyanoacrylate glues (42). If the surgeon believes that the sutures will pull out, an encircling procedure should be considered. When a band is placed over an explant, it takes some of the pressure off the sutures. Silicone sponges are less likely to intrude into the eye through thin sclera than are solid silicone explants. When a true staphyloma exists, the surgeon must be careful not to raise the intraocular pressure too high during the procedure, or the globe may rupture.

Inadvertent Perforation of the Globe

If the needle accidentally perforates the choroid while sutures are being placed, SRF may drain, causing hypotony (10). The suture should be removed and its replacement suture positioned so the accidental drainage site will later fall under the buckle. Pressure with a cotton-tipped applicator over the accidental drainage site may make the eye firm enough for proper placement of the remaining sutures. If too much fluid has drained, even this procedure will not suffice, and an intraocular injection of saline solution will be necessary to restore the intraocular pressure. If a deep suture perforates attached retina, the area should be treated with cryotherapy and SB.

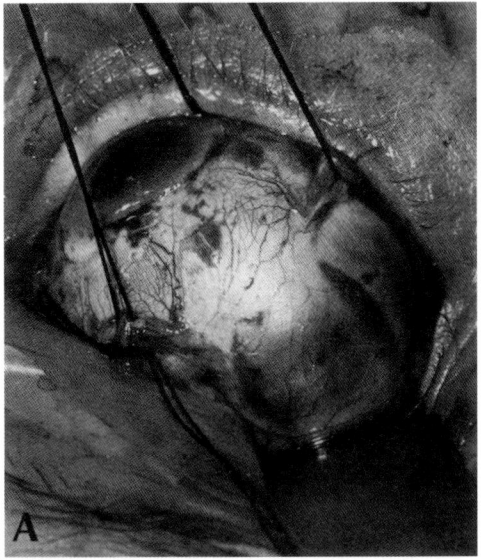 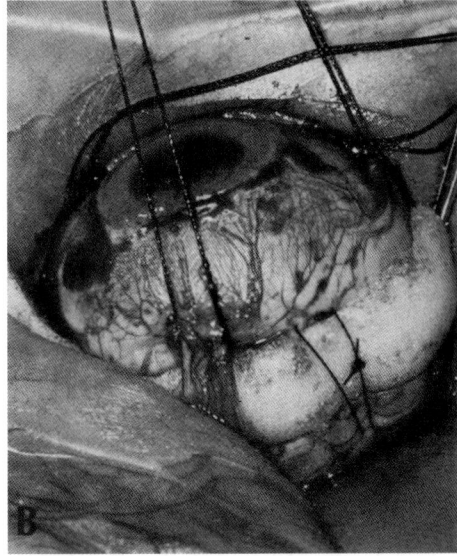

FIGURE 7-27. A: Staphylomatous sclera in which sutures for a radial explant cannot be placed. **B:** Circumferential 7.5-mm sponge anchored by a mattress suture placed in thicker sclera anterior and posterior to the staphyloma.

Increased Intraocular Pressure

As the surgeon ties the scleral sutures, the intraocular pressure must be constantly monitored. An estimate can be obtained by palpation ("finger tension") or by indentation with a muscle hook. More accurate readings can be taken with the Shiotz or Perkins tonometers. If the pressure is high, the optic disc should be inspected to see whether the central retinal artery is either pulsating or occluded. If the media are hazy, the best way to confirm arterial patency is to induce pulsations while pressing gently on the eye. If pulsations cannot be produced, the artery may be occluded.

If, during the tying of the scleral sutures, the central retinal artery is occluded or is in danger of occluding, the surgeon must lower the intraocular pressure before tying the rest of the sutures. Several maneuvers can be tried. If the patient's eyelids have been pushed behind the globe, decreasing the available orbital space, they should be pulled forward and the globe reposited. If the pressure is still high, anterior chamber paracentesis is usually effective in adequately lowering it. Caution should be exercised when performing paracentesis in aphakic eyes because vitreous may be engaged and become incarcerated into the limbal needle tract. The risk of this problem can be minimized by keeping the bevel of the needle facing upward and positioned over the iris inferiorly. If these measures are insufficient to lower the pressure, the surgeon can loosen some of the sutures or decrease the constriction of the encircling band if it has already been tied. A last resort is vitreous aspiration.

Fishmouth Phenomenon

Scleral buckling may result in a meridional fold formed by redundant retina on the posterior slope of the buckle (Fig. 7-28). The buckle, in this case, actually prevents reattachment. It keeps the break open and allows free passage of SRF posteriorly. This phenomenon, called "fishmouthing," is more likely to occur with circumferential than with radial buckling (50,61). If the break is superiorly located, an intravitreal injection of air or gas may close it. If the superior break remains open or if the break is inferior, the

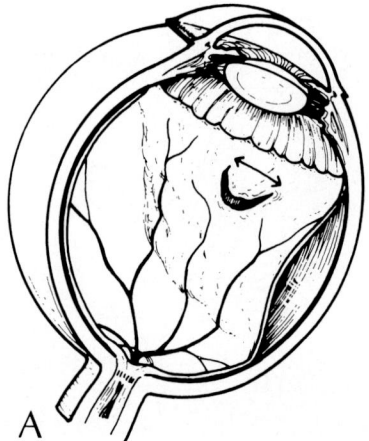
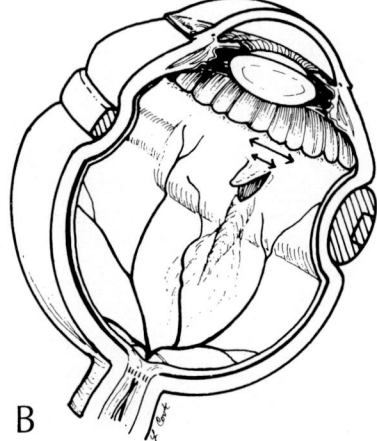

FIGURE 7-28. The fishmouth phenomenon. **A:** Flap tear in detached retina. The *solid line* indicates width of the tear. **B:** A circumferential buckle *(between arrows)* compresses the tear (the *large line* indicates original width), keeping its posterior edge open.

meridional folding can be reduced by decreasing the height of the buckle (by loosening the sutures). Alternatively, a radial element can be placed under and perpendicular to the circumferential buckle.

CLOSURE

After the SRF has been drained (if performed), the surgeon ties the sutures holding the explants (Fig. 7-29). The tighter the sutures are tied, the higher the indentation of the buckle. We like to use slipknots until the final ophthalmoscopic inspection confirms that the buckling effect is adequate because this facilitates any explant repositioning that may be needed. It is also best not to trim the explant close to the mattress sutures until after adequate closure of the retinal break has been confirmed.

If an encircling band is used, it is tightened at this time, and the ends are tied together using a suture, clip, or silicone (Watzke) sleeve (Fig. 7-30). As mentioned previously, the surgeon must avoid excessive tightening of the encircling band. The amount of tension applied with a band is best judged ophthalmoscopically. An indentation of 1 to 2 mm is usually sufficient.

If all the SRF has been drained, it is easy to determine whether the scleral buckle has been correctly placed. If SRF remains under the hole, the surgeon can push gently on the scleral buckle while observing the retinal break with the indirect ophthalmoscope. The increased indentation helps to assess the buckle's relation to the break.

If a circumferential explant is not properly placed anteriorly or posteriorly, the surgeon must replace the original suture with a correctly located suture. If the posterior edge of an encircling element is close to, but not fully buckling, the break, a trimmed piece of

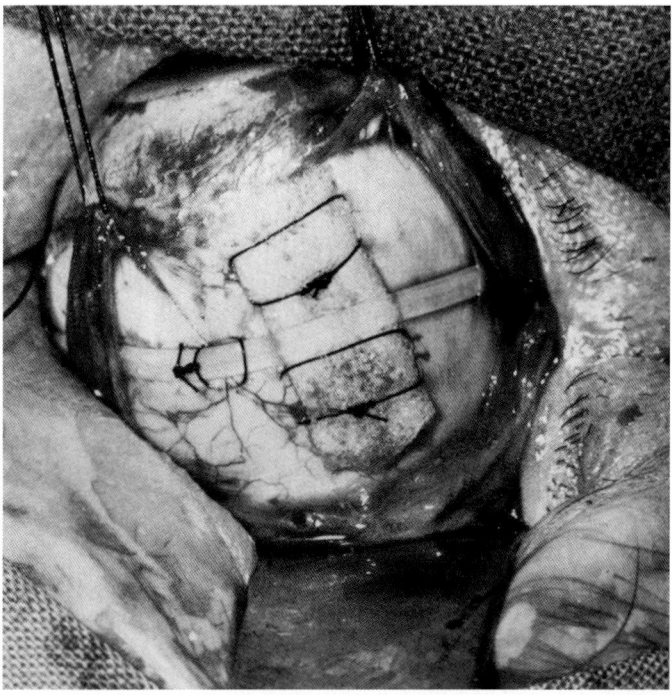

FIGURE 7-29. Radial silicone sponge explant combined with an encircling band.

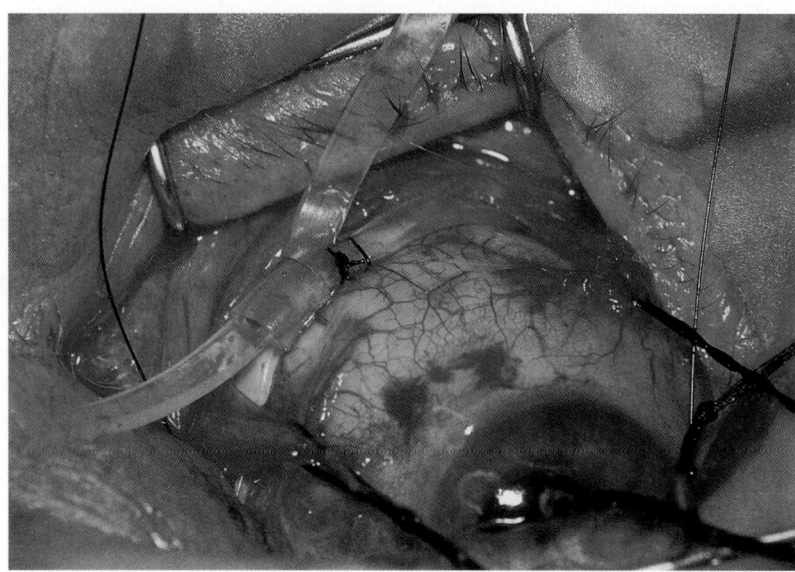

FIGURE 7-30. The ends of the encircling band are secured together at the appropriate tension with a Watzke sleeve.

sponge can be slipped under the encircling band perpendicular to it. This technique is particularly helpful when fishmouthing of the posterior edge of the break is noted.

If a radial explant has not been properly placed posteriorly or anteriorly, an additional suture can easily be placed. However, if it has not been placed in the proper radial meridian, one must replace the original mattress sutures. Usually, it is best to place the new scleral sutures before removing the old ones. This will maintain the intraocular pressure until the new sutures can be safely placed.

Once the surgeon has ascertained that the scleral buckle has been properly placed (Fig. 7-31), that no drainage site complications have occurred, and that the intraocular pressure is not unduly elevated, the temporary knots are then made permanent, and both suture ends and excess explant material are trimmed. After this, we typically irrigate the periocular space with an antibiotic solution. For operations performed with the patient under general anesthesia, we also infuse the posterior sub-Tenon's space with a long-acting local anesthetic agent such as 0.5% bupivacaine to maximize postoperative comfort (24,30).

Explants should be covered by a thick layer of Tenon's capsule to prevent late extrusion. To this end, Tenon's capsule is pulled up and is either draped over or anchored to the tendon of the rectus muscle in each quadrant. The overlying conjunctiva is secured back into anatomic position near the limbus using fast-absorbing, small-caliber suture (Fig. 7-32). For peritomies performed at the limbus, several interrupted sutures in the 3:00 and 9:00 positions (where the radial relaxing incisions were made) are all that is usually needed.

Subconjunctival injections of corticosteroid and antibiotic solutions are administered after the closure is complete. Atropine solution and antibiotic ointment are then instilled, and the eye is patched with a semipressure dressing to reduce postoperative eyelid edema.

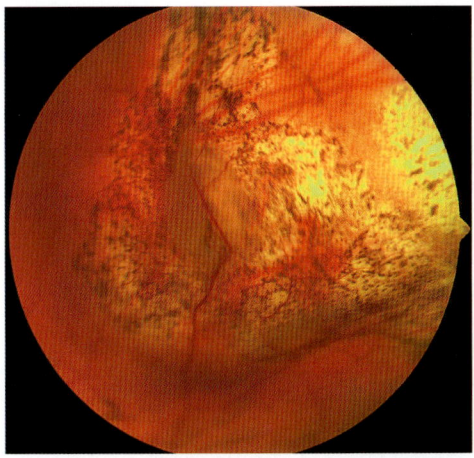 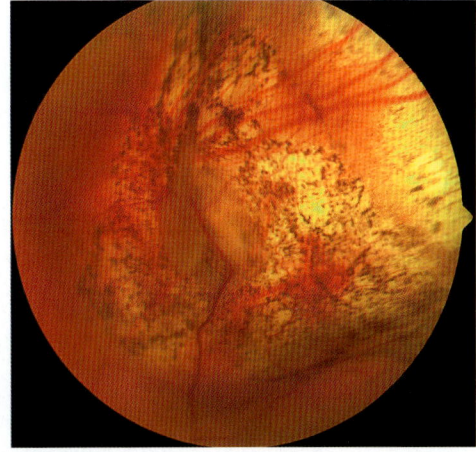

FIGURE 7-31. Postoperative photograph of flap tear correctly placed on the scleral buckle (in stereoscopic view). The underlying pigment disruption represents the cryotherapy-induced chorioretinal scar.

ROUTINE POSTOPERATIVE MANAGEMENT

Postoperatively, patients are mobilized as quickly as possible. Hair brushing and washing, as well as shaving and bathing, are permitted. However, if an air or gas bubble is present in the vitreous cavity, the patient is kept on bed rest and is positioned so the gas rises against the break to tamponade it. The eye that has had surgery is patched for the first week; bilateral patches are occasionally used for the first few days after nondrainage procedures to immobilize the eye and to facilitate settling of the retina. Atropine (1%) or scopolamine (0.25%) solution is instilled twice daily. An antibiotic–corticosteroid mixture is instilled four times daily. The severity of postoperative pain varies widely. Many patients are comfortable with mild analgesics. Others require strong, even intramuscular, analgesics, especially after lengthy procedures or reoperations.

Patients can usually return home the day of the operation, sometimes the day after. Regardless, they are examined the first postoperative day and 5 to 7 days later. Most patients return to full activities after the 1-week check because no evidence indicates that, by this time, fully active patients are more likely to have a repeat retinal detachment than are those patients whose activity remains restricted (8).

Patients with intraocular gas, even as little as 0.25 cc, should not travel in airplanes because the cabins are only pressurized to an altitude of about 8,000 feet. The gas bubble expands, raising the intraocular pressure enough to close the central retinal artery in some patients (21). For the same reason, patients should not travel to mountains higher than 4,000 feet.

SURGICAL RESULTS

Anatomic Reattachment

With current techniques, 90% to 95% of all RRDs can be successfully reattached with one or more operations (12,19,32–34,40,56,69,75,76,78). Specifically, for SB, the

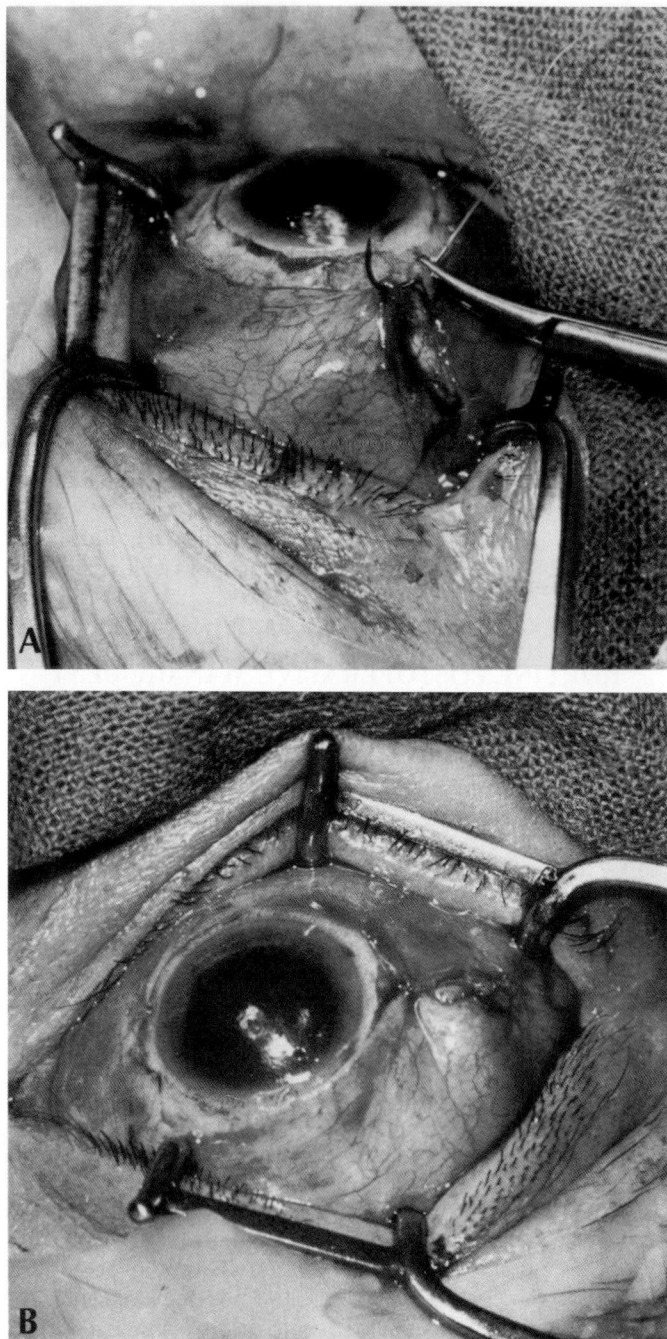

FIGURE 7-32. The ends of a relaxing incision are brought together **(A)** and are sutured closed **(B)**. Interrupted or running sutures can be used. Usually, no additional sutures are required elsewhere along the peritomy to approximate the cut edge of the conjunctiva to the limbus.

single operation success rate averages about 85% and increases to over 90% with buckle revisions (34,69). Success rates for different types of retinal detachment vary as follows:

1. Excellent prognosis (nearly 100%):
   - Detachments due to dialysis (36)
   - Detachments due to small or round holes (6)
   - Detachments with demarcation lines (7)
   - Detachments with minimal SRF
2. Slightly poorer prognosis (95%):
   - Aphakic or pseudophakic detachments (19,40,78)
   - Total detachments
   - Detachments with associated detachment of the nonpigmented epithelium of the pars plana (12)
   - Detachments caused by flap tears (6)
3. Poor prognosis (50% to 70%):
   - Detachments with associated choroidal detachment (31,68,69)
   - Detachments with giant retinal tears (45,57,77)
   - Detachments with significant PVR or hemorrhage (34,53,69)
   - Detachments in patients with Stickler's syndrome
   - Detachments caused by various forms of retinitis (23,63)

Visual Acuity Outcomes

Overall, approximately 40% to 50% of patients regain a visual acuity of 20/50 (6/15) or better; 25%, 20/60 to 20/100 (6/18 to 6/30); and 25%, 20/200 (6/60) or worse (13,59,75,76,79). Postoperative visual acuity chiefly depends on whether and for how long the macula was detached before surgery (13,35,75). When the macula has been detached, degeneration of photoreceptors may prevent good postoperative visual acuity. Seventy-five percent of patients with a macular detachment of less than 1 week's duration obtain a final visual acuity of 20/70 (6/21) or better, as opposed to 50% with a macular detachment of 1 to 8 weeks' duration (35). After successful surgery, patients should not be discouraged if their visual acuity is initially poor, because as the retina recovers, vision may continue to improve for up to a year or more (2,26).

The prognosis for vision is far better when the macula has not detached. Approximately 90% maintain their preoperative vision (76,79). The others lose some vision from macular pucker, cystoid macular edema (CME), or recurrent retinal detachment (35,65,76,79). Obviously, intraoperative complications also affect the final visual acuity.

REFERENCES

1. Ahn JC, Stanley JA. Subarachnoid injection as a complication of retrobulbar anesthesia. *Am J Ophthalmol* 1987;103:225–230.
2. Anderson DH, Guerin CJ, Erickson PA, Stern WH, Fisher SK. Morphological recovery in the reattached retina. *Invest Ophthalmol Vis Sci* 1986;27:168–183.
3. Arora R, Verma L, Kumar A, Tewari HK, Khosla PK. Peribulbar anesthesia in retinal reattachment surgery. *Ophthalmic Surg* 1992;23:499–501.
4. Axer-Siegel R, Yassur Y, Ben-Sira I. Surgical management of retinal detachment without cryopexy. *Am J Ophthalmol* 1981;91:474–479.
5. Aylward GW, Orr G, Schwartz SD, Leaver PK. Prospective, randomised, controlled trial comparing suture needle drainage and argon laser drainage of subretinal fluid [see comments]. *Br J Ophthalmol* 1995;79:724–727.

6. Benson WE, Morse PH. The prognosis of retinal detachment due to lattice degeneration. *Ann Ophthalmol* 1978;10:1197–2000.
7. Benson WE, Nantawan P, Morse PH. Characteristics and prognosis of retinal detachments with demarcation lines. *Am J Ophthalmol* 1977;84:641–644.
8. Bovino JA, Marcus DF. Physical activity after retinal detachment surgery. *Am J Ophthalmol* 1984;98:171–179.
9. Bovino JA, Marcus DF, Nelsen PT. Argon laser choroidotomy for drainage of subretinal fluid. *Arch Ophthalmol* 1985;103:443–444.
10. Brown P, Chignell AH. Accidental drainage of subretinal fluid. *Br J Ophthalmol* 1982;66:625–626.
11. Burton RL, Cairns JD, Campbell WG, Heriot WJ, Heinze JB. Needle drainage of subretinal fluid: a randomized clinical trial. *Retina* 1993;13:13–16.
12. Burton TC. Preoperative factors influencing anatomic success rates following retinal detachment surgery. *Trans Am Acad Ophthalmol Otolaryngol* 1977;83:499–505.
13. Burton TC. Recovery of visual acuity after retinal detachment involving the macula. *Trans Am Ophthalmol Soc* 1982;80:475–497.
14. Campochiaro PA, Kaden IH, Vidaurri-Leal J, Glaser BM. Cryotherapy enhances intravitreal dispersion of viable retinal pigment epithelial cells. *Arch Ophthalmol* 1985;103:434–436.
15. Charles ST. Controlled drainage of subretinal and choroidal fluid. *Retina* 1985;5:233.
16. Chignell AH. Retinal detachment surgery without drainage of subretinal fluid. *Am J Ophthalmol* 1974;77:1–5.
17. Chignell AH, Fison LG, Davies EWG, et al. Failure in retinal detachment surgery. *Br J Ophthalmol* 1973;57: 525–530.
18. Chignell AH, Markham RHC. Retinal detachment surgery without cryotherapy. *Br J Ophthalmol* 1981;65: 371–373.
19. Cousins S, Boniuk I, Okun E, et al. Pseudophakic retinal detachments in the presence of various IOL types. *Ophthalmology* 1986;93:1198–1208.
20. Diddie KR, Ernest JT. Uveal blood flow after 360 degrees constriction in rabbit. *Arch Ophthalmol* 1980;98: 729–730.
21. Dieckert JP, O'Connor PS, Schacklett DE, et al. Air travel and intraocular gas. *Ophthalmology* 1986;93:642–645.
22. Duker JS, Belmont JB, Benson WE, et al. Inadvertent globe perforation during retrobulbar and peribulbar anesthesia: patient characteristics, surgical management, and visual outcome. *Ophthalmology* 1991;98: 519–526.
23. Duker JS, Blumenkranz MS. Diagnosis and management of the acute retinal necrosis (ARN) syndrome. *Surv Ophthalmol* 1991;35:327–343.
24. Duker JS, Nielsen J, Vander JF, Rosenstein RB, Benson WE. Retrobulbar bupivacaine irrigation for postoperative pain after scleral buckling surgery: a prospective study. *Ophthalmology* 1991;98:514–518.
25. Fetkenhour CL, Hauch TL. Scleral buckling without thermal adhesion. *Am J Ophthalmol* 1980;89:662–666.
26. Fitzgerald CR, Birch DG, Enoch JM. Functional analysis of vision in patients after retinal detachment repair. *Arch Ophthalmol* 1980;98:1237–1244.
27. Flindall RJ, Norton EWD, Curtin VT, et al. Reduction of extrusion and infection following episcleral silicone implants and cryopexy in retinal detachment surgery. *Am J Ophthalmol* 1971;71:835–837.
28. Freeman HM, Schepens CL. Innovations in the technique of drainage of subretinal fluid: transillumination and choroidal diathermy. *Trans Am Acad Ophthalmol Otolaryngol* 1974;78:829–836.
29. Gardner TW, Quillen DA, Blankenship GW, Marshall WK. Intraocular pressure fluctuations during scleral buckling surgery. *Ophthalmology* 1993;100:1050–1054.
30. Gottfreothsdottir MS, Gislason I, Stefansson E, Sigurjonsdottir S, Nielsen NC. Effects of retrobulbar bupivacaine on post-operative pain and nausea in retinal detachment surgery. *Acta Ophthalmol* 1993;71:544–547.
31. Gottlieb F. Combined choroidal and retinal detachment. *Arch Ophthalmol* 1972;88:481–486.
32. Greven CM, Sanders RJ, Brown GC, et al. Pseudophakic retinal detachments: anatomic and visual results. *Ophthalmology* 1992;99:257–262.
33. Griffith RD, Ryan EA, Hilton GF. Primary retinal detachments without apparent breaks. *Am J Ophthalmol* 1976; 81:420–427.
34. Grizzard WS, Hilton GF, Hammer ME, Taren D. A multivariate analysis of anatomic success of retinal detachments treated with scleral buckling. *Graefes Arch Clin Exp Ophthalmol* 1994;232:1–7.
35. Grupposo SS. Visual acuity following surgery for retinal detachment. *Arch Ophthalmol* 1975;93:327–330.
36. Hagler WS, North AW. Retinal dialyses and retinal detachment. *Arch Ophthalmol* 1968;79:376–388.
37. Haller JA, Lim JI, Goldberg MF. Pilot trial of transscleral diode laser retinopexy in retinal detachment surgery. *Arch Ophthalmol* 1993;111:952–956.
38. Harris MJ, Blumenkrantz MS, Wittpenn J, et al. Geometric alterations produced by encircling scleral buckles: biometric and clinical considerations. *Retina* 1987;7:14–19.
39. Hilton GF. The drainage of subretinal fluid: a randomized controlled clinical trial. *Trans Am Ophthalmol Soc* 1981;79:517–540.
40. Ho PC, Tolentino FI. Pseudophakic retinal detachment: surgical success rate with various types of IOL's. *Ophthalmology* 1984;91:847–852.
41. Holekamp TLR, Arribas NP, Boniuk I. Bupivicaine anesthesia in retinal detachment surgery. *Arch Ophthalmol* 1979;97:109–111.
42. Hung JY, Hilton GF. Scleral buckling with cyanoacrylate tissue adhesive. *Retina* 1982;2:179.

43. Ibanez HE, Bloom SM, Olk RJ, et al. External argon laser choroidotomy versus needle drainage technique in primary scleral buckle procedures: a prospective randomized study. *Retina* 1994;14:348–350.
44. Javitt JC, Addiego R, Friedberg HL. Brain stem anesthesia after retrobulbar block. *Ophthalmology* 1987;94:718.
45. Kanski JJ. Giant retinal tears. *Am J Ophthalmol* 1975;79:846–852.
46. King LM, Schepens CL. Limbal peritomy in retinal detachment surgery. *Arch Ophthalmol* 1974;91:295–298.
47. Kreissig I, Rose D, Jost B. Minimized surgery for retinal detachments with segmental buckling and nondrainage: an 11-year follow-up. *Retina* 1992;12:224–231.
48. Laqua H, Machemer R. Repair and adhesion mechanisms of the cryotherapy lesion in experimental retinal detachment. *Am J Ophthalmol* 1976;81:833–846.
49. Lincoff, H. Should retinal breaks be closed at the time of surgery? In: *Controversy in Ophthalmology,* edited by Brockhurst RJ, Boruchoff SA, Hutchinson BT, Lessell S. Philadelphia: WB Saunders; 1977:582–598.
50. Lincoff H, Kreissig I. Advantages of radial buckling. *Am J Ophthalmol* 1975;79:955–957.
51. Lincoff H, Kreissig I. The treatment of retinal detachment without drainage of subretinal fluid (modifications of the Custodis procedure. VI). *Trans Am Acad Ophthalmol Otolaryngol* 1972;76:1121–1133.
52. Lincoff H, Kreissig I, Jakobiec F, et al. Remodeling of cryosurgical adhesion. *Arch Ophthalmol* 1981;99:1845–1849.
53. Machemer R, Allen AW. Retinal tears 180 degrees and greater: management with vitrectomy and intravitreal gas. *Arch Ophthalmol* 1976;94:1340.
54. McHugh DA, Schwartz S, Dowler JG, Ulbig M, Blach RK, Hamilton PA. Diode laser contact transscleral retinal photocoagulation: a clinical study. *Br J Ophthalmol* 1995;79:1083–1087.
55. Mein CE, Flynn HW Jr. Augmentation of local anesthesia during retinal detachment surgery. *Arch Ophthalmol* 1989;107:1084.
56. Meredith TA, Reeser FH, Topping TM, Aaberg TM. Cystoid macular edema after retinal detachment surgery. *Ophthalmology* 1980;87:1090–1095.
57. Michels RG, Rice TA, Blankenship G. Surgical techniques for selected giant retinal tears. *Retina* 1983;3:139.
58. Michels RG, Thompson JT, Rice TA, et al. Effect of scleral buckling on vector forces caused by epiretinal membranes. *Am J Ophthalmol* 1986;102:449–451.
59. Norton EWD. Retinal detachments in aphakia. *Trans Am Ophthalmol Soc* 1963;61:770.
60. O'Connor PR, 1973. Absorption of subretinal fluid after external scleral buckling without drainage. *Am J Ophthalmol* 1973;76:30–34.
61. Pruett RC. The fishmouth phenomenon. II. Wedge scleral buckling. *Arch Ophthalmol* 1977;95:1782.
62. Ramsay RC, Knobloch WH. Ocular perforation following retrobulbar anesthesia for retinal detachment surgery. *Am J Ophthalmol* 1978;86:61–64.
63. Regillo CD, Vander JF, Duker JS, Fischer DH, Belmont JB, Kleiner R. Repair of retinitis-related retinal detachments with silicone oil in patients with acquired immunodeficiency syndrome. *Am J Ophthalmol* 1992;113:21–27.
64. Robertson DM. Delayed absorption of subretinal fluid after scleral buckling procedures. *Am J Ophthalmol* 1979;87:57–64.
65. Sabates NR, Sabates FN, Sabates R, Lee KY, Ziemianski MC. Macular changes after retinal detachment surgery. *Am J Ophthalmol* 1989;108:22–29.
66. Schepens CL, Acosta F. Scleral implants: an historical perspective. *Surv Ophthalmol* 1991;35:447–453.
67. Scott JD. Retinal detachment surgery without drainage. *Trans Ophthalmol Soc U K* 1970;90:57.
68. Seelenfreund MH, Kraushar MF, Schepens CL, Freilich DB. Choroidal detachment associated with primary retinal detachment. *Arch Ophthalmol* 1974;91:254–258.
69. Sharma T, Challa J, Ravishanka KV, Murugesan R. Scleral buckling for retinal detachment, predictors for anatomic failure. *Retina* 1994;14:338–343.
70. Simcock PR, Raymond GL, Lavin MJ, Whitley CL. Combined peribulbar injection and blunt cannula infiltration for vitreoretinal surgery. *Ophthalmic Surg* 1994;25:232–235.
71. Smith RB, Carl B, Linn JG, Nemoto E. Effect of nitrous oxide on air in the vitreous. *Am J Ophthalmol* 1974;78:314–320.
72. Stevens JD, Franks WA, Orr G, Leaver PK, Cooling RJ. Four-quadrant local anaesthesia technique for vitreoretinal surgery. *Eye* 1992;6:583–586.
73. Stinson TW, Donlon JV. Interaction of intraocular air and sulfur hexafluoride with nitrous oxide: a computer simulation. *Anesthesiology* 1982;56:385–388.
74. Sullivan KC, Brown GC, Forman AR. Retrobulbar anesthesia and retinovascular obstruction. *Ophthalmology* 1983;90:373–377.
75. Tani P, Robertson DM, Langworthy A. Prognosis for central vision and anatomic reattachment in rhegmatogenous retinal detachment with macula detached. *Am J Ophthalmol* 1981;92:611–620.
76. Tani P, Robertson DM, Langworthy A. Rhegmatogenous retinal detachment without macular involvement treated with scleral buckling. *Am J Ophthalmol* 1980;90:503–508.
77. Vidaurri-Leal J, deBustros S, Michels RG. Surgical treatment of giant retinal tears with inverted posterior retinal flaps. *Am J Ophthalmol* 1984;98:463–466.
78. Wilkinson CP. Pseudophakic retinal detachments. *Retina* 1985;5:1–4.
79. Wilkinson CP. Visual results following scleral buckling for retinal detachments sparing the macula. *Retina* 1981;1:113–116.

80. Wilkinson CP, Bradford RH Jr. The drainage of subretinal fluid. *Trans Am Ophthalmol Soc* 1983;81:162–171.
81. Wilkinson CP, Bradford RHJ. Complications of draining subretinal fluid. *Retina* 1984;4:1–4.
82. Wittpenn JR, Rapoza P, Sternberg P. Respiratory arrest following retrobulbar anesthesia. *Ophthalmology* 1986; 93:867–870.
83. Yoshizumi MO, Friberg T. Erosion of implants in retinal detachment surgery. *Ann Ophthalmol* 1983;15:430–434.
84. Zauberman H, Rosell FG. Treatment of retinal detachment without inducing chorioretinal lesions. *Trans Am Acad Ophthalmol Otolaryngol* 1975;79:835–844.

8
Pneumatic Retinopexy

In the mid-1980s, Hilton and Dominguez independently introduced the procedure now most commonly known as pneumatic retinopexy (PR) (5,10). As the name implies, this basic technique consists of treating the retinal break (retinopexy), followed by injecting a gas bubble into the vitreous cavity (pneumatic). Postoperatively, the patient is positioned so the gas tamponades the retinal break. This, in turn, allows for the resorption of the subretinal fluid (SRF) and formation of an adequate chorioretinal adhesion around the break to ensure long-lasting retinal attachment (Fig. 8-1).

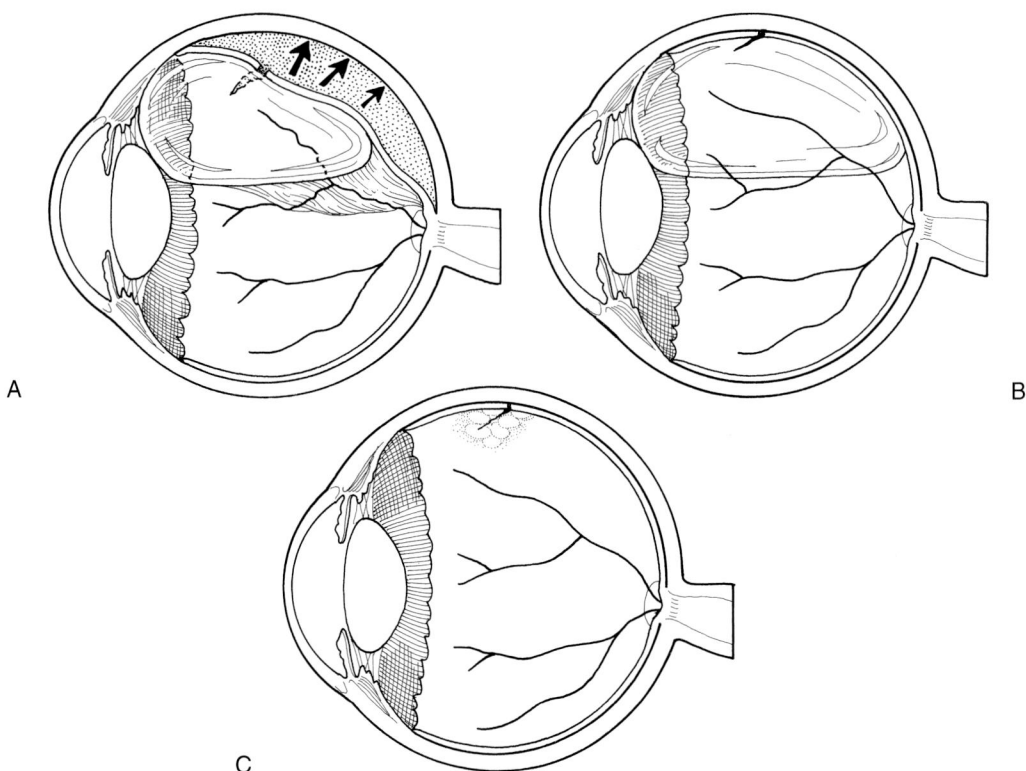

FIGURE 8-1. A: The patient's head is positioned immediately after the intravitreal gas injection so the gas bubble rises to tamponade the retinal break. **B:** The fully expanded gas bubble eliminates access of liquid vitreous through the retinal break, and the subretinal fluid spontaneously resorbs. **C:** With the break flattened, a firm chorioretinal adhesion is allowed to form, and long-lasting retinal attachment is achieved.

This minimally invasive procedure does not require any incisions and can be performed in the office setting with the operative field under local anesthesia. Reports to date have indicated an overall reattachment success rate for repairing selected retinal detachments approaching that of scleral buckling (SB) but with comparatively lower postoperative ocular morbidity (11,12,26,27). The relative ease and convenience of an office-based procedure combined with the favorable surgical results of PR account for its rapid gain in popularity for repairing selected retinal detachments over the past decade. Furthermore, from the standpoint of medical economics, the argument has been made to manage eligible retinal detachment cases first with PR rather than with SB, because PR may represent a significant savings in health care expenditure.

PATIENT SELECTION

Investigators have estimated that 30% to 50% of all primary rhegmatogenous retinal detachments (RRD) can be readily managed with PR (9). Patient selection, however, is critical in maximizing surgical success. Because closure of the retinal break with the gas bubble relies on prolonged patient positioning, it is reserved for eyes with retinal detachments caused by breaks located in the superior 8 clock hours (25). Some surgeons further restrict its use to those cases with breaks at or above the horizontal meridian (i.e., the superior 6 clock hours). Furthermore, PR is best reserved for retinal detachments in which the retinal break is less than 1 clock hour in size and, for multiple breaks, within 1 clock hour of each other (Fig. 8-2) (25).

The procedure, of course, should not be attempted in patients who cannot strictly adhere to the postoperative positioning requirements. Because of greater likelihood of failure, PR should *not* be used in cases with any limitation to the view of the peripheral retina (e.g., lens or capsule opacities), more than just minimal vitreous hemorrhage, any significant proliferative vitreoretinopathy (PVR), or extensive (more than 3 clock hours of) lattice degeneration (Table 8-1). It should also be avoided in cases that have tears with bridging vessels because the gas bubble may tear the vessel and cause a vitreous hemorrhage. Special caution should be exercised when performing PR in patients with glaucoma because the transient but sometimes high intraocular pressure rises that can

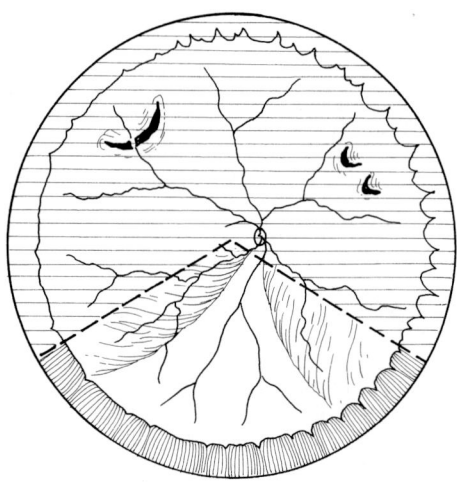

FIGURE 8-2. Retinal detachments with a single retinal tear or a group of tears less than 1 clock hour in size and located in the superior two-thirds (or 8 clock hours) of the retinal periphery are potentially amenable to pneumatic retinopexy.

TABLE 8-1. *Contraindications to pneumatic retinopexy*

Poor understanding of or inability to perform postoperative positioning
Retinal breaks larger than 1 clock hour in size
Multiple retinal breaks larger than 1 clock hour apart
Retinal breaks in the inferior one-third of the retina
Extensive (larger than 3 clock hours) lattice degeneration
Vitreous hemorrhage
Proliferative vitreoretinopathy (PVR)
Obscured view of the peripheral retina
Retinal tear with a large bridging vessel

occur during or after PR can potentially result in optic nerve damage, particularly if the glaucoma is advanced.

Although nearly all cases of RRD that are approachable with PR are also readily amenable to SB, detachments with relatively posterior breaks or breaks directly under the superior rectus muscle may be more suitably treated with PR. For patients with glaucoma whose eyes have a functioning filtering bleb or may need one in the future, PR may be the preferred technique. Furthermore, selected cases of persistent or recurrent retinal detachment after SB may be more easily approached with PR, instead of attempting to revise the scleral buckle or proceeding to vitrectomy. Regardless of whether PR is used to treat primary or secondary retinal detachments, the technique is similar and is described in detail in this chapter.

ANESTHESIA

Generally, the type of local anesthesia used for PR is a peribulbar block or subconjunctival injection. If more than a few applications of cryotherapy are needed, peribulbar or retrobulbar anesthesia is likely to be preferred because subconjunctival anesthesia often does not completely eliminate the pressure or pain sensation that is experienced during freezing. However, if the amount of retinopexy is not too extensive, many surgeons will opt for just subconjunctival anesthesia because it is theoretically safer, better tolerated, and allows for complete preservation of ocular motility, which often facilitates both examination and treatment.

Rarely, a patient may be too apprehensive for local anesthetic techniques and may require general anesthesia. If general anesthesia needed, nitrous oxide should not be used as part of the general anesthetic mixture during this short procedure. As described in the section on SB, nitrous oxide quickly diffuses into the bubble during the procedure, causing a possible excessive rise in intraocular pressure intraoperatively, and rapidly diffuses out of the bubble postoperatively, potentially resulting in a bubble that is inadequately small (9,23,24).

RETINOPEXY

The fundus should be reinspected by indirect ophthalmoscopy and scleral depression to verify the location of the breaks and other vitreoretinal disease to be treated (e.g., patches of lattice degeneration). The causative retinal breaks are treated with cryotherapy in a fashion similar to that used to treat tears during SB (Fig. 8-3). The neurosensory retina and RPE immediately around the tear are treated in a confluent fashion, avoiding any freezing to bare RPE or the overlying vitreous.

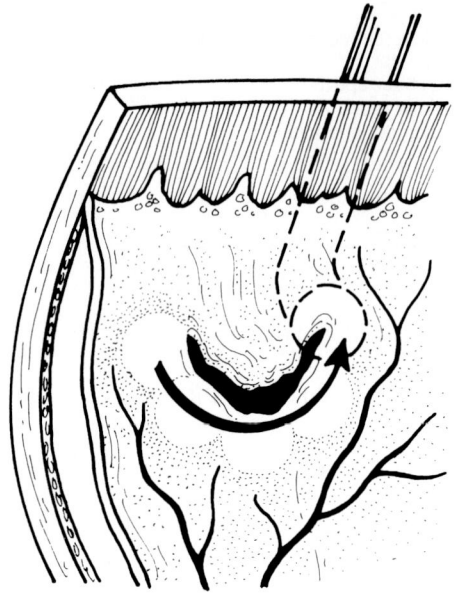

FIGURE 8-3. Transcleral cryotherapy is applied in a contiguous fashion completely around the retinal break. The best chorioretinal adhesion forms if retinal uptake (whitening) is seen in the surrounding detached retina.

In extremely elevated retinal detachments, it may not be possible to obtain any visible freezing affect to the detached retina. Although freezing the underlying retinal pigment epithelium (RPE) alone can result in some degree of adhesion after the layers are reapposed, the scar is not as strong as if both retina and RPE layers are frozen, and the risk of late reopening of the tear with redetachment is likely to be increased (13,16). Therefore, in such circumstances, supplemental cryotherapy (or laser photocoagulation) to the area around the break is recommended in the immediate postoperative period, after the gas is in place and has flattened that portion of retina.

Relatively posterior retinal breaks may be difficult to reach with the cryoprobe because of the limit of the conjunctival cul-de-sac. In such cases, one may make a small incision in the overlying conjunctiva to allow the probe to pass more posteriorly. Alternatively, the procedure can be staged with injection of the gas first and then, after positioning for 24 to 72 hours to allow the retina to reattach, treatment of the area around the flattened retinal break with laser photocoagulation (see later).

Either laser photocoagulation or cryotherapy should be applied to any significant peripheral vitreoretinal disorder such as lattice degeneration or small, incidental retinal breaks located outside the area of detachment. Treatment should be performed *before* injecting gas for two main reasons. First, the bubble may impede visualization of these lesions. Second, the scleral depression that occurs with treatment, especially cryotherapy, further softens the eye and either permits using a larger gas bubble or allows one to avoid paracentesis. Some clinicians prefer using laser rather than cryotherapy for these incidental lesions in uninvolved retina because, in experimental models, photocoagulation produces a relatively fast adhesion (6,29).

Laser photocoagulation alone can also be used in lieu of cryotherapy, but the procedure needs to be staged (7). As described earlier in the discussion of posterior breaks and supplemental treatment, the gas is injected first, and then the laser applied to the region of the tear in the postoperative period, once the retina is flat in that area. It is best to apply the laser within the first 3 postoperative days. The laser indirect ophthalmoscope delivery system is usually used, with laser directed either through or around the

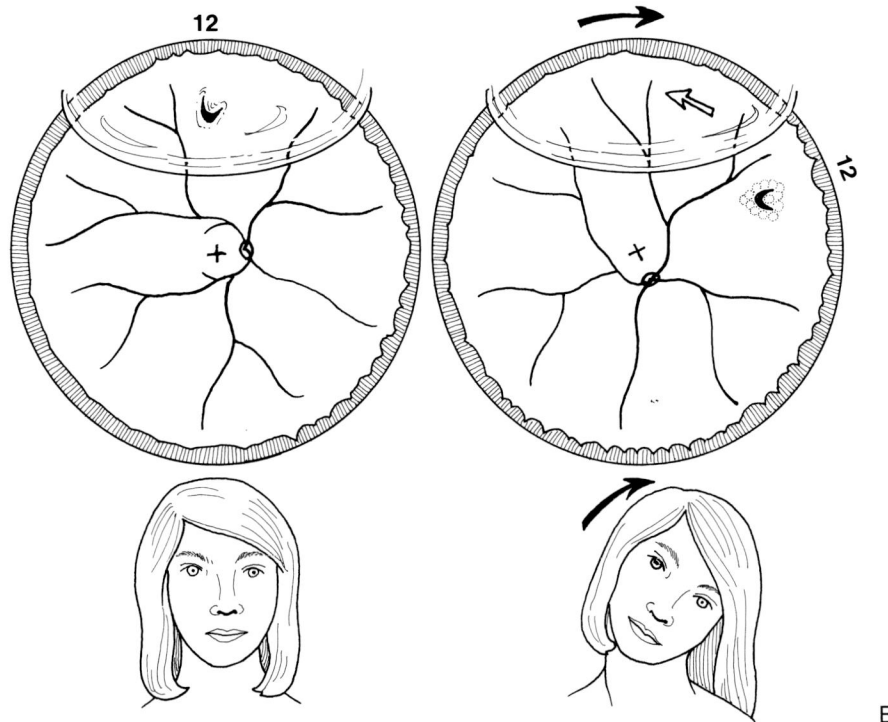

FIGURE 8-4. In pneumatic retinopexy, to treat the retinal break with laser photocoagulation, the gas bubble must be injected first and the retina around the break reattached. Using the laser indirect ophthalmoscope delivery system, the break can then be treated through the gas bubble **(A)** or around it **(B)**. Depending on the location of the tear, the patient's head may need to be rotated one way or another to put the break in the desired position with respect to the gas bubble.

bubble (Fig. 8-4). The edge of the bubble can interfere with viewing of the break and the uptake of laser around it. Depending on where the break is located and the position of the patient, one may have to tilt the patient's head to bring the bubble either well over or well away from the tear site, to apply all the treatment easily that may be needed.

When we use laser in this setting, however, we prefer to have the gas bubble shifted *away* from the break for two main reasons. First, it may be difficult to see the break through the gas bubble. Second, because gas has a greater insulating effect than liquid-vitreous, applying laser to the tissue under the gas is more likely to result in excessively heavy burns and secondary retinal holes.

Whether using cryotherapy or laser to treat the causative break, applying several rows of laser spots between the equator and posterior vitreous base region for 360 degrees has been advocated to help increase the single operation success rate, particularly in eyes that are pseudophakic with open capsules or have multiple breaks (Paul Tornambe, M.D., personal communication). The effectiveness of this type of supplemental treatment, however, has not been definitively demonstrated.

PARACENTESIS

Anterior chamber paracentesis is needed in most cases to prevent a prolonged, excessive rise in intraocular pressure from the injected gas. We routinely perform this procedure before rather than after the gas injection. Performing the paracentesis first prevents a marked rise in intraocular pressure and the associated ocular discomfort. It also is safer this way if the eye has advanced glaucoma or recently underwent operation. Furthermore, injecting the gas into a soft globe appears to help to minimize "fish egg" formation (see later).

GAS INJECTION

The ideal gas bubble for PR should be large enough to cover the breaks completely and also to provide a reasonable margin of safety for small changes or inaccuracies in patient positioning. Furthermore, the bubble should maintain this size for at least 1 week to maximize the chances for an effective retinopexy seal to take place. Gas bubbles that are much larger or last considerably longer would not be expected to be more efficacious and may only add to potential complications such as secondary breaks or cataract promotion (17). Empirically, an ultimate gas bubble size of about 1 cc works well for most cases (25). Computed tomography of gas bubbles in human eyes has shown that a 0.3-mL bubble covers almost 60 degrees of peripheral retina and a 1.2-mL bubble covers 80 to 90 degrees of peripheral retina (10).

Air is not typically used because it dissipates too quickly. The half-life of an air bubble in a phakic eye is only about 1½ days; it lasts in the eye only 3 or 4 days at the most (15). Furthermore, without expansile properties, the volume of air that would need to be injected for adequate tamponade of the break would be relatively large. Because not much more than 0.15 to 0.20 mL of aqueous fluid can be drawn off at one time in a phakic eye, paracentesis alone would not sufficiently mitigate against the dangerously high intraocular pressure elevation that would occur after injecting the necessary amount of air.

Sulfur hexafluoride (SF_6) gas has a more favorable expansile and longevity profile and is the most commonly used gas for PR. A pure (undiluted) SF_6 gas bubble doubles in size (within the first 36 hours after injection) and lasts about 10 to 14 days in the eye (Table 8-2) (17). The usual volume of SF_6 injected for PR is about 0.5 mL. Occasionally, a larger or longer lasting bubble is desired, such as with multiple breaks, breaks located around the horizontal meridian, and breaks in larger (highly myopic) eyes. In such cases, *perfluoropropane* (C_3F_8) is preferred. It quadruples in volume within the first 3 days and lasts about 4 to 8 weeks in the eye (see Table 8-2) (14,15,17). The usual amount of pure C_3F_8 injected is about 0.3 mL. Because animal models showed varying degrees of cataract promotion with long-acting gases in the vitreous cavity, many surgeons originally restricted the use of C_3F_8 gas to pseudophakic or aphakic eyes (17). In clinical practice, however, this has not been shown to occur to any significant degree with PR, and its use appears to be just as safe in phakic eyes in this setting (27). Nonetheless, patients with intraocular gas should not sleep on their backs, to avoid any prolonged gas–lenticular touch.

A few minutes before injecting the gas, half-strength or full-strength (5% to 10%) povidone–iodine solution (Betadine) is instilled for endophthalmitis prophylaxis. Using a 1- or 3-mL sterile syringe, the selected gas is then drawn up from the tank through a

TABLE 8-2. *Inert gases currently approved for intraocular use*

Gas type	Expansion	Average duration	Volume used for pneumatic retinopexy
Sulfur hexafluoride (SF_6)	2×	10–14 d	0.5 mL
Perfluoropropane (C_3F_8)	4×	30–45 d	0.35 mL

0.22-μm Millipore filter. (This filter effectively sterilizes the gas as it passes into the syringe.) A half-inch, 30-gauge needle is placed on the syringe, and the excess gas is discarded. Aiming toward the middle of the vitreous cavity, the needle is introduced into the vitreous cavity through the pars plana, 3.5 to 4.0 mm posterior to the limbus. It is best to inject in a region away from large, open breaks and away from an area in which the pars plana epithelium is detached, thereby minimizing the chances that gas bubbles will migrate or infuse directly into the subretinal space. Directly visualizing the needle tip in the eye with indirect ophthalmoscopy before or during the injection is not necessary. However, after injecting, the fundus should be reinspected with ophthalmoscopy to make sure the gas bubble is freely mobile in the vitreous and is not trapped at the injection site or anterior hyaloidal space.

For effective tamponade and to minimize the chances that bubbles will migrate subretinally through open breaks, a single, large intraocular gas bubble, rather than multiple small bubbles or "fish eggs," is the goal. Turning the patient's head to one side to place the injection site uppermost and to allow the needle to be vertically oriented during injection is probably the most important maneuver for achieving a single intraocular bubble (Fig. 8-5). Inserting the needle first about 6 mm or more into the vitreous cavity (to make sure it clears the pars plana epithelium) and then, before injecting, pulling back so about 3 mm of needle remains in the eye also appears to help in making a single gas bubble. Furthermore, injecting the gas in a smooth, brisk fashion is better than injecting slowly or in spurts. To avoid any escape of gas from the eye or into the subconjunctival space, the injection site should be covered temporarily with a cotton-tipped applicator immediately on withdrawal of the needle. It can be removed once the patient's head is rotated to the opposite side, a maneuver that brings the gas bubble away from the site.

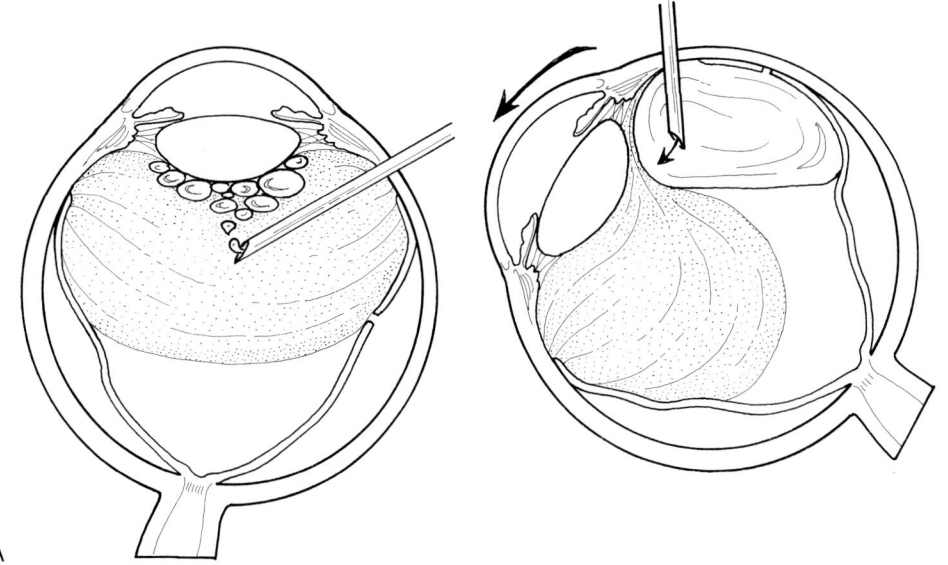

FIGURE 8-5. A: Incorrect orientation of the needle during gas injection resulting in multiple, small gas bubbles or "fish eggs." **B:** Correct orientation of the needle being in the uppermost part of the eye, vertical with respect to the ground, and pulled back slightly. A single gas bubble is obtained.

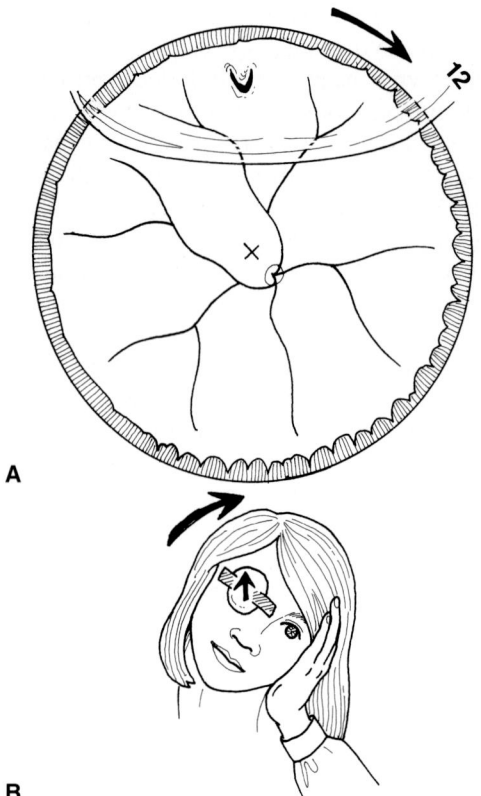

FIGURE 8-6. A: Ophthalmoscopic observation to confirm the correct head positioning for the gas to tamponade the retinal break. **B:** An arrow can be drawn on the eye patch such that it points to the ceiling when the head is in proper position.

Whether the paracentesis is performed before or after the gas injection, the central retinal artery needs to be inspected by ophthalmoscopy at the conclusion of the procedure to make sure that it is not occluded, as is done in SB procedures. If the central retinal artery is occluded and fails to become patent within 5 to 10 minutes, repeat paracentesis should be performed.

Once patency of the artery is confirmed, a combination antibiotic–steroid ointment can then be instilled, and the eye can be patched lightly. This is a good time to review with the patient the proper positioning that will be needed. An arrow that points to the ceiling when the patient's head position is oriented properly can be drawn on the eye patch to help the patient maintain the positioning at home (Fig. 8-6).

It is safe for the patient to go home after patching and counseling. Although the gases used for PR expand at the greatest rate within the first 6 hours after injection into the eye (1), the globe, mainly through increased aqueous outflow facility, compensates well during this time, and intraocular pressure rises are not typically seen (9). Therefore, checking the intraocular pressure over the hours immediately after the procedure is not necessary.

INTRAOPERATIVE PROBLEMS

Subretinal Gas

In most cases, subretinal gas is the result of small bubbles or "fish eggs" created at the time of injection with migration of the bubbles through a relatively large retinal tear during or immediately after the procedure (see Fig. 8-5). It is a rare and, in most cases, avoidable complication, encountered about 1% of the time, based on a compilation of early PR reports (9). First, the chance of creating "fish eggs" can be minimized by following the guidelines mentioned in the section on gas injection. To reemphasize, the patient should be in the supine position and the head rotated 45 degrees to one side. This makes the injection site the most superior portion of the eye and allows for the needle to enter the pars plana safely, vertical with respect to the floor (12). Furthermore, having the needle in the eye only about 3 mm and injecting briskly in a soft eye (i.e., after paracentesis) will help to maximize single bubble formation.

Should "fish eggs" come about despite following the recommended injection technique, the surgeon should keep the patient's head positioned with the bubbles away from the break (i.e., not allow the break to be uppermost) and should gently tap the globe with an index finger once or twice over where the bubbles are located. If this fails to produce a single bubble, the patient should maintain this head positioning for the first 24 hours because spontaneous coalescence of the bubbles usually occurs within this time.

If gas bubbles are seen in the subretinal space, one should first determine whether or not they appear to be holding the break open. Small bubbles under the retina that are away from the break usually are not a problem, and, therefore, no intervention is needed. If, however, the gas bubble is interfering with break closure and retinal reattachment, it will need to be removed from this location. The surgeon should first try to express it through the break with massage-like scleral depression in combination with appropriate head positioning (12,25). Should this fail, invasive maneuvers such as needle aspiration or vitrectomy surgery are required (21).

Gas under the pars plana epithelium may result from lack of complete penetration of the pars plana ciliary epithelium with the needle during gas injection (11). This complication is also readily avoidable by first entering with the needle at least 6 mm into the eye (and then pulling the needle back as described earlier) before injecting and avoiding areas where the retinal detachment has extended into the pars plana region. Nonetheless, should this be encountered, the gas bubble will need to be removed, unless it is extremely small. This procedure can be done by reintroducing a needle of slightly larger diameter (e.g., 25- or 27-gauge) on a syringe without the plunger back through the original injection site until the bubble is reached (25). Filling the syringe halfway with sterile balanced saline solution allows the surgeon to know precisely when the gas pocket is first entered with the needle. After removal, intravitreal gas injection should be performed somewhere away from this site.

Trapped Intraocular Gas

Rarely, the intraocular gas bubble can be trapped in the space bordered by the pars plana epithelium, the anterior hyaloid face, and the posterior surface of the lens, the canal of Petit (12). Characteristically, the gas bubble does not move with changes in head position and assumes a semicircular shape. This complication can also be avoided by initially passing the needle deep into the vitreous cavity, at least 6 mm, as described previously. However, if trapped or immobile gas is observed, it can be evacuated using the same needle technique described before with sub–pars plana gas. Alternatively, the patient can be instructed to maintain facedown positioning for the next 24 hours. Usually, the gas bubble spontaneously breaks through the anterior hyaloid face and becomes mobile within the vitreous cavity over that period.

Induced Macular Detachment

Displacement of SRF into the macula after injection of the gas can occur and is of potential concern if the macula was attached preoperatively (Fig. 8-7) (20,28). Only eyes with extremely bullous superior (or temporal) detachments that come close to the macula are at risk. In these eyes, the "steamroller" maneuver is recommended to help avoid this complication, the clinical or functional significance of which is uncertain (11,12,25).

Immediately after the gas is injected, the patient's head is turned to face the ground, and the turning should be performed so the gas bubble goes over the attached retina as it migrates toward the posterior pole (9). Over the next 15 minutes or so, the patient's head position is changed so the bubble moves over detached retina toward the retinal break, pushing some of the SRF out through the break (Fig. 8-8). Overall, the maneuver works better and faster with larger breaks.

The maneuver may also be considered if one is concerned that the bubble may result in shifting SRF into an area of an attached retina with an incidental break. It may also be used to reduce the amount of retinal elevation to achieve better cryotherapy uptake or better to view the central retinal artery at the optic nerve head, such as when the detachment overhangs the nerve.

Miscellaneous

Various other, rare, intraoperative complications have been described. Subretinal and vitreous hemorrhage can occur but is usually limited, and no reports of these complications affecting visual outcomes in PR have been published (12). The source of the blood, particularly when subretinal, appears to be from cryotherapy-induced freeze fracturing of retinal vessels near the tear and is not unique to PR. Hemorrhage can also be from the pars plana injection, and this complication can be minimized by avoiding the horizontal meridians where the anterior ciliary vessels are located.

Both vitreous and iris incarceration into the paracentesis tract has been observed (12). The use of a small needle (e.g., 30-gauge) for the paracentesis rather than a large needle or a surgical blade should prevent any iris incarceration to the limbal tract. Vitreous incarceration would only be seen in cases with an open capsule and vitreous gel in the anterior chamber. Avoiding paracentesis altogether by using a smaller volume of gas with

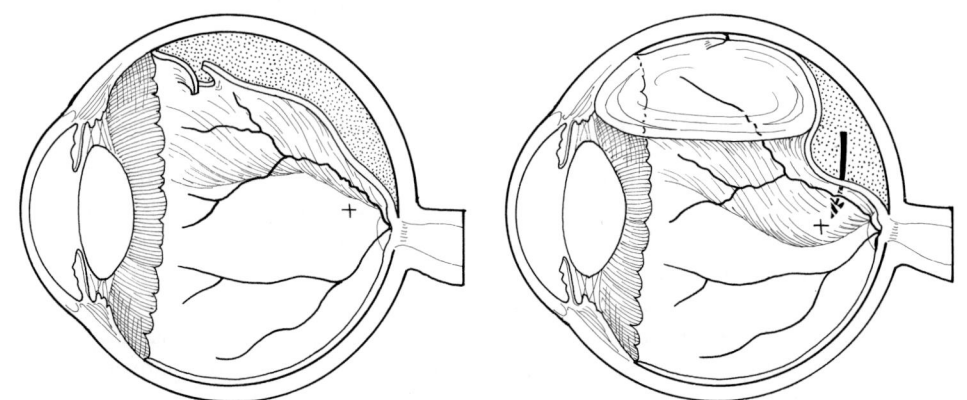

FIGURE 8-7. A: Superior retinal detachment extending close to but not involving the macula. **B:** Postoperative displacement of subretinal fluid by the gas bubble into the macula.

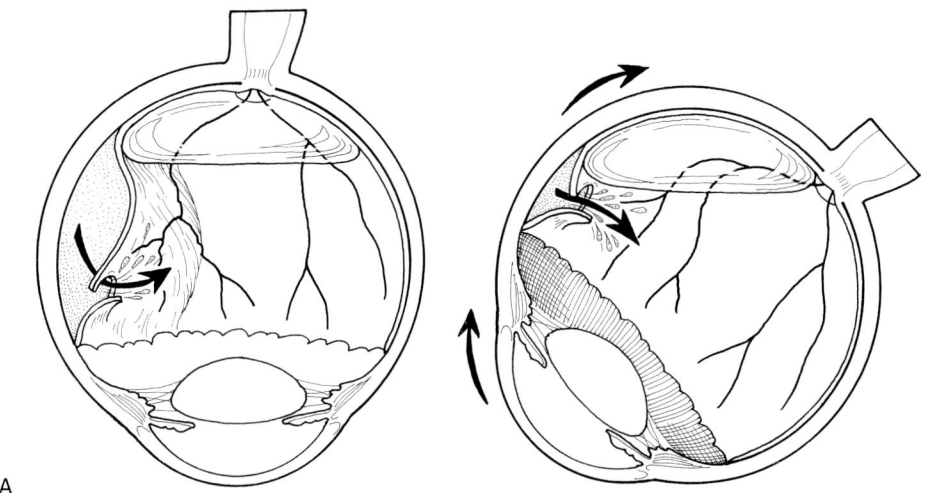

FIGURE 8-8. "Steamroller" maneuver. **A:** Immediately after the intravitreal gas injection, the patient's head is turned face down in such a way that the gas bubble reaches the posterior pole by traversing attached retina. **B:** The head is then slowly repositioned so the gas bubble moves across detached retina toward the retinal tear, "steamrolling" the retina flat.

greater expansile properties (e.g., C_3F_8 instead of SF_6) is the easiest solution. If paracentesis is needed in an eye that has undergone cataract extraction, it is best to minimize the chances of engaging vitreous gel in the needle by performing the paracentesis inferiorly (away from the old cataract incision) and keeping the bevel of the needle over iris and facing upward. Care must be taken not to strike the iris. One case of hyphema and anterior lens touch was observed in the large, multicenter, controlled PR trial (26).

Subconjunctival gas, a minor and clinically insignificant finding, can be encountered on withdrawal of the gas injection needle from the pars plana (11). A small bead of formed vitreous at the injection site has also been reported (7). Both complications can be averted by using a small needle (30-gauge) for gas injection and by placing a cotton-tipped applicator on the site immediately after removing the needle.

ROUTINE POSTOPERATIVE MANAGEMENT

The patient is sent home from the office to be at relative rest and to adhere to the appropriate positioning of the head for most of the day and through the night, while sleeping, during the first 5 postoperative days. The patch is discontinued on the first day, and a steroid–antibiotic combination drop is used four times a day over the first week or so. Unless cryotherapy was extensive, the degree of ocular discomfort is usually minimal, and acetaminophen or other oral nonsteroidal antiinflammatory medications alone are all that is typically needed for the first 24 to 48 hours. The patient may watch television but should refrain from reading because the eye motions may cause breakup of the gas bubble into smaller ones, rendering the bubble less effective. Until the gas bubble is gone (or extremely small), the patient is restricted from any high-altitude (higher than 4,000 feet) travel, including any airplane travel, because the cabin is pressurized to an equivalent of 8,000 feet of altitude. Otherwise, the patient's usual daily routine, including work-related activities, can be resumed typically by 2 weeks after the procedure.

Close follow-up is recommended. The eye should be examined on the first postoperative day, 3 to 4 days later, and then every 2 to 4 weeks for the first 3 months, similar to SB procedures. Subretinal fluid should start to resorb within the first 24 to 48 hours, and the retina is usually completely attached within the first 3 to 5 days. The SRF of chronic detachments can take longer to resorb.

If the detachment is persisting or increasing, then either the original break is not well sealed, or new or missed breaks are open. Depending on the location of the breaks, repeat (supplemental) retinopexy with or without another gas injection (depending on how much of the original gas remains), followed by additional positioning, is often successful in obtaining retinal reattachment. However, new breaks located inferiorly or in multiple quadrants and the emergence of significant PVR is best handled by proceeding to SB (with or without vitrectomy) next to achieve retinal reattachment after the failed PR procedure.

SURGICAL RESULTS

Using the general eligibility criteria outlined earlier in the section on patient selection, large uncontrolled (2,9,11,12,18) and controlled (26,27) series showed a single-procedure reattachment success rate of PR of around 80%. Furthermore, in the only study that compared the procedure directly with SB in a randomized, controlled fashion, the single-procedure reattachment rate in this selected patient population was not statistically significantly different (26,27). This clinical trial also indicated that initial PR failures that later required additional procedures of various types (e.g., repeat PR, SB, or vitrectomy) to achieve eventual reattachment did not compromise anatomic or visual outcome, compared with similar cases first approached with SB (26,27). (The ultimate reattachment rate with one or more procedures in both groups was comparable at around 98%.) These findings, coupled with the knowledge that PR typically is better tolerated and perhaps has a lower complication rate than SB, have prompted many surgeons to perform PR routinely as the primary procedure for uncomplicated primary or recurrent retinal detachment with small or localized breaks in the superior retinal quadrants.

As with SB, the reattachment success rate varies according to the presence or absence of certain preoperative ocular features. In general, in patients with eyes that otherwise meet the strict PR selection criteria but have extensive retinal detachments, aphakia or pseudophakia (especially with open posterior capsules), multiple breaks, or other vitreoretinal disorders such as lattice degeneration or early PVR, anatomic outcomes are worse (3,4,8,19,27). In contrast, in patients with phakic eyes with a single, small, superior tear, a limited area of detachment, and no other peripheral retinal abnormalities, single-procedure success rates are good, probably averaging more than 90%.

Failure of the procedure to achieve retinal reattachment is typically seen soon after the procedure is performed, with 86% of failures occurring within the first month (8). Failure usually is the result of either new or missed breaks or treated breaks that either never closed or reopened as the gas dissipated. The rate of new or missed breaks is in the range of about 7% to 15% for most large series (8,9,11,12,26). Although new breaks and detachments definitively do occur after PR (22), many of the cases in this category probably represent missed breaks, and the percentage of these cases should be able to be minimized with meticulous preoperative and intraoperative examination and avoiding PR in eyes with less than optimal visualization of the peripheral retina. Cases with breaks that never closed are usually the result of inadequate treatment or positioning. Cases with tears that reopen later may either be from inadequate initial treatment (and manifest as the gas bubble is nearly gone) or from the formation of PVR, which comes about after

PR about 3% to 4% of the time (9,26). Many of the missed, new, or reopened breaks remain amenable to repeat PR either in full or in part (e.g., supplemental cryotherapy and repositioning without repeat gas injection if the original bubble is still adequate).

With regard to functional results, PR has an overall visual acuity outcome comparable to that of SB for similar retinal detachment presentations (see chapter 7, Scleral Buckling Procedure). As with all retinal detachment repair techniques, final visual acuity mainly depends on the preoperative status of the macula, that is, whether or not the macula is detached and, if so, for how long. In the PR multicenter controlled clinical trial, SB and PR had equally good final visual acuity results for detachments that spared the macula preoperatively (27). However, when the macula was detached for up to 2 weeks before the initial surgical intervention, the percentage of eyes that had a final visual acuity of 20/50 or better was higher in the PR group compared with the SB group (89% vs. 67%), and this difference was statistically significant (27). This difference may be at least partially explainable by the greater percentage of eyes that went on to significant cataract formation in patients in the SB group or perhaps to chronic, postoperative cystoid macular edema (CME) either directly from SB or from later cataract surgery.

REFERENCES

1. Abrams GW, Edelhauser H, Aaberg TM, et al. Dynamics of intravitreal sulfur hexafluoride. *Invest Ophthalmol* 1974;13:863–868.
2. Algvere P, Hallnas K, Palmqvist BM. Success and complications of pneumatic retinopexy. *Am J Ophthalmol* 1988;106:400–404.
3. Boker T, Schmitt C, Mougharbel M. Results and prognostic factors in pneumatic retinopexy. *Ger J Ophthalmol* 1994;3:73–78.
4. Chen JC, Robertson JE, Coonan P, et al. Results and complications of pneumatic retinopexy. *Ophthalmology* 1988;95:601–608.
5. Dominguez DA. Cirugia precoz y ambulatoria del desprendimiento de retina. *Arch Soc Esp Oftal* 1985; 48:47–54.
6. Folk JC, Sneed SR, Folberg R, Coonan P, Pulido JS. Early retinal adhesion from laser photocoagulation. *Ophthalmology* 1989;96:1523–1525.
7. Friberg TR, Eller AW. Pneumatic repair of primary and secondary retinal detachments using a binocular indirect ophthalmoscope laser delivery system. *Ophthalmology* 1988;95:187–193.
8. Grizzard WS, Hilton GF, Hammer ME, Taren D, Brinton DA. Pneumatic retinopexy failures: cause, prevention, timing, and management. *Ophthalmology* 1995;102:929–936.
9. Hilton GF, Brinton DA. Pneumatic retinopexy and alternative techniques. In: Ryan SJ, Glaser BM, eds. *Retina*, 2nd ed. St Louis: CV Mosby, 1994:2093–2112.
10. Hilton GF, Grizzard WS. Pneumatic retinopexy: a two-step outpatient operation without conjunctival incision. *Ophthalmology* 1986;93:626–641.
11. Hilton GF, Kelly NE, Salzano TC, Tornambe PE, Wells JW, Wendel RT. Pneumatic retinopexy: a collaborative report of the first 100 cases. *Ophthalmology* 1987;94:307–314.
12. Hilton GF, Tornambe PE. Pneumatic retinopexy: an analysis of intraoperative and postoperative complications. The Retinal Detachment Study Group. *Retina* 1991;11:285–294.
13. Laqua H, Machemer R. Repair and adhesion mechanisms of the cryotherapy lesion in experimental retinal detachment. *Am J Ophthalmol* 1976;81:833–846.
14. Lincoff A, Haft D, Liggett P, Reifer C. Intravitreal expansion of perfluorocarbon bubbles. *Arch Ophthalmol* 1980; 98:1646.
15. Lincoff H, Coleman J, Kreissig I, Richard G, Chang S, Wilcox LM. The perfluorocarbon gases in the treatment of retinal detachment. *Ophthalmology* 1983;90:546–551.
16. Lincoff H, Kreissig I, Jakobiec F, et al. Remodeling of cryosurgical adhesion. *Arch Ophthalmol* 1981;99: 1845–1849.
17. Lincoff H, Mardirossian J, Lincoff A, Liggett P, Iwamoto T, Jakobiec F. Intravitreal longevity of three perfluorocarbon gases. *Arch Ophthalmol* 1980;98:1610–1611.
18. Lowe MA, McDonald HR, Campo RV, Boyer DS, Schatz H. Pneumatic retinopexy: surgical results. *Arch Ophthalmol* 1988;106:1672–1276.
19. McAllister IL, Meyers SM, Zegarra H, Gutman FA, Zakov ZN, Beck GJ. Comparison of pneumatic retinopexy with alternative surgical techniques. *Ophthalmology* 1988;95:877–883.
20. McAllister IL, Zegarra H, Meyers SM, et al. Treatment of retinal detachments with multiple breaks by pneumatic retinopexy. *Arch Ophthalmol* 1987;105:913–916.

21. McDonald HR, Abrams GW, Irvine AR, et al. The management of subretinal gas following attempted pneumatic retinal reattachment. *Ophthalmology* 1987;94:319–326.
22. Poliner LS, Grand MG, Schoch LH, et al. New retinal detachment after pneumatic retinopexy. *Ophthalmology* 1987;94:315–318.
23. Smith RB, Carl B, Linn JG, Nemoto E. Effect of nitrous oxide on air in the vitreous. *Am J Ophthalmol* 1974;78:314–320.
24. Stinson TW, Donlon JV. Interaction of intraocular air and sulfur hexafluoride with nitrous oxide: a computer simulation. *Anesthesiology* 1982;56:385–388.
25. Tornambe PE. Pneumatic retinopexy. *Surv Ophthalmol* 1988;32:270–281.
26. Tornambe PE, Hilton GF. Pneumatic retinopexy: a multicenter randomized controlled clinical trial comparing pneumatic retinopexy with scleral buckling. The Retinal Detachment Study Group. *Ophthalmology* 1989;96:772–783.
27. Tornambe PE, Hilton GF, Brinton DA, et al. Pneumatic retinopexy: a two-year follow-up study of the multicenter clinical trial comparing pneumatic retinopexy with scleral buckling. *Ophthalmology* 1991;98:1115–1123.
28. Yeo JH, Vidaurri-Leal J, Glaser BM. Extension of retinal detachments as a complication of pneumatic retinopexy. *Arch Ophthalmol* 1986;104:1161–1163.
29. Yoon YH, Marmor MF. Rapid enhancement of retinal adhesion by laser photocoagulation. *Ophthalmology* 1988;95:1385–1388.

9
Alternative Techniques for the Treatment of Retinal Detachment

TEMPORARY BALLOON BUCKLING

In 1979, Lincoff and associates proposed using an inflatable balloon as a temporary buckle to treat retinal detachments (23). Like pneumatic retinopexy (PR), it is a relatively quick, minimally invasive, office-based technique that can be used for uncomplicated retinal detachments associated with either a single break or a closely grouped cluster of breaks. Unlike PR, however, it can also be used for detachments caused by an inferior break.

The device consists of a silicone balloon located at the end of a 9.0- or 12.5-cm soft silicone catheter. The balloon is inflated by injecting saline or water. In the inflated position, the balloon is ovoid and therefore assumes the appropriate configuration to act as a radial buckle (Fig. 9-1). The other end of the catheter where the fluid-filled syringe attaches has a valve to retain the fluid and to keep the balloon at a constant size once the syringe is removed. A wire stylet runs the entire length of the balloon catheter and serves to stiffen the device and to facilitate placement in the sub-Tenon's space. The stylet is removed once the balloon catheter is in position.

The balloon is positioned on the surface of the sclera, under both Tenon's capsule and conjunctiva. The epibulbar tissue and bony orbit provide the countertraction necessary for the inflated balloon to create a localized area of eyewall indentation (Fig. 9-2). No scleral sutures over the balloon are needed. It is well tolerated and has little tendency to dislodge even with extraocular movements (23). With the retinal break effectively tamponaded externally, the subretinal fluid (SRF) spontaneously resorbs, and the retinal break seals from cryotherapy or laser photocoagulation applied as part of the procedure. The balloon is deflated and removed after about 1 week or so. The basic steps of the procedure are described in the next section.

Technique

Anesthesia is usually achieved with a subconjunctival, posterior sub-Tenon's, or retrobulbar injection. Subconjunctival anesthesia using 2% lidocaine suffices for most cases and allows for adequate pain control yet also the retention of ocular motility throughout the procedure.

The retinal tear is treated with transcleral cryotherapy in the usual fashion under ophthalmoscopic visualization. (Laser photocoagulation can also be used for retinopexy but, like PR, must be administered in the postoperative period, once the retina has flattened.) The location of the break is then marked on the conjunctiva with a marking pen.

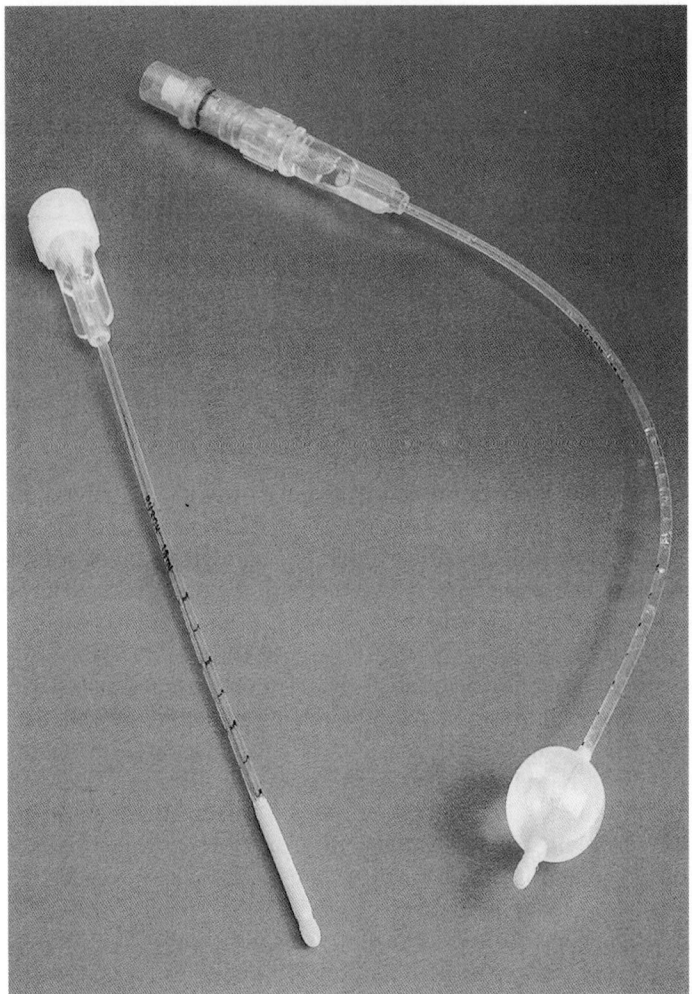

FIGURE 9-1. The temporary balloon buckling device. The balloon prior to *(left)* and after *(right)* inflation. (Courtesy of Grieshaber, Inc., Kennesaw, Georgia.)

Precise localization is critical. The mark should correspond to both the exact meridian and the most posterior aspect of the break. One technique that can be used to facilitate determining this location is to make the final application of cryotherapy at this most posterior site and then mark the depression on the conjunctiva produced by the defrosting iceball. (14) Some surgeons make an additional mark at a more anterior location in the meridian where conjunctiva and Tenon's is less mobile, to ensure correct placement of the balloon catheter.

The eye is then prepared with topical povidone–iodine (Betadine). A sterile drape is also typically used around the eye. A 2-mm conjunctival–Tenon's opening is then made about 3 to 4 mm anterior to the retinal tear localization mark. Making the opening too large or in too posterior a location decreases the overlying tissue support of the balloon. A blunt probe such as a large lacrimal dilator is then inserted to create a narrow tunnel in the sub-Tenon's space up to and several millimeters beyond the mark. This technique facilitates insertion of the balloon catheter in the correct meridian.

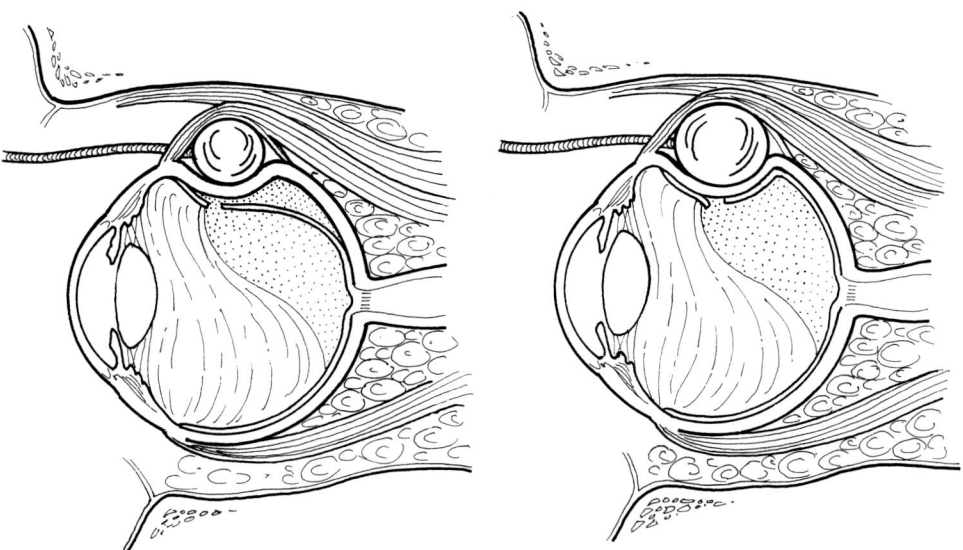

FIGURE 9-2. Schematic drawing of the balloon indenting the sclera and choroid toward a retinal break *(left)*; with the retinal break effectively closed, the subretinal fluid spontaneously resorbs *(right)*.

The surgeon should test the balloon by inflating it once immediately before using it to make sure it has no leaks. The deflated balloon is then inserted into the sub-Tenon's space and is advanced to lie over the break. The stylet is removed, and the balloon is inflated only partially at first using, about 0.25 to 0.5 mL of sterile saline or water to confirm by indirect ophthalmoscopy that it is in the correct position. (Because of the presence of scleral memory and lingering indentation effect, a deflated balloon that was initially partially filled is much more easily repositioned than one that was completely filled.) Once in precise position over the retinal break, additional saline is then injected to expand the balloon to a size that adequately supports the break. Usually about 0.75 to 1.25 mL of additional saline is all that is required. To minimize the chance of balloon rupture, the surgeon should avoid filling the balloon with more than a total of 2.5 mL of fluid.

The intraocular pressure rises during the inflation, and the central retinal artery also should be monitored at this time to ensure that it remains patent. If flow through the artery stops, one should first deflate the balloon slightly and then reinflate slowly, in small increments. Alternatively, a paracentesis can be performed to bring the intraocular pressure down and to reestablish retinal blood flow. Once the desired buckle height is achieved, the operation is completed. A subconjunctival injection of an antibiotic solution can then be administered. Although early reports described securing the silicone tube at the conjunctival opening to the surrounding conjunctiva or sclera, many surgeons have not found the suture to be necessary (14).

The exposed end of the tube is then taped to the patient's periocular skin. The tube should be positioned such that contact with the cornea is avoided, to prevent a postoperative corneal abrasion. Keeping it well away from the cornea also helps to prevent dellen formation. Antibiotic ointment is instilled, and the eye is then patched.

The patient is allowed to be up and around, but not at full activity while the catheter is in place during the first week or so. The eye is patched, and an antibiotic–steroid combination as a drop or ointment is used four times daily. Close follow-up is recommended. The eye should be examined on the first postoperative day and, if the break is flat on the area of indentation, several days later. On the first postoperative day, it is sometimes necessary to increase the buckling effect by injecting up to 0.5 mL more of sterile saline (14). Repositioning may sometimes be needed. Laser photocoagulation can be placed around the original tear to augment the cryotherapy, or it can be used as the sole retinopexy technique within the first few days after the procedure, once the retina is attached in the region of the tear.

The balloon is deflated and removed between postoperative days 7 and 10. The conjunctival opening closes spontaneously within the next couple of days, and the topical medication can then be stopped. With the retina well attached, follow-up should be about 1 week after removal of the balloon. At that time, if the status of the retina is unchanged, the patient may resume full activity. The fundus should be rechecked about every 3 to 4 weeks for the first 3 months, monitoring specifically for early and late reopening of the original tear, new tear and detachments, and proliferative vitreoretinopathy (PVR). Most of these complications manifest within the first month or so after balloon removal (19).

Surgical Results

This technique has several advantages over standard, permanent scleral buckling (SB). First, it can be easily done in 15 to 30 minutes using under local anesthesia and in the office setting. Second, because no implant or explant remains under a rectus muscle, the risk of persistent postoperative diplopia is minimized. Third, no sharp instruments are used on the sclera; the risk of penetrating the eyewall posteriorly and producing complications such as subretinal bleeding or retinal perforation is negligible. Fourth, no long-term risk of orbital or intraocular infection exists. Fifth, no late extrusion or intrusion of an explant can occur. Sixth, no permanent changes in refractive error occur (20,23,29).

An advantage over PR is that the globe is never entered, and, therefore, no risk of intraocular infection exists. Furthermore, potential problems related to intraocular gas such as subretinal bubbles, anteriorly trapped gas, and maybe even cataract promotion or secondary breaks are avoided. Last, no special postoperative patient positioning is needed for the procedure to work, and inferior breaks can be effectively managed.

Overall, most series have reported a reattachment success rate between approximately 80% and 90% (4,14,19,21,23,29). As with PR, these were selected, uncomplicated, primary rhegmatogenous retinal detachments (RRD) using the criteria of retinal break size and involvement noted previously. Most cases in the series published to date were phakic eyes, which usually have better success rates, regardless of the retinal detachment repair approach (10,14,24,29,35). In a series that used the balloon in aphakic detachments, the rate of sustained retinal attachment after balloon removal was only 69% (22). Furthermore, many of the studies, particularly those that report higher initial success rates, included eyes that required postoperative repositioning of the balloon or supplemental cryotherapy or photocoagulation in the "single-procedure success" group (14,19,29). As with studies on PR, retinal reattachment rates, starting with the balloon technique and going on to other procedures such as SB or vitrectomy in case of balloon failure, ultimately increase to about 92% to 99% (14,19,21).

Anatomic failures with the balloon technique are most often the result of significant vitreoretinal traction to the retinal tear that either keeps it open with the balloon in place or, more commonly, reopens the tear, despite apparently good retinopexy, after the balloon is removed (Table 9-1) (14,19,21,29). Failures can also result from balloon malpositioning or malfunction of the balloon with spontaneous, premature deflation (14,19). The meridional location of the break does not appear to be related to success or failure (14).

In common with all retinal detachments and repair techniques, long-term reattachment failure can also be related to PVR, inadequate cryotherapy or laser retinopexy to the primary tear, and new or missed breaks (19). The rate of PVR or significant macular epiretinal membrane formation associated with the balloon technique is low and has been reported to be in the range of up to 2% or 3% (14). This rate is comparable to that with SB and PR for similar, initially uncomplicated retinal detachments (33). The rate of new tear formation has been variable among the balloon studies reported to date, ranging from 1.5% to 17% (4,14,19). Data on "new" breaks after any retinal detachment (or even just retinal tear without detachment) are difficult to interpret because one can never be certain what is actually new versus missed, whether any real cause-and-effect relationship exists between the intervention and the new tear, and, if so, what specific component of the intervention, such as cryotherapy or gas injection, may have led to the break. Various retinal procedures, both invasive and noninvasive, have been "associated" with new breaks, and the rate can be as high as 9% with just cryotherapy or laser to treat tears without any detachment (30).

Functional (visual) outcomes reported to date have been favorable and, as expected, mainly a function of the preoperative status of the macula. In the two largest series to date, final visual acuity was within two lines of the original acuity in about 95% of patients whose eyes had the macula attached at presentation (14,19). Reasons for a significant visual loss in this group included failure to reattach the retina with a single procedure, macular pucker, macular hole, macular degeneration, cataract, and vitreous hemorrhage (from a bridging vessel). In patients whose macula initially was detached, 84% to 88% of eyes had a two or more line improvement of visual acuity (14,19).

Overall, the temporary balloon technique seems to be an excellent method for repairing selected retinal detachments. Few complications occur (see Table 9-1). Some surgeons have reported difficulty in performing reoperations because of excessive scar tissue (13), but others have not found this to be a problem (20–23). Reasons that it has not gained much popularity to date may be, in part, related to the relative paucity of clinical

TABLE 9-1. Reported complications of temporary balloon buckling*

Relatively common
Corneal abrasion or dellen*
Balloon malposition*
Reopening of retinal tear (after planned deflation)*
New or missed retinal breaks
Temporary diplopia (balloon in place)
Rare
Balloon malfunction (e.g., spontaneous deflation)*
Choroidal detachment
Macular hole
Macular pucker
Vitreous hemorrhage (from a bridging vessel)
Proliferative vitreoretinopathy
Persistent diplopia

*Unique to this specific retinal detachment repair technique

PRIMARY VITRECTOMY (WITHOUT SCLERAL BUCKLING)

series reported until recently and also to its temporarily unavailability in the United States in the early 1990s. It is likely that more and more surgeons will use this approach to repair selected retinal detachments, particularly detachments with inferior breaks.

Pars plana vitrectomy without SB is another technique that can be used for repairing a primary, uncomplicated retinal detachment. The general technique consists of performing a vitrectomy, internally draining the SRF with a fluid–gas exchange, and treating the retinal break with cryotherapy or laser photocoagulation (Fig. 9-3). The vitrectomy allows for direct access to and, theoretically, relief of vitreoretinal traction holding open the retinal tear. The gas that fills the posterior segment serves as temporary internal postop-

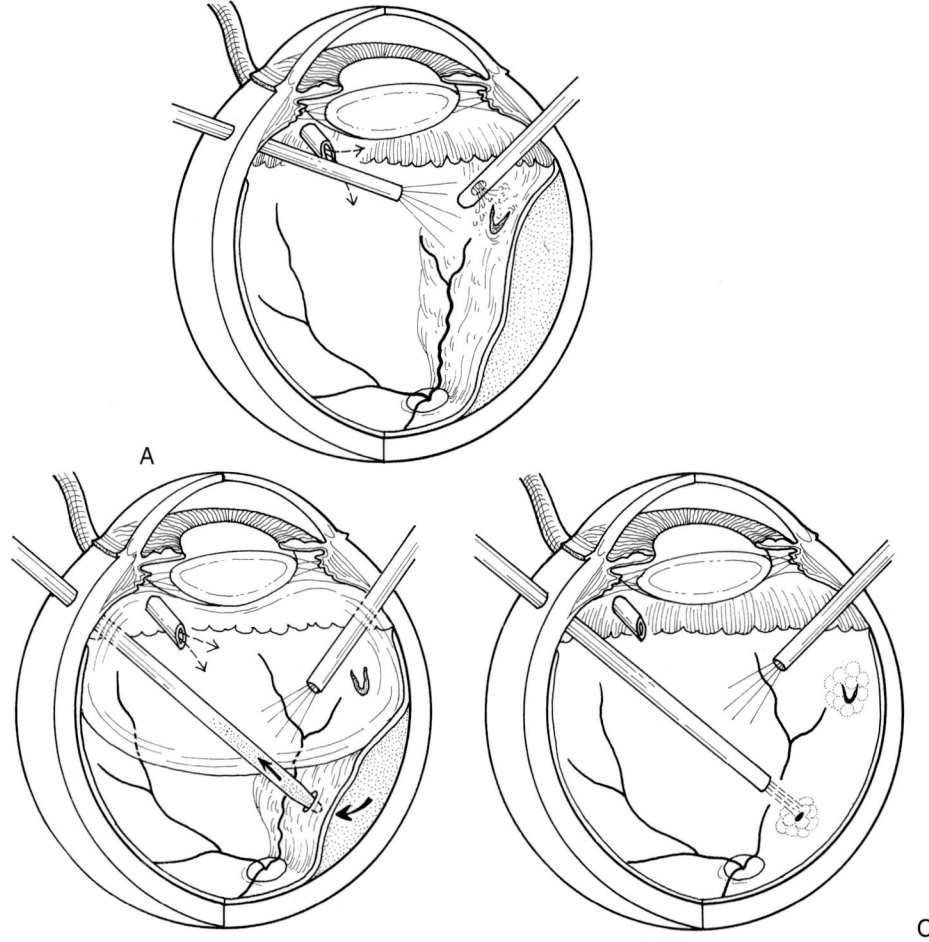

FIGURE 9-3. The basic steps of pars plana vitrectomy for repair of an uncomplicated retinal detachment. **A:** After performing the core vitrectomy, the vitreous base is trimmed in the region of the retinal tear to relieve vitreoretinal traction. **B:** A complete fluid-air exchange is then carried out with draining of the subretinal through either the peripheral retinal break or, as shown in this diagram, through a posterior retinotomy. **C:** With the retina completely attached under air, laser photocoagulation is applied around all retinal breaks.

erative tamponade of the retinal break, whereas the retinopexy performed intraoperatively takes hold over the first week after the procedure, as with PR.

Because there is minimal extraocular muscle manipulation and no significant scleral wall deformation, the potentially disturbing postoperative motility and refraction changes that sometimes accompany SB would not be expected to be encountered with vitrectomy. Unlike PR or temporary balloon buckling, the vitrectomy approach is not restricted by the size or location of the associated retinal breaks. Vitrectomy may be a particularly attractive alternative for otherwise uncomplicated retinal detachments that are extremely bullous and have large posterior breaks. Certainly, cases with significant vitreous media opacities (e.g., blood), PVR, and other complicating features are typically first managed with vitrectomy with or without combining with SB (see chapter 10, Surgery of Complicated Cases). This section, however, deals specifically with the use of vitrectomy without SB for primary, uncomplicated detachments, ones that are technically approachable with SB alone, and, in many cases, also potentially amenable to PR or temporary balloon buckling.

Technique

Because this is a relatively advanced surgical technique, the details of a three-port, pars plana vitrectomy are beyond the scope of this text. However, the general steps are worth mentioning to appreciate what is involved compared with the other methods available to repair a retinal detachment. This procedure is performed using either general or local anesthesia, with the latter in the form of a peribulbar or retrobulbar block. The eye is prepared and draped in the usual manner for intraocular surgery. The standard operating room microscope and various special contact lenses are needed to view parts of the posterior segment during the operation.

Small openings are created in the conjunctiva and Tenon's capsule in the superior and inferotemporal quadrants. Full-thickness eyewall incisions (sclerotomies) are made in each of the three quadrants using a 20-gauge microvitreoretinal blade and are positioned either 4.0 mm or 3.5 mm posterior to the limbus, depending on whether the eye is phakic or pseudophakic/aphakic, respectively. The inferotemporal sclerotomy is made first because this is the location where the infusion canula is inserted and secured in place. The vitreous cutting–aspirating instrument and the fiberoptic endoilluminator probe are inserted through each of the two superior sclerotomies.

A complete posterior vitrectomy is performed (see Fig. 9-3A). The vitreous base, particularly in the region of the retinal tear is then trimmed; as much vitreous as possible is removed from around the retinal tear to relieve vitreous traction holding open the break. This is more easily accomplished in pseudophakic or aphakic eyes. The retinal tear can be treated either at this point with transcleral cryotherapy, while the retina is still detached, or after the fluid–air exchange, once the retina is reattached, with either cryotherapy or laser photocoagulation.

A complete fluid-air exchange is performed to flatten the retina and to drain the SRF internally simultaneously. Subretinal fluid is aspirated out through either the original peripheral break or a posterior retinotomy (see Fig. 9-3B). It is ideal to be able to drain the fluid through the peripheral break and to avoid making new retinal openings. For eyes with extremely peripheral tears, especially if phakic, draining through the peripheral tear directly is difficult, and the surgeon risks striking the lens and causing rapid cataract formation. In such cases, the options are to either make the posterior retinotomy or to instill perfluorocarbon liquid (PFCL) as an intermediary step in the fluid–air exchange.

PFCLs are clear, heavier-than-water, inert liquids that can be used to steamroller the retina flat in a controlled posterior-to-anterior direction (see chapter 10, Surgery of Complicated Cases) (6,8,28,32). As they are instilled, they displace the SRF out through the original peripheral retinal break and all other fluid out the open sclerotomies such that one is left with posterior segment that is nearly completely filled with just the PFCL. With the retina attached, the PFCL is then exchanged with the air such that the posterior segment is ultimately completely filled with air and all PFCL is removed from the eye. The peripheral retinal break can be treated with laser photocoagulation with the retina attached under either PFCL or air. Laser photocoagulation is delivered with either the endoprobe or the indirect ophthalmoscope delivery system.

Whether or not PFCL is used as an intraoperative tool to help reattach the retina, the eye eventually has a complete air fill and an attached retina. Under air, any untreated retinal openings need to be addressed and at this point treated (see Fig. 9-3C). Endolaser photocoagulation is used to treat any posterior retinotomies, and peripheral breaks can be treated with either laser photocoagulation or cryotherapy, as mentioned previously.

Because air dissipates quickly from the eye postoperatively, it is, in turn, fully exchanged with one of the available inert, relatively long-lasting gases approved for intraocular use such as sulfur hexafluoride (SF_6) or perfluoropropane (C_3F_8) gas (see chapter 8, Pneumatic Retinopexy). Unlike with PR, there is a complete posterior segment fill of gas and, therefore, only *nonexpansile* mixtures of these gases are used in this setting. A nonexpansile mixture is approximately 20% for SF_6 and 14% for C_3F_8 (1,7). Once the air–gas exchange is complete, the sclerotomies and overlying conjunctival openings are closed with 7-0 or 8-0 dissolvable (e.g., Vicryl) sutures.

Postoperatively, specific head positioning is usually needed to tamponade the retinal breaks most effectively. With a much larger volume of gas than that used for PR, positioning may not need to be as strict, and multiple breaks in different locations are often adequately closed with one position. Supine positioning, however, should be avoided for most patients, particularly if the operated eye is phakic or has required a posterior drainage retinotomy. As with other procedures that use intraocular gas, patients are restricted from high-altitude travel until the gas is completely dissipated.

Surgical Results

In the late 1970s and early 1980s, Kloti first reported on the use of vitrectomy with air for repairing uncomplicated retinal detachments (16,17). In 1985, Escoffery and associates used a similar approach in an uncontrolled series of cases with uncomplicated retinal detachments and achieved complete retinal reattachment in 23 of 29 (79%) after one operation and 27 of 29 (93%) with two operations (12). Causes of surgical failure included new or missed breaks, PVR, and insufficient postoperative gas bubble size. Visual results were comparable to those expected after routine SB repair. Since then, other investigators have had even more favorable results, with a single-procedure reattachment rate as high as 87% to 94% (3,34). Perhaps improvements in vitreoretinal surgical instrumentation and techniques that came about in the 1990s such as PFCL and wide-angle operating microscope viewing systems have allowed a better success rate with vitrectomy in this setting (3). However, no controlled studies are available that compare vitrectomy alone with SB alone for such retinal detachments.

Of all the techniques described for repairing retinal detachments, vitrectomy is the most invasive approach. It carries significant potential complications such as cataracts, new retinal breaks and detachments, and endophthalmitis (2,9,11,18,26,27,31). In particular, cataract formation is accelerated in most phakic eyes after vitrectomy, particularly in older patients. Even with vitrectomy for less involved indications such as macular pucker in which gas is not used, significant nuclear sclerosis becomes evident in up to 70% of eyes within a few years after the surgery (11,27). The rate is even higher when vitrectomy is combined with fluid–gas exchange (5,15,31). Because of this possibility, many surgeons will not consider the use of vitrectomy as a primary approach for uncomplicated retinal detachments in patients with phakic eyes.

In summary, comparing the potential risks and benefits of all the approaches available to repair retinal detachment, most would agree that vitrectomy should be reserved for those detachments associated with vitreous hemorrhage, PVR, or other complicating factors. If the aim is to avoid SB, PR or temporary balloon buckling would be preferred over primary vitrectomy for most cases because these procedures are simpler, safer, and probably have similar results in many cases (34). Furthermore, they are probably associated with less total cost to perform than vitrectomy.

LASER PHOTOCOAGULATION

In managing selected retinal detachments, another option is to wall the detachment off with laser photocoagulation instead of attempting to reattach it completely. The technique merely serves to prevent progression of the detachment. This is a reasonable option when the detachment is limited in extent and the patient is either too ill or unwilling to undergo one of the reattachment procedures. In addition to standard retinal tears associated with posterior vitreous detachments (PVD), this approach has been used successfully in the setting of limited rhegmatogenous detachments related to cytomegalovirus retinitis (25).

To be effective, a continuous, firm chorioretinal adhesion needs to be formed completely around the detachment. This is accomplished by applying two or three rows of nearly confluent, moderate-intensity laser spots to the attached retina that borders the detachment and extending the laser barrier all the way to the ora serrata. Laser is delivered with either the slit-lamp or indirect ophthalmoscope delivery system. Care must be taken not to apply spots that are too hot because new retinal breaks may be created at the edge of such laser burns.

With a limited (less than one to two disc diameters), shallow detachment, applying laser (or cryotherapy) to the edges of the tear once flattened by indentation can sometimes lead to resolution of the detachment and sealing of the tear. This may be attempted instead of or in addition to just applying the laser spots around the area of detachment as described earlier. The exact mechanism that leads to resorption of the SRF with just retinopexy alone is not known.

REFERENCES

1. Abrams GW, Edelhauser H, Aaberg TM, et al. Dynamics of intravitreal sulfur hexafluoride. *Invest Ophthalmol* 1974;13:863–868.
2. Bacon AS, Davison CR, Patel BC, Frazer DG, Ficker LA, Dart JK. Infective endophthalmitis following vitreoretinal surgery. *Eye* 1993;7:529–534.
3. Bartz-Schmidt KU, Kirchhof B, Heimann K. Primary vitrectomy for pseudophakic retinal detachment. *Br J Ophthalmol* 1996;80:346–349.
4. Binder S. Repair of retinal detachments with temporary balloon buckling. *Retina* 1986;6:210–214.
5. Blodi BA, Paluska SA. Cataract after vitrectomy in young patients. *Ophthalmology* 1997;104:1092–1095.
6. Chang S. Low viscosity liquid fluorochemicals in vitreous surgery. *Am J Ophthalmol* 1987;103:38–43.
7. Chang S, Lincoff HA, Coleman DJ, Fuchs W, Farber ME. Perfluorocarbon gases in vitreous surgery. *Ophthalmology* 1985;92:651–656.
8. Chang S, Ozmert E, Zimmerman NJ. Intraoperative perfluorocarbon liquids in the management of proliferative vitreoretinopathy. *Am J Ophthalmol* 1988;106:668–674.

9. Cohen SM, Flynn HW Jr, Murray TG, Smiddy WE. Endophthalmitis after pars plana vitrectomy: the Postvitrectomy Endophthalmitis Study Group. *Ophthalmology* 1995;102:705–712.
10. Cousins S, Boniuk I, Okun E, et al. Pseudophakic retinal detachments in the presence of various IOL types. *Ophthalmology* 1986;93:1198–1208.
11. de Bustros S, Thompson JT, Michels RG, et al. Nuclear sclerosis after vitrectomy for epiretinal membranes. *Am J Ophthalmol* 1988;105:160–164.
12. Escoffery RF, Olk RJ, Grand MG, Boniuk I. Vitrectomy without scleral buckling for primary rhegmatogenous retinal detachment. *Am J Ophthalmol* 1985;99:275–281.
13. Fetherston T, Eagling EM. The use of Lincoff balloons in the management of retinal detachment. *Trans Ophthalmol Soc U K* 1982;102:230.
14. Green SN, Yarian DL, Masciulli L, Leff SR. Office repair of retinal detachment using a Lincoff temporary balloon buckle. *Ophthalmology* 1996;103:1804–1810.
15. Heimann H, Bornfeld N, Friedrichs W, et al. Primary vitrectomy without scleral buckling for rhegmatogenous retinal detachments. *Graefes Arch Clin Exp Ophthalmol* 1996;234:561–568.
16. Kloti R. Amotio-Chirurgie ohne Skleraeindellung: primare Vitrektomie. *Klin Monatsbl Augenheilkd* 1983;182:474–478.
17. Kloti R. Management of retinal detachments after vitrectomy: internal drainage–air tamponade. *Mod Probl Ophthalmol* 1979;20:188.
18. Kreiger AE. Wound complications in pars plana vitrectomy. *Retina* 1993;13:335–344.
19. Kreissig I, Failer J, Lincoff H, Ferrari F. Results of a temporary balloon buckle in the treatment of 500 retinal detachments and a comparison with pneumatic retinopexy. *Am J Ophthalmol* 1989;107:381–389.
20. Lincoff HA, Kreissig I. Additional indications for a temporary balloon buckle. *Trans Ophthalmol Soc U K* 1980;100:550.
21. Lincoff HA, Kreissig I. Results with a temporary balloon buckle for the repair of retinal detachment. *Am J Ophthalmol* 1981;92:245–251.
22. Lincoff HA, Kreissig I, Farber M. Results of 100 aphakic detachments treated with a temporary balloon buckle: a case against routine encircling operations. *Br J Ophthalmol* 1985;69:798–804.
23. Lincoff HA, Kreissig I, Hahn YS. A temporary balloon buckle for the treatment of small retinal detachments. *Ophthalmology* 1979;86:586–596.
24. McAllister IL, Meyers SM, Zegarra H, Gutman FA, Zakov ZN, Beck GJ. Comparison of pneumatic retinopexy with alternative surgical techniques. *Ophthalmology* 1988;95:877–883.
25. McCluskey P, Grigg J, Playfair TJ. Retinal detachments in patients with AIDS and CMV retinopathy: a role for laser photocoagulation. *Br J Ophthalmol* 1995;79:153–156.
26. Michels RG. Vitreous surgery for macular pucker. *Am J Ophthalmol* 1981;92:628–639.
27. Poliner LS, Olk RJ, Grand MG, et al. Surgical management of premacular fibroplasia. *Arch Ophthalmol* 1988;106:761–764.
28. Regillo CD, Brown DC. Perfluorocarbon liquids and vitreous surgery. *Ophthalmic Pract* 1994;12:236–241.
29. Schoch LH, Olk RJ, Arribas NP, et al. The Lincoff temporary balloon buckle. *Am J Ophthalmol* 1986;101:646–649.
30. Smiddy WE, Flynn HW Jr, Nicholson DH, et al. Results and complications in treated retinal breaks. *Am J Ophthalmol* 1991;112:623–631.
31. Thompson JT, Glaser BM, Sjaarda RN, et al. Progression of nuclear sclerosis and long-term visual results of vitrectomy with transforming growth factor beta-2 for macular holes. *Am J Ophthalmol* 1995;119:48–54.
32. Tornambe PE, Hilton GF. Office repair of retinal detachment [Letter]. *Ophthalmology* 1997;104:1059–1060.
33. Tornambe PE, Hilton GF. Pneumatic retinopexy: a multicenter randomized controlled clinical trial comparing pneumatic retinopexy with scleral buckling. The Retinal Detachment Study Group. *Ophthalmology* 1989;96:772–783.
34. van Effenterre G, Haut J, Larricault P, et al. Gas tamponade as a single technique in the treatment of retinal detachment: is vitrectomy needed? *Graefes Arch Clin Exp Ophthalmol* 1987;225:254.
35. Wilkinson CP. Pseudophakic retinal detachments. *Retina* 1985;5:1–4.

10

Surgery of Complicated Cases

MACULAR HOLES

Macular holes rarely cause retinal detachment unless they are in eyes that are highly myopic or have suffered blunt trauma (55). They are responsible for 0.5% to 0.7% of all retinal detachments (55).

Many rhegmatogenous retinal detachments (RRD) can have severe cystoid macular edema (CME) with a relatively large central foveal "cyst" that has extremely thin walls. Even with the aid of slit-lamp biomicroscopy with a fundus contact lens and fluorescein angiography, an experienced examiner may be unable to differentiate such a "cyst" from a full-thickness macular hole in this setting (55). For this reason alone, one should conduct a careful search for peripheral breaks, and all of these must be closed before a suspected macular hole is treated (Fig. 10-1). Furthermore, even if an unequivocal full-thickness macular hole accompanies a peripheral retinal break, adequately treating the peripheral break often cures the detachment, even though the macular hole itself is not directly treated (Fig. 10-2) (55,77). If all the peripheral breaks have been treated and the detachment persists, or if no accompanying peripheral breaks are present, the macular hole must be treated. In years past, various techniques for buckling the macula were devised, but these have been rendered obsolete by methods that approach the hole from the inside rather than from the outside of the eye.

The simplest technique is to remove some aqueous from the anterior chamber and inject pure sulfur hexafluoride (SF_6) or perfluoropropane (C_3F_8) into the vitreous cavity in amounts similar to what is used in pneumatic retinopexy (PR) (see chapter 8, Pneumatic Retinopexy) (5,51,56). Alternatively, these gases can be directly exchanged with liquid vitreous (4). Postoperatively, the patient is positioned face down so the gas rises against the macula, tamponading the hole (Fig. 10-3). The subretinal fluid is absorbed, and for reasons that are not yet known, the retina remains attached in many cases even though no thermal scar is induced. As with PR, these long-lasting gases are preferred to air because they remain in the eye longer and allow the normal retinal–retinal pigment epithelium (RPE) relationship to reestablish itself. If the retina is initially reattached, but then redetaches, the procedure can be repeated, with the exception that photocoagulation of the hole is performed when the retina is flat.

The foregoing procedures may not reattach the retina in some cases if traction exists around the macular hole from adherent cortical vitreous or epiretinal membranes. Unfortunately, the presence of such traction cannot always be easily determined preoperatively. Therefore, to maximize the chances of both reattaching the retina and com-

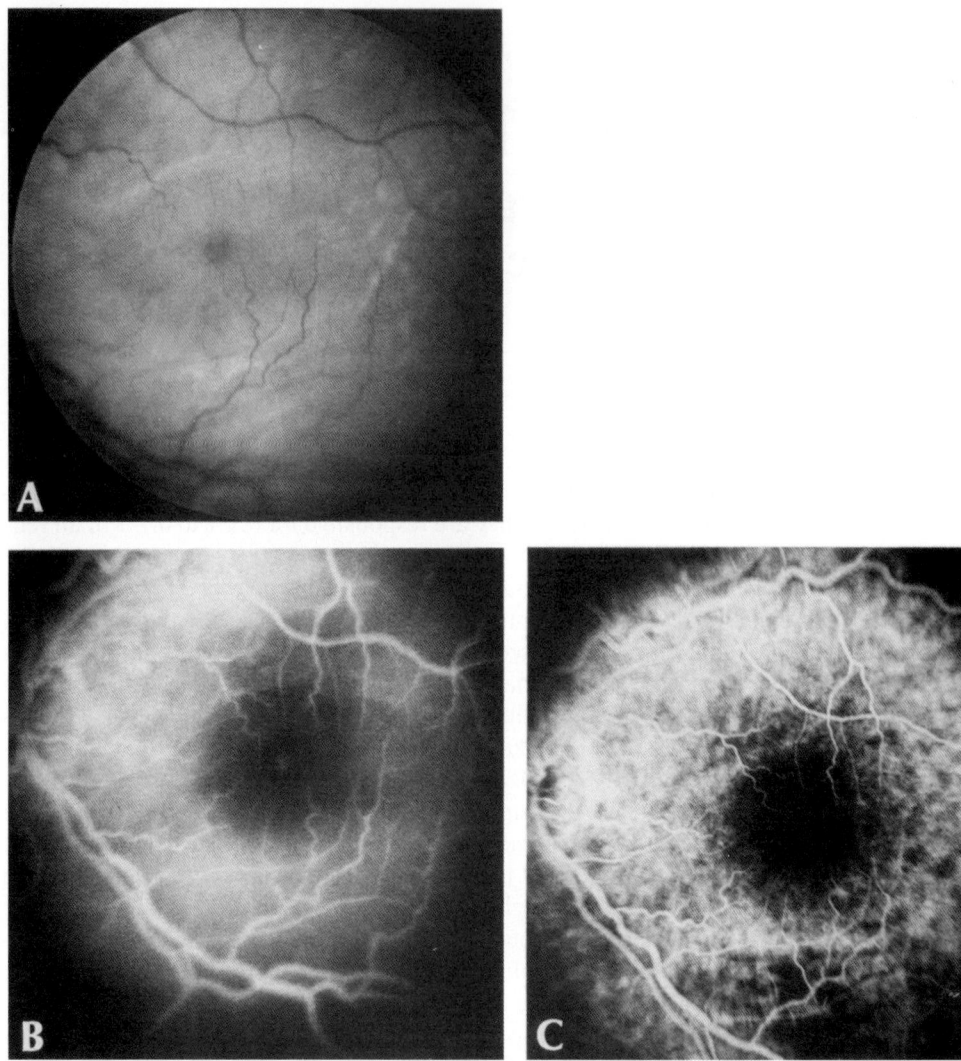

FIGURE 10-1. A: Temporal retinal detachment with a thin macula. Clinically, the patient was thought to have a full-thickness macular hole. **B:** Fluorescein angiogram. Increased transmission of background fluorescence through the macula is consistent with the misdiagnosis of full-thickness macular hole. **C:** A peripheral retinal break was found and closed. The retina is reattached. Visual acuity is 6/15 (20/50). No macular hole is present. The fluorescein angiogram is normal.

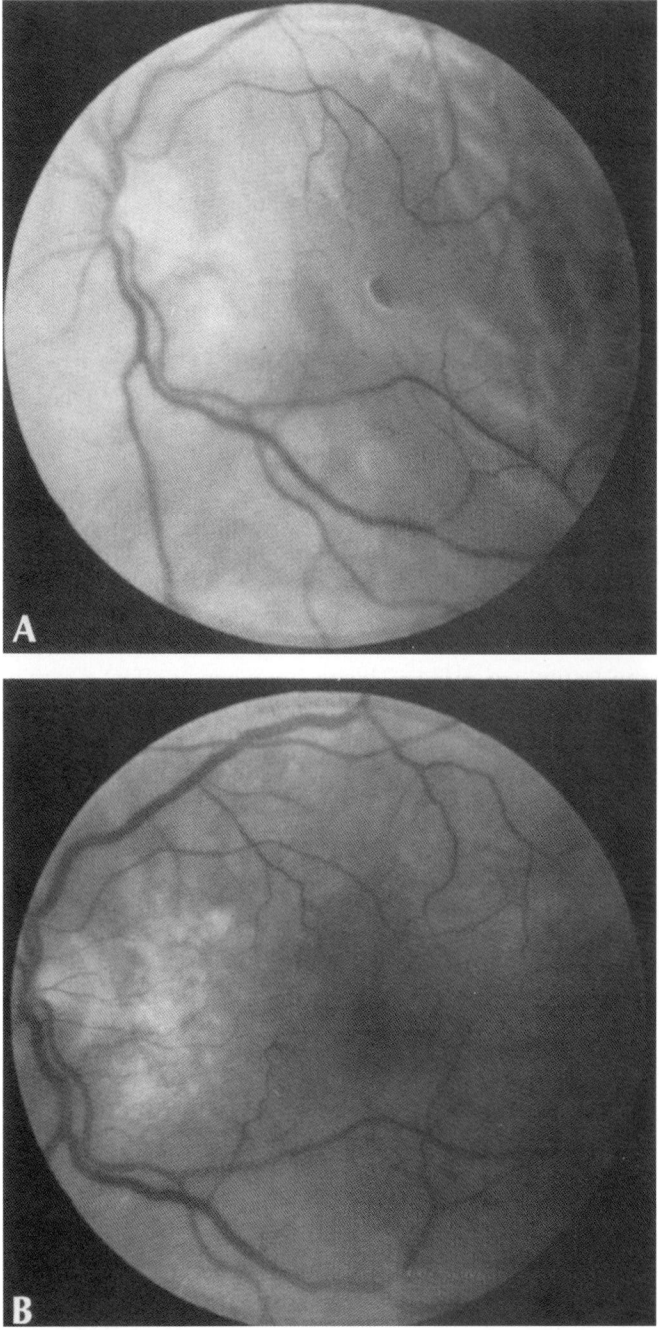

FIGURE 10-2. A: Retinal detachment with a full-thickness macular hole. **B:** Peripheral breaks were closed by a scleral buckling procedure. The retina is reattached, even though the macular hole has not been treated.

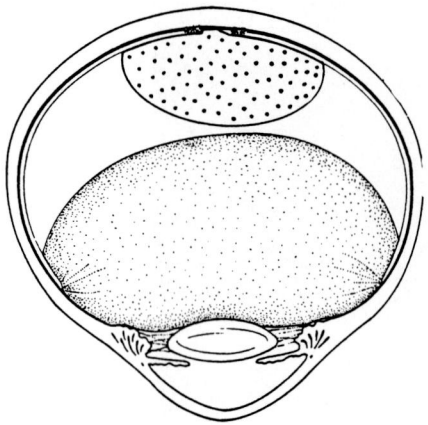

FIGURE 10-3. In many cases, injecting a gas bubble and positioning the patient face down may effect a permanent cure.

pletely closing the hole, many surgeons prefer to approach these cases by performing a pars plana vitrectomy with membrane or hyaloid peeling around the hole, effecting complete intraoperative drainage of the subretinal fluid internally through the hole with an air–fluid exchange, and then fully exchanging the air with a nonexpansile mixture of one of the long-lasting gases (34). This technique may effect a cure even in patients with posterior staphyloma (Fig. 10-4). Nonetheless, some retinas may still redetach, and reoperation with laser photocoagulation to the edges of the hole will be needed (41,61).

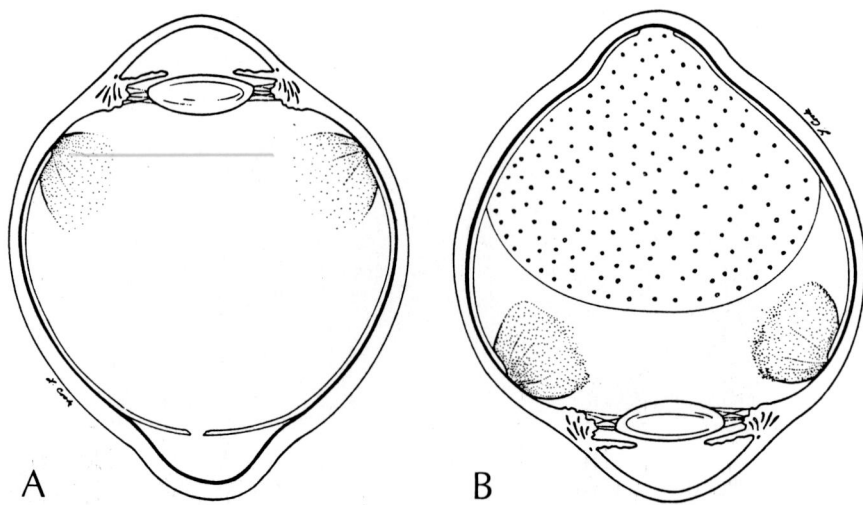

FIGURE 10-4. A: In some cases with a large posterior staphyloma or with posterior vitreous adhesions, a vitrectomy is necessary to allow the placement of a much larger volume of gas. **B:** The patient is positioned to tamponade the break. The macular hole may be sealed in spite of a posterior staphyloma.

GIANT RETINAL TEARS

By definition, giant retinal tears are those tears that are 3 clock hours (90 degrees circumferentially) or larger in size. Some degree of retinal detachment and rolling over of the posterior margin of the break is usually present (Fig. 10-5). Eyes with giant retinal tears have a high risk of developing proliferative vitreoretinopathy (PVR), which can further complicate their management.

Until recently, the techniques available to unroll the retina and keep it in position without slipping posteriorly were relatively difficult and time-consuming. After complete vitreous gel removal, a combination of laborious stroking maneuvers with various instruments and cumbersome patient repositioning during the fluid–air exchange was needed to reattach the retina properly (63). However, with the advent of perfluorocarbon liquids (PFCL) such as perfluorooctane and perfluorophenanthrene in the late 1980s and early 1990s, intraoperative retinal reattachment in cases with giant retinal tears was greatly simplified (7,13,31,45,47,64,87).

As described in the vitrectomy section of chapter 9, the heavier-than-water characteristic of PFCL allows one to steamroller a retina flat in a controlled posterior-to-anterior direction (Fig. 10-6) (68,71). PFCL is instilled over the optic nerve head, and, as it fills the eye, it simultaneously unrolls and reattaches the retina with displacement of the subretinal fluid through the large peripheral retinal opening and all other fluid out the open sclerotomies. One is left with a posterior segment that is nearly completely filled with the PFCL and the retina back in anatomic position. Under PFCL, the tear is then treated with laser photocoagulation, applied with either the endoprobe or the indirect ophthalmoscope delivery system. The PFCL is then completely exchanged with the air, and the air, in turn, is exchanged with either a long-acting gas or silicone oil (7,43,47).

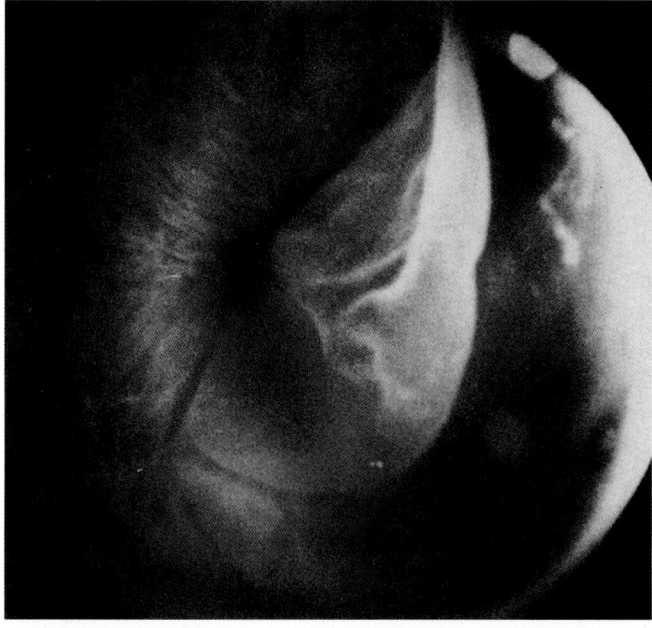

FIGURE 10-5. Giant retinal tear with a rolled-over retina. (Courtesy of L.K. Sarin, M.D.)

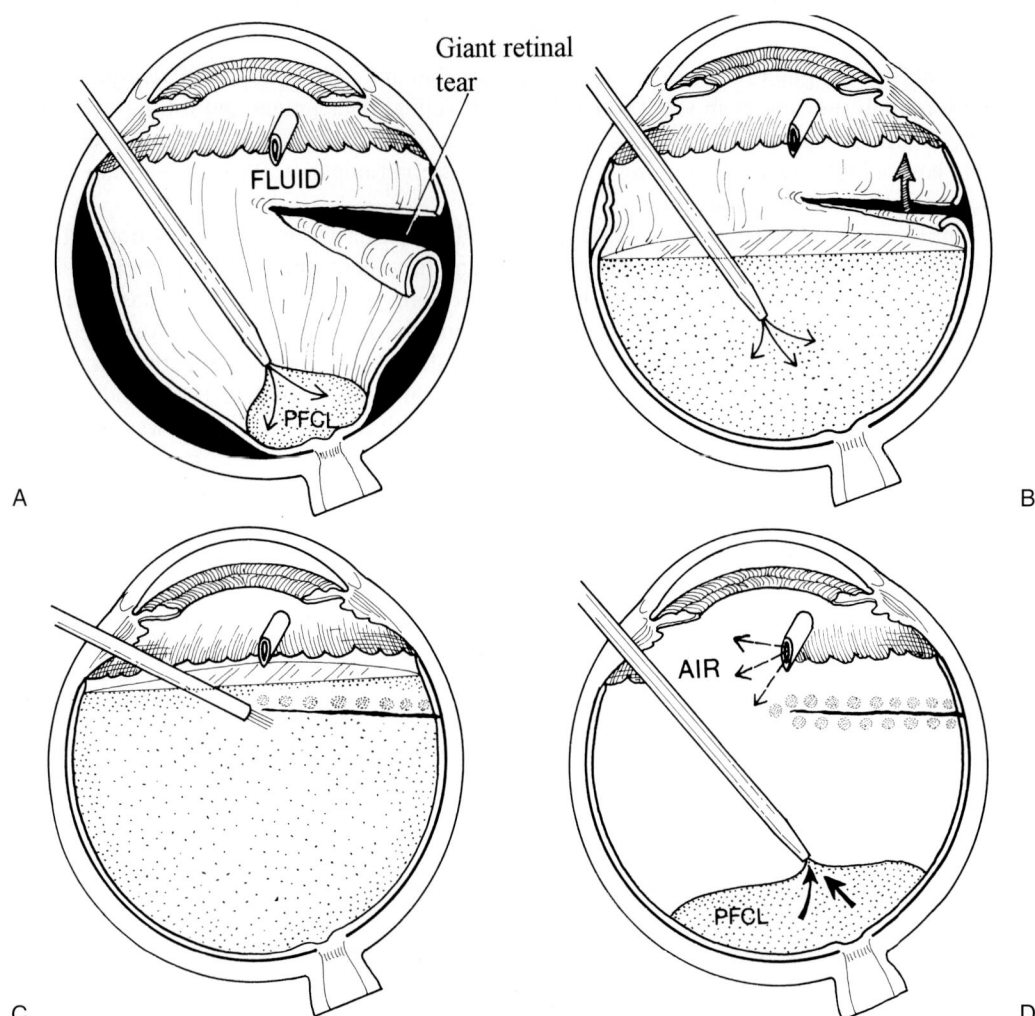

FIGURE 10-6. Giant retinal tear and the use of perfluorocarbon liquid. **A:** After performing a complete vitrectomy, PFCL is slowly instilled over the optic disc. **B:** As the eye is filled with PFCL, the subretinal fluid is displaced out through the tear, and the retina unravels as it reattaches. **C:** Laser photocoagulation is applied around the flattened tear. **D:** An air–fluid exchange is performed, completely filling the eye with air and removing all PFCL.

Because these eyes are at high risk for developing PVR postoperatively, laser is preferred over cryotherapy to treat such large breaks (32). Furthermore, many surgeons also encircle these eyes prophylactically. The native lens often can be preserved if the patient has no significant PVR at the time of surgery (91).

If PVR is seen at the initial presentation, it is particularly important to not only remove any preretinal membranes, but also meticulously to trim the entire vitreous base. If the eye is phakic, the lens probably will need to be removed. It is also best to use a relatively broad scleral buckle with encircling in these cases. Last, many surgeons prefer the use of silicone oil over one of the long-lasting gases when the PVR is significant from the beginning. With these techniques, detachments with giant retinal tears and PVR can be reattached up to 90% of the time, but multiple reoperations may still be necessary to achieve anatomic success (31).

PROLIFERATIVE VITREORETINOPATHY

In advanced cases of PVR, a scleral buckling (SB) procedure alone cannot reattach the retina. As discussed in detail in chapter 2 on retinal detachment pathophysiology, the more severe forms of PVR cause significant inward or anteriorly directed vitreoretinal traction that either keeps retinal breaks open or creates new breaks. Furthermore, the preretinal or subretinal membranes that are typically present stiffen and contract the retina. Together, a relatively immobile retinal detachment results (Fig. 10-7).

The vitrectomy approach allows for direct relief of the various vitreoretinal traction forces. The vitreous cutting–aspirating instrument is used first to remove as much of the vitreous gel as possible, including close shaving of the vitreous base region, as mentioned earlier with giant retinal tears (Fig. 10-8). To mobilize the retina further, various retinal picks and forceps are used to peel away epiretinal (or subretinal) membranes

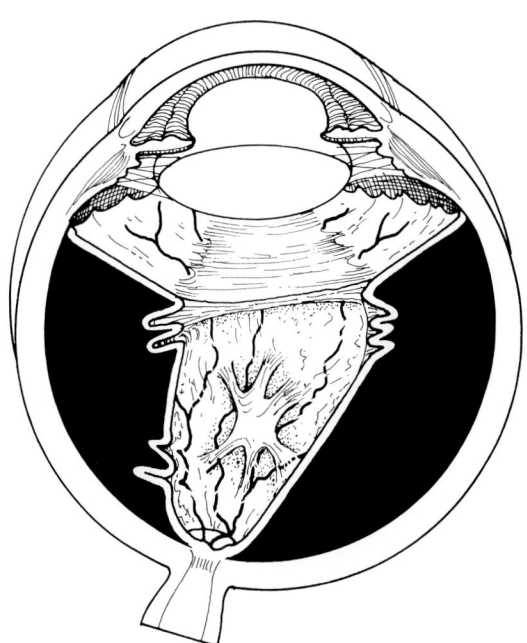

FIGURE 10-7. Total retinal detachment with advanced proliferative vitreoretinopathy. The vitreous gel is pulling the peripheral retina inward and anteriorly. Preretinal membranes are present posteriorly, causing fixed, star-like folds and further stiffening the retina.

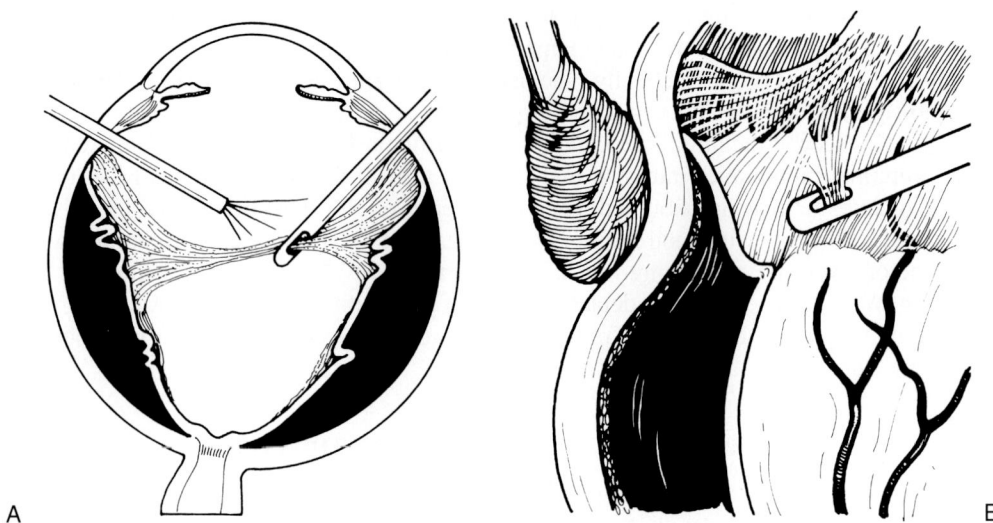

FIGURE 10-8. Pars plana vitrectomy for advanced proliferative vitreoretinopathy. Vitreoretinal traction is relieved by carrying out a complete vitrectomy **(A)**, including trimming the vitreous base **(B)**.

(Fig. 10-9). Sometimes, peripheral ("relaxing") retinotomies are also needed to achieve adequate retinal mobilization and intraoperative reattachment (Fig. 10-10) (53). This is either because preretinal membranes are too adherent to remove without tearing retina or because the retina appears foreshortened despite removal of all visible abnormal vitreoretinal tissue. If significant anterior PVR is present, the lens will need to be removed. Furthermore, a broad encircling element is also used to counter residual or recurrent vitreous base contracture. PFCL is a valuable intraoperative tool in patients with PVR to

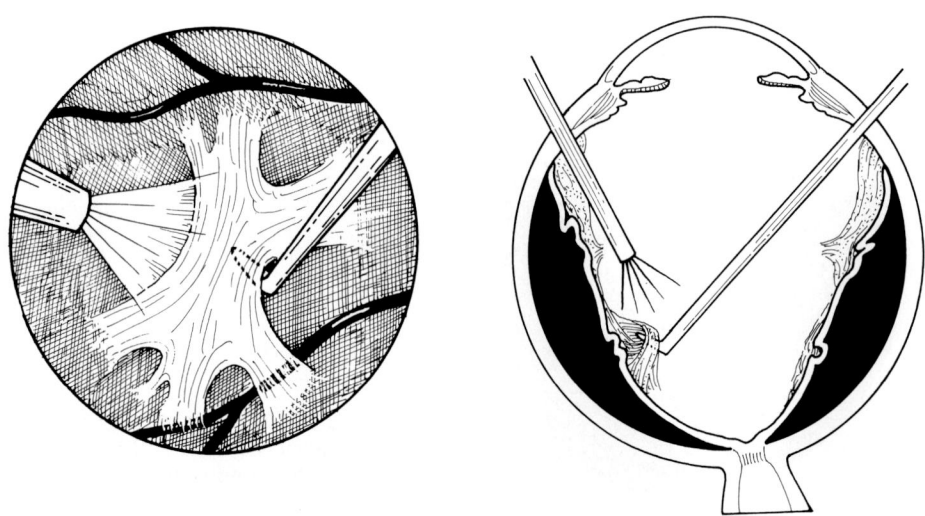

FIGURE 10-9. Preretinal membranes are peeled away from the retina using various retinal picks and forceps.

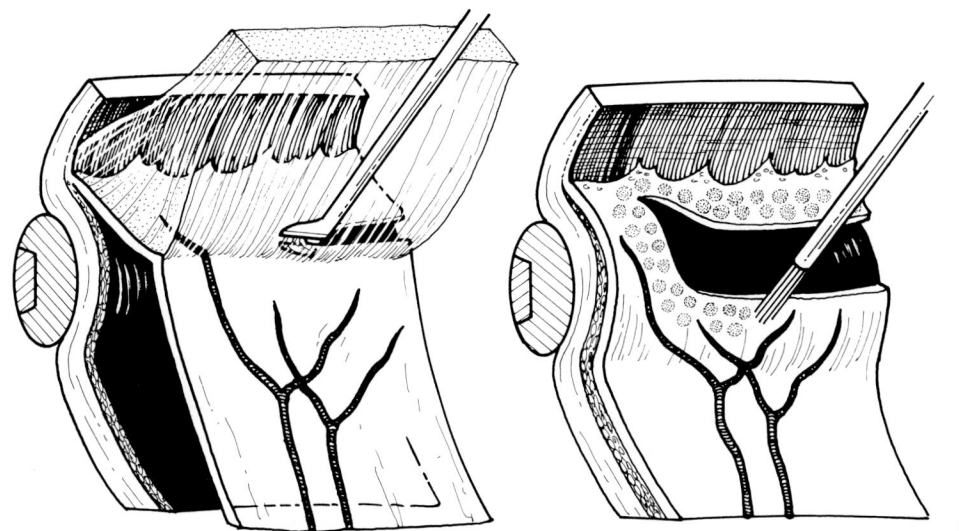

FIGURE 10-10. Relaxing retinotomy. The foreshortened retina is cut peripherally **(A)**. The retina is then able to attach, and the cut edge is sealed with laser photocoagulation **(B)**.

stabilize the retina for better dissection of anteriorly located membranes and to achieve a controlled, intraoperative retinal reattachment while minimizing the amount of retinal cutting (15,17,68,71,85).

A relatively long-lasting, internal tamponade of the retina is needed while waiting for the retinopexy around all the breaks to take hold and the PVR process to abate. C_3F_8 gas and silicone oil are the preferred agents. Other gases can be used, but extremely short-acting ones such as SF_6 have been shown to be less effective in managing severe PVR (83). A nonexpansile mixture of C_3F_8 (14% to 15%) is used and lasts approximately 6 to 8 weeks in the eye (14). Silicone oil lasts indefinitely, and, therefore, its use necessitates another vitrectomy procedure to remove it. This is usually performed 3 to 4 months after the complete retinal reattachment. Either 1,000 centistoke (cs) or 5,000 cs silicone oil is available, but the more viscous (5,000 cs) preparation is preferable to minimize oil-related complications such as emulsification (75,84). The Silicone Study Group has demonstrated that silicone oil and C_3F_8 perform equally well in cases with severe PVR (C3 or more) in terms of achieving retinal attachment and final visual acuity of 5/200 or better (1,82).

Overall, retinal reattachment can be achieved with the above vitrectomy techniques in 61% to 93% of eyes with retinal detachment and varying degrees of PVR (18,19,27,33, 40,49,82,93). The rate of reattachment is inversely correlated with the degree of PVR, and multiple operations are often needed to achieve long-lasting retinal attachment (40,52). More recent studies tend to show better anatomic success rates. This is probably a result of both a better understanding of the disease process and improved instrumentation or techniques, including the availability of PFCL and wide-angle viewing systems (17). Failed procedures are usually the result of recurrent or persistent proliferation, particularly anterior PVR (48,49). Although for most cases, C_3F_8 and silicone oil have comparable anatomic outcomes, patients with severe anterior PVR or hypotony preoperatively may do better with silicone oil (23).

When long-term retinal attachment is achieved in patients with PVR, the rate of obtaining ambulatory visual acuity (e.g., 5/200 or better) can be as high as 88%, although most series report rates in the range of about 60% to 70% (18,27,40,52,82). Patients whose eyes require multiple operations for anatomic success or have persistent hypotony have worse final visual outcomes (17,58). Because the macula is involved with most complicated PVR detachments, the chances of obtaining visual acuity of better than 20/80 is low (17). Subjectively, however, many patients report that the modest improvement in peripheral vision is beneficial, and undergoing multiple procedures is worthwhile (57,90).

Despite recent advances in surgical technique, single-operation failure rates remain relatively high and, in most cases, this is the result of recurrent proliferation. Research has focused on developing pharmacologic treatments to either inhibit proliferation or neutralize a key factor in the process (11). Agents currently being investigated include 5-fluorouracil (6,8), daunomycin (46,70,92), corticosteroids (12), vitamin A and E preparations (26,65), minoxidil derivatives (38), and suramin (22). For drugs that prove useful, it is likely that devices that permit direct intraocular administration in a controlled, sustained-release fashion will need to be used to maximize efficacy and to minimize toxicity.

PENETRATING INJURIES

Patients with penetrating injuries involving the posterior segment have a high risk of developing complicated retinal detachments (21,69). Initially, one often sees some degree of vitreous hemorrhage, choroidal detachment, and direct retinal disruption. Soon after the injury, an exuberant, wound-like healing response occurs with intraocular fibrovascular proliferation that typically starts along the path of the foreign body (see Fig. 3-3). The vitreous fibers act as a scaffold on which the tissue grows (78). The transvitreal membranes that result can contract and cause traction or combined traction–RRDs. Secondary retinal tears are usually seen 90 to 180 degrees from the site of penetration (Fig. 10-11) (3).

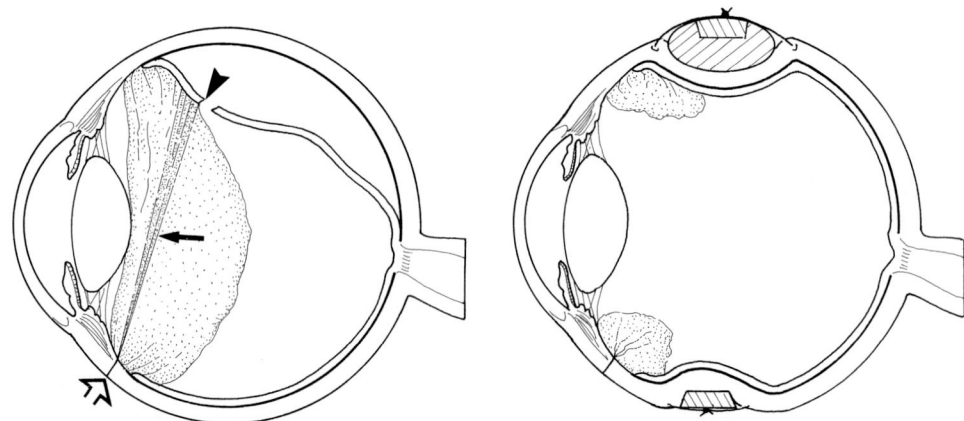

FIGURE 10-11. A: Retinal tear *(arrowhead)* and detachment caused by fibrovascular tissue *(arrow)* proliferating through the entry wound *(open arrow)* of a foreign body. **B:** The fibrous tissue and associated vitreous gel are excised by vitrectomy; the break and vitreous base region are supported by a scleral buckle and an encircling band, respectively.

Vitrectomy is usually necessary to clear the vitreous media and to relieve vitreoretinal traction, and to maximize anatomic success, complete vitreous and membrane removal is advocated (62,78). This may require extensive membrane peeling or dissection and lens removal. Because some degree of vitreous gel remains adherent in the vitreous base region, an encircling SB procedure is also typically performed (see Fig. 10-11) (78). As with patients with PVR, a long-acting gas or silicone oil is often used if retinal detachment is extensive. PFCLs can facilitate intraoperative retinal reattachment (16). Although the exact timing of surgical intervention for posterior segment complications of trauma has always been controversial, most surgeons wait at least 3 to 5 days after the initial injury to allow uveal congestion to diminish and a spontaneous posterior vitreous separation to occur, both of which will make vitrectomy surgery safer and easier (78).

Despite our improved understanding of the pathobiology of ocular trauma and more refined surgical techniques, the visual potential for eyes that sustain severe penetrating trauma remains limited. Although the incidence of enucleation has decreased over the years, the percentage of eyes that achieve ambulatory visual acuity (5/200) or better remains similar at about 60% (69). Factors that adversely influence visual outcome include the initial presence of poor visual acuity, afferent pupillary defect, significant vitreous hemorrhage, large or posterior wound sites, blunt mechanism of injury, and lens involvement (21,69).

PROLIFERATIVE DIABETIC RETINOPATHY

Vitreous traction associated with proliferative diabetic retinopathy usually causes pure traction retinal detachment. Occasionally, a combined traction–rhegmatogenous detachment can occur with the breaks most commonly stretch-like in nature and located near the focus of fibrovascular proliferation (44). With either type of detachment, if the macula is directly involved or is threatened to become involved, vitrectomy is indicated to preserve vision.

These cases have anteroposterior traction on the retina from the vitreous gel that remains adherent to and pulls on the areas of retinal fibrovascular proliferation. Furthermore, one also typically sees some degree of tangential retinal traction from contraction of the fibrovascular foci. To restore the retinal anatomy best, both traction forces need to be relieved (Fig. 10-12). The anteroposterior traction is released by excising formed gel with the standard vitrectomy handpiece. The tangential traction is approached next and is rectified by either cutting the bridges of fibrovascular tissue that connect individual foci of neovascularization ("segmentation") or dissecting the tissue completely off the surface of the retina ("delamination"). Addressing this tangential traction is what can make these cases so challenging because this is when intraoperative retinal tears and bleeding are typically encountered. Intraocular gas tamponade is not used in patients with diabetic vitrectomy unless retinal tears are present. When both retinal tears and PVR are present, long-acting gases or even silicone oil may be indicated (9,76,93).

In diabetic traction retinal detachments, reattachment of the macula is the primary objective, and this can be obtained in 65% to 80% of cases (42,86). Improvement in visual acuity ranges in reports from 26% to 65% (42,86). The prognosis for recovery of useful vision is worst in cases with chronic macular detachments (more than 6 months' duration), extensive retinal detachment, severe fibrovascular proliferation, vitreous hemorrhage, and lack of any preoperative panretinal photocoagulation (42).

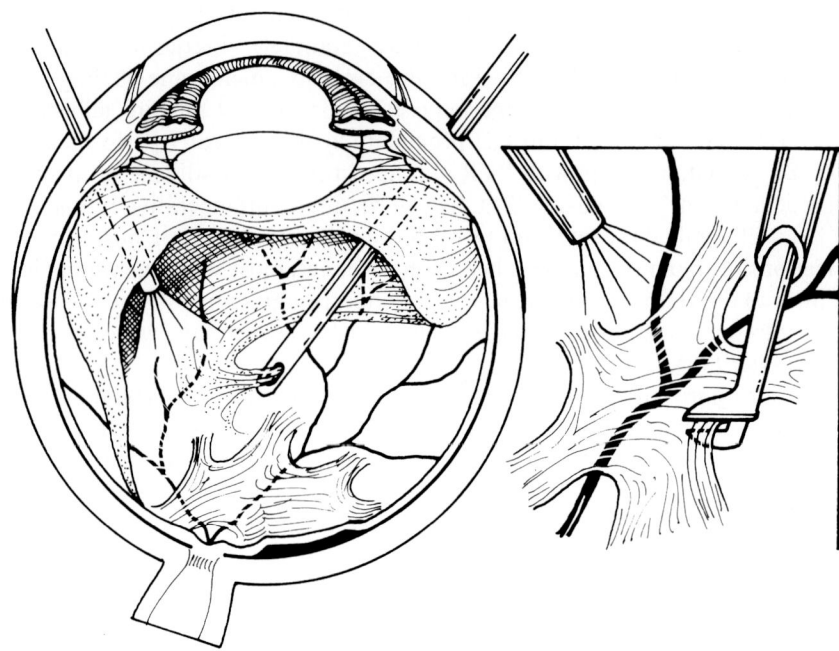

FIGURE 10-12. Proliferative diabetic retinopathy and traction retinal detachment. The anteroposterior traction is first addressed by trimming away the vitreous gel from the posterior fibrovascular membranes. Tangential traction is then relieved by segmenting **(inset)** or delaminating the adherent preretinal tissue.

RETINITIS-RELATED RETINAL DETACHMENTS

Necrotizing infections of the retina can result in retinal breaks and RRD. This is most commonly encountered in patients who are infected with the human immunodeficiency virus (HIV) and have cytomegalovirus retinitis (CMV) (81). Other herpes family viruses such as varicella-zoster and herpes simplex can also cause retinitis, producing the clinical picture of acute retinal necrosis (ARN), regardless of the immune status of the affected individual (25,74). Rarely, parasitic (e.g., toxoplasmosis) and bacterial infections that involve the posterior segment can also lead to retinal breaks and detachments (81).

Especially when the area of retinitis has been extensive, multiple and often posteriorly located holes are typically encountered (28). Furthermore, the involved retina is atrophic and friable, so finding the breaks and obtaining a good chorioretinal adhesion to the underlying RPE with laser or cryotherapy is difficult. Because of these characteristics, cases originally approached with SB or vitrectomy with temporary gas tamponade not uncommonly failed. With the HIV epidemic, a sharp rise in retinitis-related detachments was seen in the late 1980s and early 1990s, and it soon became apparent that primary vitrectomy with permanent silicone oil tamponade was needed to maximize long-term success in these cases (24,30,50,74). In patients who are HIV positive, PVR is not often a complicating feature, and, therefore, the surgical procedure does not need to be combined with any SB (30,66,74).

RETINOSCHISIS-RELATED RETINAL DETACHMENTS

Rhegmatogenous retinal detachments can come about from holes in the walls of schisis cavities associated with either X-linked ("juvenile") retinoschisis or degenerative ("senile") retinoschisis. Although the underlying conditions are different, when they result in retinal detachment, they both may be associated with schisis-related breaks that are multiple, posterior, and difficult to find. These features make successful reattachment difficult with standard first-line approaches such as SB, PR, or temporary balloon buckling. Therefore, vitrectomy with internal drainage of subretinal fluid and gas tamponade sometimes may be needed. Because the cortical vitreous is frequently adherent to the inner layer of the schisis cavity in both conditions, inner layer retinectomy may be needed in some cases to facilitate retinal reattachment, particularly in the juvenile form of retinoschisis (72,73,89).

MISCELLANEOUS CONDITIONS

Colobomas

Colobomas of the choroid are congenital defects that result from faulty closure of the embryonal fissure. Although the defect is rare, it may lead to RRD in about 20% to 40% of affected persons at some point in their lifetimes (10). The detachments typically result from one or more breaks in the intercalary membrane, the thin, glial sheet over the coloboma that is continuous with the neurosensory retina (10,35,79).

Without the RPE and choroid to provide good contrast, the breaks are difficult to visualize. The breaks may also be multiple and relatively posterior in location. For these reasons, vitrectomy with internal drainage of the subretinal fluid and internal tamponade is usually needed to reattach the retina. Also of note with these cases is that a firm chorioretinal adhesion directly around the break with either cryotherapy or laser photocoagulation cannot be achieved. Therefore, the colobomatous defect has to be "isolated" from the rest of the retina by applying laser along the entire border of the coloboma (36,59). Alternatively, cyanoacrylate glue can be used to seal the breaks directly (39).

Pediatric Proliferative Diseases

Retinopathy of prematurity (ROP) and familial exudative vitreoretinopathy (FEV) are similar in that both conditions potentially can result in peripheral fibrovascular proliferation and secondary traction or combined traction–RRDs at a young age (2). Incontinentia pigmenti is another disease of early childhood that can have a similar presentation.

Because the traction on the retina in these conditions is peripherally located, the associated retinal detachments are often approachable with SB. However, if fibrous proliferation is extensive and severe traction draws the retina inward, vitrectomy techniques are usually used either alone or in combination with SB (60). A two-port, lens-sparing vitrectomy technique may be preferred when the proliferation and detachment are not advanced (54), but when the detachment assumes a narrow or closed-funnel configuration and there is extensive retrolental fibrous tissue, a more complete vitrectomy (closed or open-sky) with lensectomy is needed (20,60).

Of these conditions, the most experience with retinal detachment surgery has been with ROP. In selected cases, successful retinal reattachment with SB can be obtained in 40% to 70% of cases, being on the higher side with subtotal (stage 4A or 4B) detachments and on the lower side with total (stage 5) detachments (37,67,88). Reattachment results range from 35% to 60% in more advanced stage 5 disease approached by various vitrectomy techniques, with most series reporting a success rate averaging around 40% (29,60). Unfortunately, even when the retina is successfully attached, visual results are often disappointing (29,67,80).

REFERENCES

1. Abrams GW, Azen SP, McCuen BW, et al. Vitrectomy with silicone oil or long-acting gas in eyes with severe proliferative vitreoretinopathy: results of additional and long-term follow-up: Silicone Study Report 11. *Arch Ophthalmol* 1997;17:335–344.
2. Benson WE. Familial exudative vitreoretinopathy. *Trans Am Ophthalmol Soc* 1995;93:473–521.
3. Benson WE, Machemer R. Severe penetrating injuries treated with pars plana vitrectomy. *Am J Ophthalmol* 1976;81:728–732.
4. Blankenship GW, Ibanez-Langlois S. Treatment of myopic macular hole and detachment: intravitreal gas exchange. *Ophthalmology* 1987;94:333–336.
5. Blodi CF, Folk JC. Treatment of macular hole retinal detachments with intravitreal gas. *Am J Ophthalmol* 1984;98:811.
6. Blumenkrantz M, Hernandez E, Ophir A, et al. 5-Fluorouracil: new applications in complicated retinal detachment for an established antimetabolite. *Ophthalmology* 1984;91:122–129.
7. Boker T, Schmitt C, Mougharbel M. Results and prognostic factors in pneumatic retinopexy. *Ger J Ophthalmol* 1994;3:73–78.
8. Borhani H, Peyman GA, Rahimy MH, Thompson H. Suppression of experimental proliferative vitreoretinopathy by sustained intraocular delivery of 5-FU. *Int Ophthalmol* 1995;19:43–49.
9. Brourman ND, Blumenkranz MS, Cox MS, Trese MT. Silicone oil for the treatment of severe proliferative diabetic retinopathy. *Ophthalmology* 1989;96:759–764.
10. Brown GC, Tasman WS. *Congenital Anomalies of the Optic Disc.* New York: Grune & Stratton, 1983:141–157.
11. Campochiaro PA. Pathogenic mechanisms in proliferative vitreoretinopathy. *Arch Ophthalmol* 1997;115:237–241.
12. Chandler DB, Rozakis G, de Juan E Jr, Machemer R. The effect of triamcinolone acetonide on a refined experimental model of proliferative vitreoretinopathy. *Am J Ophthalmol* 1985;99:686–690.
13. Chang S. Low viscosity liquid fluorochemicals in vitreous surgery. *Am J Ophthalmol* 1987;103:38–43.
14. Chang S, Lincoff HA, Coleman DJ, Fuchs W, Farber ME. Perfluorocarbon gases in vitreous surgery. *Ophthalmology* 1985;92:651–656.
15. Chang S, Ozmert E, Zimmerman NJ. Intraoperative perfluorocarbon liquids in the management of proliferative vitreoretinopathy. *Am J Ophthalmol* 1988;106:668–674.
16. Chang S, Reppucci V, Zimmerman NJ, Heinemann MH, Coleman DJ. Perfluorocarbon liquids in the management of traumatic retinal detachments. *Ophthalmology* 1989;96:785–791 [discussion 791–792].
17. Coll GE, Chang S, Sun J, Wieland MR, Berrocal MH. Perfluorocarbon liquid in the management of retinal detachment with proliferative vitreoretinopathy. *Ophthalmology* 1995;102:630–638 [discussion 638–639].
18. Cox MS, Trese MT, Murphy PL. Silicone oil for advanced proliferative vitreoretinopathy. *Ophthalmology* 1986;93:646–650.
19. de Bustros S, Michels RG. Surgical treatment of retinal detachments complicated by proliferative vitreoretinopathy. *Am J Ophthalmol* 1984;98:694–699.
20. de Juan E, Machemer R. Retinopathy of prematurity: surgical technique. *Retina* 1987;7:53–69.
21. de Juan E, Sternberg P, Michels RG. Penetrating ocular injuries: types of injuries and visual results. *Ophthalmology* 1983;90:1318–1322.
22. de Souza OF, Sakamoto T, Kimura H, et al. Inhibition of experimental proliferative vitreoretinopathy in rabbits by suramin. *Ophthalmologica* 1995;209:212–216.
23. Diddie KR, Azen SP, Freeman HM, et al. Anterior proliferative vitreoretinopathy in the silicone study: Silicone Study Report Number 10. *Ophthalmology* 1996;103:1092–1099.
24. Dugel PU, Liggett PE, Lee MB, et al. Repair of retinal detachment caused by cytomegalovirus retinitis in patients with the acquired immunodeficiency syndrome. *Am J Ophthalmol* 1991;112:235–242.
25. Duker JS, Blumenkranz MS. Diagnosis and management of the acute retinal necrosis (ARN) syndrome. *Surv Ophthalmol* 1991;35:327–343.
26. Fekrat S, de Juan E Jr, Campochiaro PA. The effect of oral 13-cis-retinoic acid on retinal redetachment after surgical repair in eyes with proliferative vitreoretinopathy. *Ophthalmology* 1995;102:412–418.
27. Fisher YL, Shakin JL, Slakter JS, Sorenson JA, Shafer DM. Perfluoropropane gas, modified panretinal photocoagulation, and vitrectomy in the management of severe proliferative vitreoretinopathy. *Arch Ophthalmol* 1988;106:1255–1260.
28. Freeman WR, Friedberg DN, Berry C, et al. Risk factors for development of rhegmatogenous retinal detachment in patients with cytomegalovirus retinitis. *Am J Ophthalmol* 1993;116:713–720.

29. Fuchino Y, Hayashi H, Kono T, Ohshima K. Long–term follow-up of visual acuity in eyes with stage 5 retinopathy of prematurity after closed vitrectomy. *Am J Ophthalmol* 1995;120:308–316.
30. Garcia RF, Flores-Aguilar M, Quiceno JI, et al. Results of rhegmatogenous retinal detachment repair in cytomegalovirus retinitis with and without scleral buckling. *Ophthalmology* 1995;102:236–245.
31. Glaser BM, Carter JB, Kuppermann BD, Michels RG. Perfluoro-octane in the treatment of giant retinal tears with proliferative vitreoretinopathy. *Ophthalmology* 1991;98:1613–1621.
32. Glaser BM, Vidaurri-Leal J, Michels RG, Campochiaro PA. Cryotherapy during surgery for giant retinal tears and intravitreal dispersion of viable retinal pigment epithelial cells. *Ophthalmology* 1993;100:466–470.
33. Gonvers M. Temporary silicone oil tamponade in the management of retinal detachment with proliferative vitreoretinopathy. *Am J Ophthalmol* 1985;100:239–245.
34. Gonvers M, Machemer R. A new approach to treating retinal detachment with macular hole. *Am J Ophthalmol* 1982;94:468–472.
35. Gopal L, Badrinath SS, Sharma T, Parikh SN, Biswas J. Pattern of retinal breaks and retinal detachments in eyes with choroidal coloboma. *Ophthalmology* 1995;102:1212–1217.
36. Gopal L, Kini MM, Badrinath SS, Sharma T. Management of retinal detachment with choroidal coloboma. *Ophthalmology* 1991;98:1622–1627.
37. Greven C, Tasman W. Scleral buckling in stages 4B and 5 retinopathy of prematurity. *Ophthalmology* 1990;97:817–820.
38. Handa JT, Murad S, Jaffe GJ. Inhibition of cultured human RPE cell proliferation and lysyl hydroxylase activity by hydroxy derivatives of minoxidil. *Invest Ophthalmol Vis Sci* 1994;35:463–469.
39. Hanneken AM, de Juan E Jr, McCuen BWD. The management of retinal detachments associated with choroidal colobomas by vitreous surgery. *Am J Ophthalmol* 1991;111:271–275.
40. Hanneken AM, Michels RG. Vitrectomy and scleral buckling methods for proliferative vitreoretinopathy. *Ophthalmology* 1988;95:865–869.
41. Harris MJ, de Bustros S, Michels RG. Treatment of retinal detachments due to macular holes. *Retina* 1984;4:144–147.
42. Ho T, Smiddy WE, Flynn HW Jr. Vitrectomy in the management of diabetic eye disease. *Surv Ophthalmol* 1992;37:190–202.
43. Ie D, Glaser BM, Sjaarda RN, Thompson JT, Steinberg LE, Gordon LW. The use of perfluoro-octane in the management of giant retinal tears without proliferative vitreoretinopathy. *Retina* 1994;14:323–328.
44. Kakehashi A, Trempe CL, Fujio N, McMeel JW, Schepens CL. Retinal breaks in diabetic retinopathy: vitreoretinal relationships. *Ophthalmic Surg* 1994;25:695–699.
45. Kertes PJ, Wafapoor H, Peyman GA, et al. The management of giant retinal tears using perfluoroperhydrophenanthrene. *Ophthalmology* 1997;104:1159–1165.
46. Khawly JA, Saloupis P, Hatchell DL, Machemer R. Daunorubicin treatment in a refined experimental model of proliferative vitreoretinopathy. *Graefes Arch Clin Exp Ophthalmol* 1991;229:464–467.
47. Kreiger AE, Lewis H. Management of giant retinal tears without scleral buckling. Use of radical dissection of the vitreous base and perfluoro-octane and intraocular tamponade. *Ophthalmology* 1992;99:491–497.
48. Lewis H, Aaberg TM. Causes of failure after repeat vitreoretinal surgery for recurrent proliferative vitreoretinopathy. *Am J Ophthalmol* 1991;111:15–19.
49. Lewis H, Aaberg TM, Abrams GW. Causes of failure after initial vitreoretinal surgery for severe proliferative vitreoretinopathy. *Am J Ophthalmol* 1991;111:8–14.
50. Lim JI, Enger C, Haller JA, et al. Improved visual results after surgical repair of cytomegalovirus-related retinal detachments. *Ophthalmology* 1994;101:264–269.
51. Lincoff H, Kreissig I, Brodie S, Wilcox L. Expanding gas bubbles for the repair of tears in the posterior pole. *Graefes Arch Clin Exp Ophthalmol* 1982;219:193–197.
52. Lopez R, Chang S. Long-term results of vitrectomy and perfluorocarbon gas for the treatment of severe proliferative vitreoretinopathy. *Am J Ophthalmol* 1992;113:424–428.
53. Machemer R, McCuen BW, de Juan E. Relaxing retinotomies and retinectomies. *Am J Ophthalmol* 1986;102:7–12.
54. Maguire AM, Trese MT. Lens-sparing vitreoretinal surgery in infants. *Arch Ophthalmol* 1992;110:284–286.
55. Margherio RR, Schepens CL. Macular breaks. 1. Diagnosis, etiology, and observations. *Am J Ophthalmol* 1972;74:219–232.
56. Matsumura M, Kuriyama S, Harada T, Ishigooka H, Ogino N. Surgical techniques and visual prognosis in retinal detachment due to macular hole. *Ophthalmologica* 1992;204:122–133.
57. McCormack P, Simcock PR, Charteris D, Lavin MJ. Is surgery for proliferative vitreoretinopathy justifiable? *Eye* 1994;8:75–78.
58. McCuen BWd, Azen SP, Stern W, et al. Vitrectomy with silicone oil or perfluoropropane gas in eyes with severe proliferative vitreoretinopathy. Silicone Study Report 3. *Retina* 1993;13:279–284.
59. McDonald HR, Lewis H, Brown G, Sipperley JO. Vitreous surgery for retinal detachment associated with choroidal coloboma. *Arch Ophthalmol* 1991;109:1399–402.
60. McNamara JA. Treatment of advanced stages of retinopathy of premaurity. In: Tasman W, Jaeger AE, eds. *Duane's Clinical Ophthalmology*. Philadelphia: Lippincott–Raven, 1993:1–15.
61. Mester U, Kroll P, Volker B, Kreissig I. Intraocular SF6 gas applications: treatment of retinal detachments caused by holes at the posterior pole. *Ophthalmologica* 1983;186:151–155.

62. Michels RG. Vitrectomy methods in penetrating ocular trauma. *Ophthalmology* 1980;87:629–645.
63. Michels RG, Rice TA, Blankenship G. Surgical techniques for selected giant retinal tears. *Retina* 1983;3:139.
64. Millsap CM, Peyman GA, Mehta NJ, et al. Perfluoroperhydrophenanthrene (Vitreon) in the management of giant retinal tears: results of a collaborative study. *Ophthalmic Surg* 1993;24:759–763.
65. Mojon D, Boscoboinik D, Haas A, Bohnke M, Azzi A. Vitamin E inhibits retinal pigment epithelium cell proliferation in vitro. *Ophthalmic Res* 1994;26:304–309.
66. Nasemann JE, Mutsch A, Wiltfang R, Klauss V. Early pars plana vitrectomy without buckling procedure in cytomegalovirus retinitis-induced retinal detachment. *Retina* 1995;15:111–116.
67. Noorily SW, Small K, de Juan R Jr, Machemer R. Scleral buckling for stage 4B retinopathy of prematurity. *Ophthalmology* 1992;99:263–268.
68. Peyman GA, Schulman JA, Sullivan B. Perfluorocarbon liquids in *Surv Ophthalmol* 1995;39:375–395.
69. Pieramici DJ, MacCumber MW, Humayan MU, Marsh MJ, de Juan E Jr. Open-globe injury: update on types of injuries and visual results. *Ophthalmology* 1996;103:1798–1803.
70. Rahimy MH, Peyman GA, Fernandes ML, el-Sayed SH, Luo Q, Borhani H. Effects of an intravitreal daunomycin implant on experimental proliferative vitreoretinopathy: simultaneous pharmacokinetic and pharmacodynamic evaluations. *J Ocular Pharmacol* 1994;10:561–570.
71. Regillo CD, Brown DC. Perfluorocarbon liquids and vitreous surgery. *Ophthalmic Pract* 1994;12:236–241.
72. Regillo CD, Custis PH. Surgical management of retinoschisis. *Curr Opin Ophthalmol* 1997;8:80–86.
73. Regillo CD, Tasman WS, Brown GC. Surgical management of complications associated with X-linked retinoschisis. *Arch Ophthalmol* 1993;111:1080–1086.
74. Regillo CD, Vander JF, Duker JS, Fischer DH, Belmont JB, Kleiner R. Repair of retinitis-related retinal detachments with silicone oil in patients with acquired immunodeficiency syndrome. *Am J Ophthalmol* 1992;113:21–27.
75. Riedel KG, Gabel VP, Neubauer L, Kampik A, Lund OE. Intravitreal silicone oil injection: complications and treatment of 415 consecutive patients. *Graefes Arch Clin Exp Ophthalmol* 1990;228:19–23.
76. Rinkoff JS, de Juan E Jr, McCuen BWD. Silicone oil for retinal detachment with advanced proliferative vitreoretinopathy following failed vitrectomy for proliferative diabetic retinopathy. *Am J Ophthalmol* 1986;101:181–186.
77. Riordan-Eva P, Chignell AH. Full thickness macular breaks in rhegmatogenous retinal detachment with peripheral retinal breaks. *Br J Ophthalmol* 1992;76:346–348.
78. Ryan SJ. Traction retinal detachment: XLIX Edward Jackson Memorial Lecture. *Am J Ophthalmol* 1993;115:1–20.
79. Schubert HD. Schisis-like rhegmatogenous retinal detachment associated with choroidal colobomas. *Graefes Arch Clin Exp Ophthalmol* 1995;233:74–79.
80. Seaber JH, Machemer R, Eliott D, et al. Long-term, visual results of children after initially successful vitrectomy for stage V retinopathy of prematurity. *Ophthalmology* 1995;102:199–204.
81. Sidikaro Y, Silver L, Holland GN, Kreiger AE. Rhegmatogenous retinal detachments in patients with AIDS and necrotizing retinal infections. *Ophthalmology* 1991;98:129–135.
82. Silicone Study Group. Vitrectomy with silicone oil or perfluoropropane gas in eyes with severe proliferative vitreoretinopathy: results of a randomized clinical trial. Silicone Study Report 2. *Arch Ophthalmol* 1992;110:780–792.
83. Silicone Study Group. Vitrectomy with silicone oil or sulfur hexafluoride gas in eyes with severe proliferative vitreoretinopathy: results of a randomized clinical trial. Silicone Study Report 1. *Arch Ophthalmol* 1992;110:770–779.
84. Snead MP. Ocular therapy with silicone oils. *Curr Opin Ophthalmol* 1993;4:36–43.
85. Stolba U, Binder S, Velikay M, Datlinger P, Wedrich A. Use of perfluorocarbon liquids in proliferative vitreoretinopathy: results and complications. *Br J Ophthalmol* 1995;79:1106–1110.
86. Thompson JT, de Bustros S, Michels RG, Rice TA. Results and prognostic factors in vitrectomy for diabetic traction-rhegmatogenous retinal detachment. Archives of *Ophthalmology* 1987;105:503–507.
87. Tornambe PE, Hilton GF. Office repair of retinal detachment [Letter]. *Ophthalmology* 1997;104:1059–1060.
88. Trese MT. Scleral buckling for retinopathy of prematurity. *Ophthalmology* 1994;101:23–26.
89. Trese MT, Ferrone PJ. The role of inner layer retinectomy in the management of juvenile retinoschisis. *Graefes Arch Clin Exp Ophthalmol* 1995;233:706–708.
90. van Meurs JC, Mertens DA, Peperkamp E, Post J. Five-year results of vitrectomy and silicone oil in patients with proliferative vitreoretinopathy. *Retina* 1993;13:285–289.
91. Verstraeten T, Williams GA, Chang S, et al. Lens-sparing vitrectomy with perfluorocarbon liquid for the primary treatment of giant retinal tears. *Ophthalmology* 1995;102:17–20.
92. Wiedemann P, Leinung C, Hilgers RD, Heimann K. Daunomycin and silicone oil for the treatment of proliferative vitreoretinopathy. *Graefes Arch Clin Exp Ophthalmol* 1991;229:150–152.
93. Yeo JH, Glaser BM, Michels RG. Silicone oil in the treatment of complicated retinal detachments. *Ophthalmology* 1987;94:1109–1113.

11

Postoperative Complications of Primary Retinal Detachment Repair

SCLERAL BUCKLING: EARLY COMPLICATIONS

Elevated Intraocular Pressure

Compression of veins draining the ciliary body by scleral buckling (SB) causes sufficient congestion and forward displacement of the ciliary body to close the filtration angle in up to 7% of cases (8,71,73). This situation is more commonly seen in hyperopic and aphakic eyes. Predisposing operative factors include a tight encircling band, obstruction of multiple vortex veins, and excessive cryotherapy.

The intraocular pressure elevation can be as high as 50 mm Hg and can result in pain and corneal edema. On slit-lamp biomicroscopy, the anterior chamber depth centrally is often normal, but gonioscopy confirms the diagnosis by showing the angle to be closed. Significant choroidal detachments may or may not be present. Intraocular pressure elevation from this mechanism must be distinguished from other causes such as postoperative inflammation, steroid response, pupillary block glaucoma, and, rarely, intraocular gas expansion.

Treatment for anterior ciliary body rotation-induced angle closure is directed at deepening the anterior chamber with cycloplegics and lowering the intraocular pressure with aqueous suppressants such as acetazolamide and beta blockers. Frequent applications of topical corticosteroids should also be used to help to prevent peripheral anterior synechiae.

The prognosis is generally good; most cases gradually resolve. Rarely, it may be necessary to remove or loosen the encircling element or, if present, to drain choroidal detachments and reform the anterior chamber.

Infection

Buckling elements can become infected at any time in the postoperative course. Early infections are probably the result of bacteria introduced at the time of surgery. Late infections are likely caused by bacteria entering through an erosion of the overlying conjunctiva (see later, on buckle exposure and extrusion.) The infections may remain localized, or they may spread to cause orbital cellulitis or, rarely, endophthalmitis. Although silicone sponges are more likely to become exposed late in the postoperative course (see later), early infection rates are probably comparable to those of solid silicone elements.

The incidence of *buckle infections* is around 1% to 3%, and the most common affecting organism is *Staphylococcus* (3,44,53,93,105). New or increased pain after surgery is usually one of the most important indicators of early infection. Other signs are marked chemosis and injection of the conjunctiva (Fig. 11-1). Mucopurulent discharge follows. Tenderness in the region of the buckle is frequently present. Some patients have significant anterior chamber cells. A localized subretinal exudate over a scleral buckle is a particularly ominous sign, because it may indicate early scleral necrosis, a setup for endophthalmitis.

The infection cannot be cured by topical or intravenous antibiotics alone; the explant must also be removed. If the infection is localized to the buckle, these interventions will nearly always result in a cure. Sometimes, virulent organisms such as *Pseudomonas* quickly begin to cause scleral necrosis, and debridement of the eyewall intraoperatively may also be necessary to help eradicate the infection. Experimental (26) and clinical (3,50) studies have shown that soaking sponge explants in antibiotic solution before suturing them to the sclera decreases the incidence of both early and late postoperative infections.

Removing a scleral buckle, regardless of the indication, can result in retinal redetachment; the reported incidence varies from 0% to 35% (23,36,43,53,54,85,102). Retinas that are most likely to redetach are those with significant vitreous traction on the tear, recent SB (i.e., less than 1 month) and infected buckles (85). If the retina does redetach, a reoperation can be performed 1 week after removal of the buckle, by which time the orbit will have resterilized itself.

Endophthalmitis from SB is rare (4). As mentioned earlier, it may be secondary to a buckle infection, or it may be the result of bacteria introduced directly into the eye during the surgical procedure from one of the more invasive steps such as drainage of subretinal fluid (SRF). The presence of a hypopyon or marked vitritis after SB indicates endophthalmitis until proven otherwise. As in other types of postoperative endophthalmitis, prompt intravitreal antibiotics and maybe also vitrectomy surgery are needed.

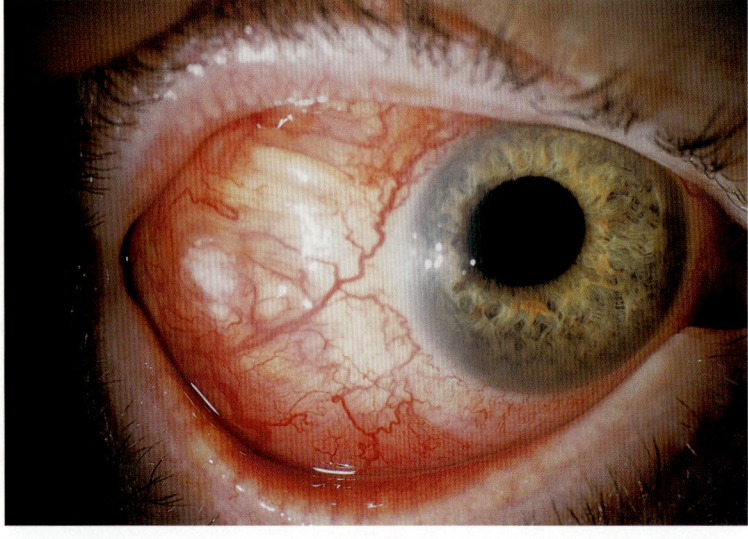

FIGURE 11-1. Infected scleral buckle with conjunctival injection, chemosis, and localized mucopurulent discharge.

Anterior Segment Ischemia

Scleral buckling procedures have the potential to compromise blood flow to or from the anterior segment and result in anterior segment ischemia. Although postmortem studies show some evidence of anterior segment necrosis in 8% of eyes that had undergone SB, clinically apparent changes are rare (104). With current techniques, anterior segment ischemia is only likely to be encountered in eyes that have been encircled or are at risk for microvascular insufficiency, such as in patients with sickle cell anemia (24,25,27,38,67,78,82,109). Extremely large, posteriorly located buckles may also contribute to compromised ocular blood flow by occluding multiple vortex veins. Intraoperative disinsertion of multiple recti muscles is another predisposing factor, but this is rarely, if ever, needed with SB (39,103).

In severe cases, the earliest finding is striate keratopathy. Later, one sees corneal stromal edema without elevated intraocular pressure. Many patients have marked chemosis, anterior chamber reaction, and some degree of eye ache. Large keratic precipitates also may be present. White flakes floating in the anterior chamber or deposited on the lens are diagnostic of the condition. Late findings are hypotony from atrophy of the ciliary processes, irregularly dilated pupil, sector iris atrophy, posterior synechiae, and cataract (Fig. 11-2). Histopathologically, one sees necrosis of the iris and ciliary body, thrombosis of the major arterial circle of the iris, and necrosis of the choroid under the buckle (27). If anterior segment necrosis is suspected, the patient should be treated with high doses of topical and systemic corticosteroids, and the encircling band, if present, should be loosened.

Ciliary Body and Iris Abnormalities

In addition to dysfunction caused by impaired circulation, cryotherapy, diathermy, and photocoagulation all can independently damage the ciliary nerves, resulting in multiple abnormalities in both the parasympathetic and the sympathetic innervation of the pupil (55,64). A picture similar to Adie's syndrome may be seen with chronic dilation, hypersensitivity to $1/8$% pilocarpine, light-near dissociation, and sector iris sphincter palsy. Ciliary nerve dysfunction also may cause a decrease in accommodation up to 7 diopters. Fortunately, full recovery usually occurs by 5 weeks (51).

Choroidal Detachments

Serous choroidal detachments are relatively common after retinal detachment surgery, especially in elderly or aphakic patients (69). They also tend to be seen in patients who have broad or posteriorly located buckles that compress multiple vortex veins and in patients who have undergone reoperations. Prolonged hypotony after drainage of SRF is believed to be a contributing factor, although choroidal detachments have also been reported after nondrainage procedures (17).

The suprachoroidal fluid characteristically accumulates during the first 3 to 4 days after surgery and then remains stable for 1 to 2 weeks. Because of decreased aqueous secretion, the intraocular pressure remains low despite apparent occlusion of the filtration angle. Some degree of associated exudative retinal detachment overlying or adjacent to large choroidal detachments is not unusual; this must not be misinterpreted as a new or recurrent rhegmatogenous detachment (see later).

Specific treatment such as systemic steroids or surgical drainage is rarely indicated. In almost all cases, these detachments spontaneously reabsorb and do not affect the final sur-

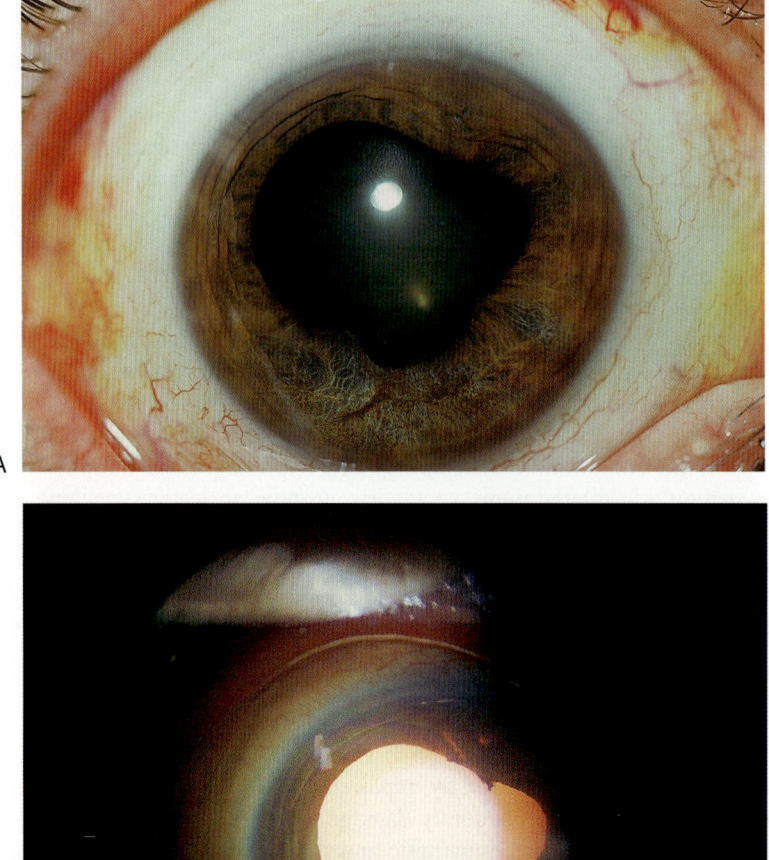

FIGURE 11-2. A: Iris atrophy and posterior synechiae after moderately severe anterior segment necrosis. **B**: Transillumination defects in the inferior half of the atrophic iris.

gical success rate. Even if the detachments are extremely large and meet in the center of the vitreous cavity, intervention is not needed in most cases; the retinal surfaces do not usually remain adherent to each other when these so-called "kissing choroidals" start to recede.

Pigment Fallout

Cryotherapy shatters pigment epithelial cells, releasing pigment into the subretinal space. The pigment accumulates in the most dependent part of the retinal detachment

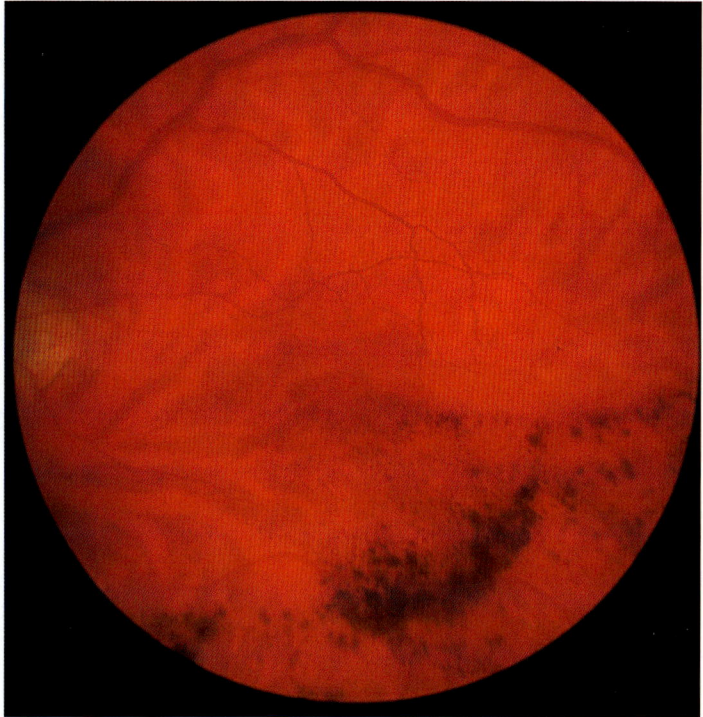

FIGURE 11-3. Pigment fallout after scleral buckle repair of a retinal detachment.

(Fig. 11-3). In limited retinal detachments, the pigment collects at the junction of attached and detached retina, causing a "pseudodemarcation line" (94). If the detachment is total, pigment may collect in the posterior pole. Hilton has shown that such a pigment accumulation does not cause a decrease in visual function (40).

Macular Hole

Full-thickness macular hole is a rare complication of otherwise successful, prompt retinal reattachment. It was first described after SB (10), but it has also been seen after pneumatic retinopexy (PR) and temporary balloon buckling (31,97). It is often first recognized within the first few weeks of retinal reattachment. We have observed the complication in cases with the macula both attached and detached preoperatively. If the macula was not detached or was detached for just a short period of time preoperatively, injection of a gas bubble or vitrectomy with gas–fluid exchange and facedown positioning should be considered to close the hole in hopes of improving the final visual result.

Slow Absorption of Subretinal Fluid

Even if all breaks have been closed, it may take weeks for complete absorption of the SRF after either nondrainage operations or operations in which the SRF has been incompletely drained (Fig. 11-4) (18,19,66,79). If the surgeon is confident that no breaks

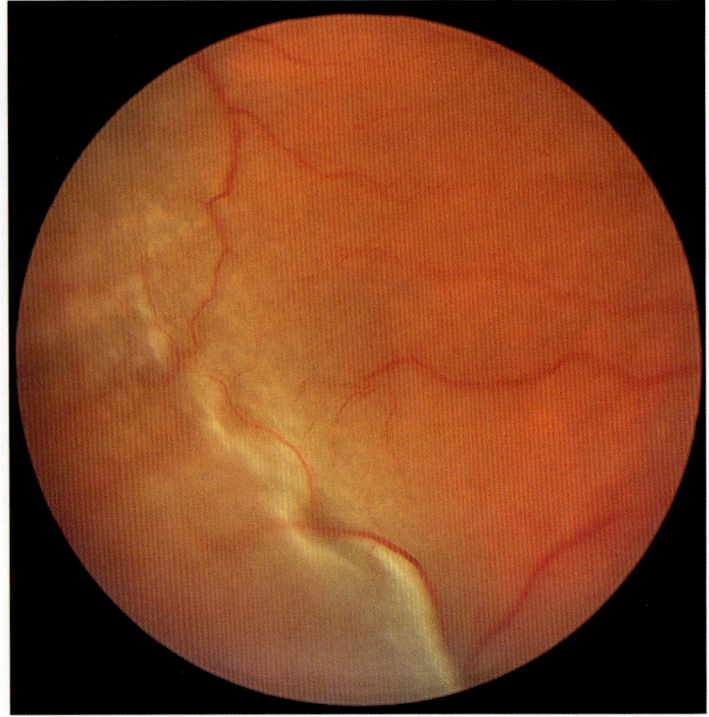

FIGURE 11-4. Persistent subretinal fluid 2 months after a scleral buckling procedure that successfully closed the retinal breaks. One month after this photograph was taken, the fluid was absorbed.

are open, then observation only is needed. If fluid begins to reaccumulate, exudative retinal detachment, a missed break, or an open break must be excluded.

Exudative Retinal Detachment

Recognizing exudative retinal detachments is important because they may be confused with reaccumulation of SRF due to an open break. In exudative detachments, the retinal breaks are successfully closed and remain closed, but 2 to 3 days postoperatively, fluid from the choroid begins to accumulate under the retina posterior to the buckle. The fluid shifts with changes in the position of the eye and is often turbid. Choroidal detachments are frequently present. Spontaneous absorption of the fluid takes up to 12 weeks, but it may be accelerated by systemic corticosteroids (1,96). When an open break is the source of the accumulating SRF, the fluid is usually clear and does not shift with changes in the position of the eye. Careful examination is necessary to locate the break, which must then be closed or, if the SRF is limited, walled off with laser photocoagulation.

Initial Retinal Reattachment Failure

Except for cases of severe proliferative vitreoretinopathy (PVR; see Late Complications, later in this chapter), all surgical failures are caused by an open retinal break. The surgeon must be familiar with all the possible causes and must rule them out in turn.

Inadequate Absorption of the Subretinal Fluid

If the retinal break is not in contact with the scleral buckle at the end of the surgical procedure, reattachment depends on spontaneous absorption of enough SRF to lower the break onto the buckle. In some cases, even with a high and properly placed buckle, the operation fails from insufficient postoperative absorption of fluid. Two major causes of such failures exist. First, certain ocular conditions are characterized by a poor absorption capability. High myopia, senile choroidopathy, and long-standing retinal detachment fall into this category. Second, incorrectly assessed vitreous traction can keep the break open and thus can prevent the absorption of fluid (65).

In other cases, a properly positioned scleral buckle can fail to close the break because it does not adequately indent the sclera (18) or because of the fishmouth phenomenon (see chapter 7, Scleral Buckling Procedure). In nondrainage procedures, it is often difficult to obtain a high buckle because tightening the scleral sutures may excessively raise the intraocular pressure. A low buckle may not close the break even after partial postoperative absorption of SRF. If the fluid had been drained, however, even this low buckle may have sufficed to close the break permanently.

If a small amount of fluid separates the retina from the buckle, reoperation may be avoided. Supplemental laser photocoagulation alone may seal the break, repairing the detachment unless the buckle is too low or vitreoretinal traction is too strong (14,20). When too much fluid remains for photocoagulation to form an adequate scar, the patient may be treated with an intravitreal injection of gas, provided the break is not inferiorly located (see chapter 8, Pneumatic Retinopexy) (48). With proper positioning of the patient, the gas bubble tamponades the break and usually effects closure and subsequent reabsorption of the SRF. If it does not, drainage of the fluid is indicated. If this fails to close the break permanently, the original buckle must be replaced by a higher one, or vitrectomy must be performed.

Misplaced Scleral Buckle

If the break is not fully closed by the buckle, the operation may fail. The most common error is failure to place the buckle far enough posteriorly. Fluid then leaks down the posterior slope of the buckle, redetaching the retina (see Fig. 6-37A). A less common reason is inadequate anterior support of the retinal break (Fig. 11-5). This permits fluid to leak anteriorly, to run along the anterior slope of the buckle, and eventually to leak posteriorly (see Fig. 6-37B). Options to rectify the situation include repositioning of the buckle, supplemental PR, or vitrectomy.

Complications of the Initial Surgery

Unrecognized or untreated surgical complications may prevent reattachment of the retina. Retinal incarceration at the drainage site (see Fig. 7-21) causes folds that may keep the original break open. Reoperation is necessary to flatten the folds and close the break. Traction from incarcerated vitreous may prevent the retina from settling, or it may reopen any initially closed retinal break. The traction must be relieved and the break closed by a high encircling buckle. Iatrogenic retinal holes, caused either by the drainage needle or by a deep scleral suture, must be found and treated. If a large break is kept open by fishmouthing, or if a small break is kept open by meridional folding, the operation will fail. Corrective measures are discussed in chapter 7.

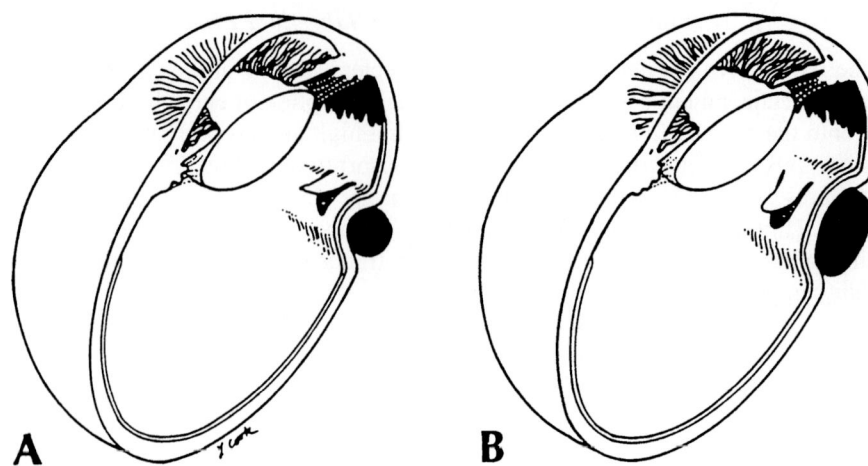

FIGURE 11-5. A: Incorrectly buckled flap tear. The break is not supported anteriorly. **B:** Correctly buckled flap tear. The entire break is supported.

Undetected or New Break

An undetected or new retinal break may be responsible for surgical failure. If the SRF has been drained, new fluid will accumulate; if it has not, the retina will not settle. The only remedy is to find and close the break.

Vitreous Traction and Early Proliferative Vitreoretinopathy

If excessive vitreous traction is present, retinal breaks closed at the time of surgery may be reopened in the early postoperative period. On reoperation, a higher scleral buckle, combined with an encircling procedure, is required (see later). In some cases, the traction must be released by vitrectomy (see chapter 10, Surgery of Complicated Cases).

SCLERAL BUCKLING: LATE COMPLICATIONS

Refractive Error

Scleral buckling can induce both spherical and astigmatic refractive errors (5,11,80,91). Encircling procedures not uncommonly produce a myopic shift, averaging 1 to 2 diopters. This increase in myopia is the result of either an increase in the globe's axial length or a forward displacement of the iris–lens diaphragm (49,80). The former effect is caused by horizontal globe constriction when the encircling band is tightened. If multiple mattress sutures are used to invaginate an encircling explant deeply into the sclera, the axial length of the globe may actually decrease (37). Nonencircling SB procedures may cause regular astigmatism. In one study, the greatest degree of induced astigmatism was seen with segmental buckles that spanned one to two quadrants (47). Sometimes irregular astigmatism, which cannot be corrected by spectacles, is seen after placement of a radial explant (11). Many patients have decreased accommodation, which may persist for several months.

The various refractive changes seen with SB are usually stable by 3 months after the operation. Spectacles or contact lenses can then be prescribed. When large refractive changes are encountered and the visual acuity is good in both eyes, patients may have difficulty adjusting to the resultant spectacle-induced anisometropia.

Strabismus

Strabismus after SB is common, observed to some degree early on in as many as 80% of cases (6,61). Fortunately, this is a transient phenomenon in most cases, and resolution of the heterotropia usually occurs within 6 to 12 weeks after the operation (61). Excessive traction on and freezing of the extraocular muscles may be contributing factors to temporary postoperative strabismus.

Significant, permanent motility disturbances after SB, however, can occur (29,61,70, 90). This may be encountered in up to one-fifth of cases, but the rate varies depending on the type of surgery and probably averages more on the order of 3% to 5%. Persistent strabismus has several possible causes in this setting (45,63,88,106,107):

- Faulty reinsertion or postoperative slippage of a temporarily disinserted extraocular muscle
- Intentional intraoperative disinsertion (partial or complete) of the superior oblique muscle
- Placement of a large explant under or near a muscle insertion
- Adhesions of muscles to Tenon's capsule or sclera
- Encircling band placed near or inadvertently under the superior oblique muscle
- Excessive scarring and shortening of Tenon's capsule, especially after reoperations
- Permanent muscle injury from intraoperative trauma

In general, persistent extraocular muscle imbalance is seen more often in cases that have encircling elements or large explants, undergo extraocular muscle disinsertion, and are reoperations.

Motility imbalances usually are a problem only if there is significant deviation in primary gaze or downgaze and if the visual acuity is relatively good in both eyes. Prisms should be tried first to correct any bothersome diplopia (29). If this fails and symptoms persist beyond 6 months after the SB procedure, then removal of the buckle or corrective muscle surgery can be considered. Botulinum toxin injections may also be useful in this setting (72).

In planning muscle surgery, the surgeon must determine whether the diplopia is caused by scar tissue preventing rotation of the eye or by the underaction of a muscle that is bound down to the globe (63,76). Forced ductions aid greatly in this determination. When the limitation in motility is caused by scar tissue, the eye cannot be forcibly rotated away from the apparently overacting muscle. To restore ocular motility, the surgeon must first dissect the scar tissue from the sclera. Tenon's capsule and the conjunctiva are then recessed to the level of the muscle insertion, and the sclera is left bare anteriorly (76). When the limitation is caused by underaction of a muscle adherent to the globe, the eye can be forcibly rotated in all directions. The adherent muscle must be freed and resected (76). The results of surgery are variable. Diplopia in primary gaze can be eliminated, but most patients have some diplopia in some fields of gaze (107). An adjustable suture technique and operating on the untreated eye may help to maximize the surgical success rate (29,63).

Extrusion or Intrusion

Conjunctiva and Tenon's layers can sometimes break down over a scleral buckle and lead to exposure ("extrusion") of the element (Fig. 11-6). This occurs more commonly with sponge, as opposed to solid silicone explants (43). Exposure can cause persistent irritation or can lead to localized infection. Pain, mucopurulent discharge, and subconjunctival hemorrhage may be the initial signs of extrusion, with or without definite infection. Even if the element is not thought to be an infected, attempts at recovering an exposed element using various grafts often fail. Therefore, exposed elements usually need to be removed. If a sponge explant has been used in addition to an encircling band and no obvious signs of infection are present, it often suffices to remove the explant alone (81). Removal of part or all of the buckling elements may lead to retinal redetachment, as discussed earlier, and, therefore, patients should be followed closely in the immediate postoperative period.

Erosion of a buckling element through the sclera and into the globe ("intrusion") is a much less common but potentially devastating complication. Encircling polyethylene tubes, which are no longer used, had a great tendency to intrude. Intrusion was also more common with the use of scleral implants (110). Now that silicone explants are used almost exclusively, this complication is rare. Predisposing factors include tight encircling elements, thin sclera, multiple operations, and glaucoma. Signs include subretinal and vitreous hemorrhage and recurrent retinal detachment. If intrusion occurs, the recommended treatment is to cut the encircling band. Removal of an intruding element should only be performed if absolutely necessary. Because ocular rupture may occur on removal of the element, a scleral patch graft should be on hand in the operating room.

Macular Pucker

Proliferation of a preretinal membrane derived from either astrocytes or retinal pigment epithelial cells causes clinically apparent wrinkling or pucker of the macula after

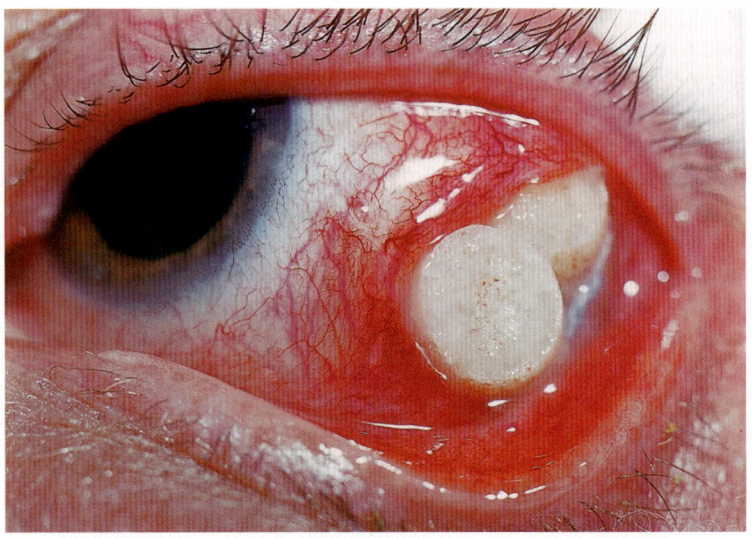

FIGURE 11-6. Extruding radial silicone sponge explants.

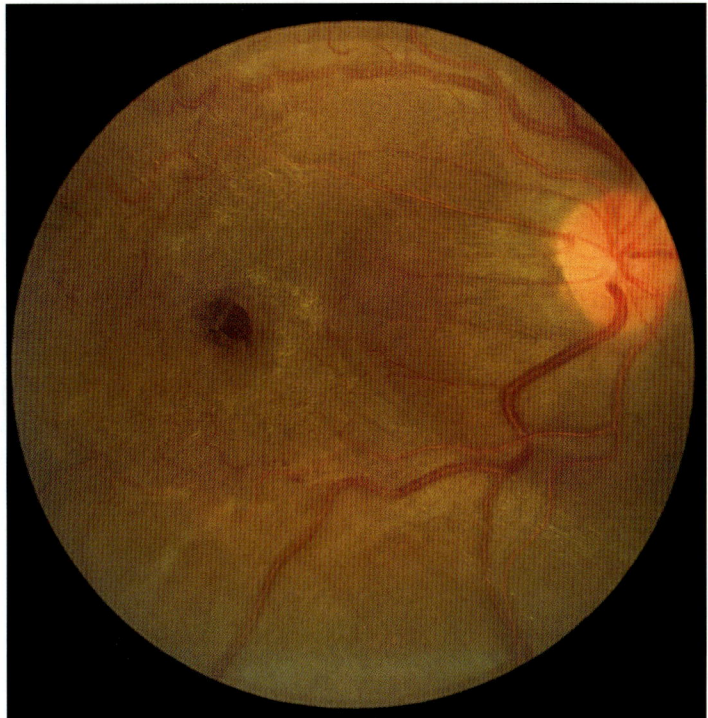

FIGURE 11-7. Severe macular pucker: Contraction of the preretinal membrane wrinkles the retina. Notice the straightening of the blood vessels between the disc and the fovea.

6% to 17% of SB procedures (Fig. 11-7) (33–35,56,60,95,101). Histopathologically, it was found in 31% of eyes that had undergone retinal detachment surgery (104). Macular pucker is usually first noted 6 to 8 weeks postoperatively. The mechanism that causes pucker is unknown. It probably represents a forme fruste of PVR, and cryotherapy may contribute to the process by promoting dispersion of viable retinal pigment epithelial cells into the vitreous cavity (12,13,101).

Macular pucker is more commonly seen in cases associated with older patient age, preoperative vitreous hemorrhage, and large retinal tears (101). Its incidence is also higher after certain intraoperative complications, such as loss of formed vitreous, retinal incarceration, subretinal hemorrhage, and vitreous hemorrhage (95). It represents one of the most common causes of late visual acuity decrease after otherwise successful SB repair (83,84). It is not, however, unique to SB because it is also encountered with an often comparable overall incidence after all the other types of retinal repair techniques (31,97,99). When it occurs to a significant degree, pars plana vitrectomy with peeling of the membrane can be offered (21,75).

Cystoid Macular Edema

Some degree of cystoid macular edema (CME) is common after SB; it is demonstrable angiographically in up to 29% and 60% of phakic and aphakic eyes, respectively (57,60,62,83). Its incidence is the same in eyes in which the macula was attached preoperatively as in those with the macula detached (57,60). Spontaneous resolution of CME usually occurs within several months of the operation. Persistent CME with a permanent decrease in vision is uncommon.

Cataract

Cataract formation or acceleration is sometimes observed after SB (68). A true cause-and-effect relationship with the procedure when no other complications are present, however, is unclear. On one hand, cataract formation is known to occur from retinal detachment itself, especially when the patient has long-standing detachment and preoperative hypotony or inflammation (86). On the other hand, in the PR trial, eyes randomized to SB had a statistically significant greater incidence of cataract formation at final follow-up (99).

Regardless of whether SB contributes to cataract formation, removal of the cataract in this setting, especially using modern phacoemulsification techniques, does not appear to increase the risk of redetachment significantly (46,92). However, it is probably best to wait at least several months after the buckling procedure to allow for maximal chorioretinal adhesion to form around the retinal breaks, for the refractive status of the eye to be stable, and for all ocular inflammation to have resolved.

Late Detachment of the Retina

If an initially reattached retina redetaches after a period of 6 weeks or longer, the case is typically considered a late redetachment, rather than a surgical failure. Redetachment results from either the development of a new tear or the reopening of the original break.

New Retinal Tears

In an unpublished series at Wills Eye Hospital in Philadelphia, the most common cause of late redetachment (16 of 19 cases) was a new retinal tear resulting from increased vitreous traction. Of the 16 cases, the new tear was located posterior to an encircling band in 9, on an encircling band in 3, and in previously unbuckled quadrants in 4. The prognosis for successful reattachment is excellent in these cases: 15 of the 16 detachments were repaired.

New tears that overlie a buckle can often be closed by photocoagulation alone (87). New tears elsewhere can be approached in various ways, depending on the exact location of the tear, the original surgical procedure performed, and the presence of PVR. Most cases can be effectively managed by adding cryotherapy and a new buckling element to close the break. If the patient has early PVR, an encircling band is added if it was not used originally (see Appendix, Fig. A-13). Alternative approaches include PR for superiorly located breaks (see Appendix, Fig. A-14), temporary balloon buckling for breaks located away from permanent buckling elements, and vitrectomy for breaks located extremely posteriorly. Vitrectomy is the procedure of choice, often in combination with revising the scleral buckle, in the presence of more advanced PVR.

Reopening of the Original Break

Increased vitreous traction on a flap tear can extend the tear through an area of cryotherapy and allow anterior leakage of SRF (7,22). This problem can be avoided if the cryotherapy of flap tears is extended to the ora serrata. If this has not been done initially and detachment results, photocoagulation may close the break. If the increased traction has extended the tear beyond the original scleral buckle, either a broader buckle must be substituted at the time of supplemental treatment or, if the break is located in the superior quadrants, PR can be used.

Proliferative Vitreoretinopathy

PVR is the most common cause of primary failure of retinal detachment surgery in general, and depending on how advanced it is at the initial operation or how rapidly it develops to a significant degree, it may be either an early or a late complication. If mild PVR reopens the original break, repair can often be effected by a higher scleral buckle used in combination with an encircling procedure. Reapplication of cryotherapy or adding laser photocoagulation is also required. As mentioned previously, more advanced cases necessitate vitrectomy (see also chapter 10, Surgery of Complicated Cases).

Decreased or Displaced Scleral Buckle

Occasionally, a suture erodes out of the sclera. This may either decrease the height of the buckle or cause it to shift its position. Vitreous traction can then reopen the retinal break. Most of these detachments can be cured by repeating the original operation, or, if the break is located in a superior quadrant, PR can be used.

Removal of the Scleral Buckle

Redetachment after removal of a scleral buckle is discussed on page 176. Occasionally, scleral buckles must be removed for severe postoperative pain, exposure (extrusion), or infection. If the buckle is infected and the retina redetaches immediately after its removal, the reoperation must be delayed 1 week to allow the orbit to resterilize itself.

PNEUMATIC RETINOPEXY: EARLY AND LATE COMPLICATIONS

As a minimally invasive, incisionless technique, PR has much fewer postoperative complications than SB. In a multicenter, controlled clinical trial comparing primary scleral buckling with PR in selected retinal detachments, PR was shown to have significantly lower rates of cataract formation, choroidal detachment, and myopic shift (97). Without conjunctival or extraocular muscle manipulation, PR does not cause symblepharon or postoperative strabismus. Anterior segment ischemia is also not a potential problem. Of course, exposure or infection of foreign materials is not an issue with PR.

Intraocular Pressure Elevation

Maximum intraocular pressure elevation occurs immediately after the gas injection. If the pressure were left high, optic nerve damage or central retinal artery occlusion could theoretically occur. Whether paracentesis is performed before or after the gas injection, as long as the central retinal artery is perfused by the end of the procedure, then such complications are not encountered. Although the gas expands postoperatively, the globe is able to compensate well, and no significant rise in intraocular pressure occurs during this period; there have been no reports of delayed central retinal artery closure or optic neuropathy (41).

Subretinal Gas

Migration of gas bubbles under the retina is a rare complication of PR (42,59,97). It usually occurs within the first 24 hours of the procedure. The risk of subretinal gas is greatest if the retinal tear is large and if small bubbles or "fish eggs" are encountered when the gas is injected.

In general, this is a preventable complication for two main reasons. First, "fish eggs" can almost always be avoided by using the proper injection technique, as described in chapter 8 (see Fig. 8-5). Second, even if they do occur, the patient should maintain a head position with the bubbles away from the retinal break for the first 24 hours, during which time the bubbles typically coalesce (42). Once coalescence is confirmed by ophthalmoscopy on the first postoperative day, the patient's head position then can be changed to allow the bubble to tamponade the break.

In rare instances, a single gas bubble obtained at the time of injection breaks up in the first 24 hours. This is possibly the result of rapid eye movements during sleep. This complication should be looked for and managed on the first postoperative day.

A small, subretinal bubble that does not hold the tear open is not typically detrimental and can be observed (42). Large bubbles near or under the tear, however, are likely to prevent it from settling and will require removal with vitrectomy surgery if they cannot be massaged out with scleral depression (59).

New or Missed Retinal Breaks

New or missed breaks after PR occur in about 13% of cases, with a reported range in the literature of 0% to 29% (42). This complication is not unique to PR because it has been reported with all other retinal detachment repair methods (9,18,31,52,58,77). Whether or not the rate is higher with PR is debatable.

The rate of missed breaks may be higher for procedures performed in the office compared with those performed in the operating room because the latter setting may allow for more extensive scleral depression. New breaks could be either the result of natural history in eyes that are predisposed to having retinal breaks or induced from direct or indirect effects on the vitreous gel from the expanding intraocular gas or the cryotherapy, respectively (30,74,89). Last, a "new" break may also represent a known (treated or untreated) flat break that opened because of a shift in the SRF into uninvolved retina after the gas bubble was injected.

Whether the breaks are new or missed, they usually manifest within the first month after the procedure (97). Because many of these breaks are located within 3 clock hours of the initial break, repeat PR often works to establish complete, long-term retinal reattachment. In general, about one-half of patients who undergo PR that fails because of new or missed breaks eventually require SB (99).

Minimizing this complication requires meticulous, systematic ophthalmoscopic examination of the entire fundus to locate all vitreoretinal disease. Any patient in whom the peripheral retina is not completely visualized is not a good candidate for PR. Laser photocoagulation applied in a scatter fashion between the ora serrata and the equator for 360 degrees once the retina is flat after PR may help to decrease the rate of redetachment from new or missed breaks further (Paul Tornambe, M.D., personal communication).

Reopened Retinal Breaks

Rarely, the original retinal break can reopen after the gas bubble has dissipated or the patient stops special head positioning (42,97). This complication should be differentiated from breaks that were never completely closed. The former situation is the result of either inadequate initial retinopexy or extension of the tear from excessive or increased vitreoretinal traction. The latter situation is more likely caused by improper head positioning or inadequate gas bubble volume. Reopened breaks can often be managed by repeating the PR procedure, extending the retinopexy beyond the area originally covered, and making sure that treatment extends at least two disc diameters beyond the edge of the break (42).

Shift of Subretinal Fluid

Some shifting of SRF can occur shortly after the gas bubble is injected. This is only a problem if the fluid is displaced into the macula or into an area that has a preexisting flat peripheral retinal break (16,58,100,108). Detaching a previously flat macula can, of course, compromise the final visual outcome. In cases with bullous superior detachments that come close to or are within the superotemporal arcade, the "steamroller maneuver" is recommended to minimize chance of detaching the macula (see chapter 8, Pneumatic Retinopexy). To minimize squeezing subretinal pigment debris into the vitreous cavity and thereby possibly promoting PVR, the retinal break should be treated after performing the maneuver (32,98).

Similarly, if any flat retinal breaks are present inferior to the detachment, there is a risk of opening the break and causing a new or persistent retinal detachment with a significant shift of the SRF. First, all uninvolved retinal breaks should be treated with laser photocoagulation before the gas is injected. Then, if any are located near the border of the SRF, a steamroller maneuver should be used.

Hemorrhage

Vitreous or subretinal hemorrhage is rarely encountered (97). Hemorrhage into the vitreous cavity is either from bleeding at the pars plana injection site or from cryotherapy-induced fracturing of a retinal blood vessel (42). Subretinal hemorrhage is more likely to be the result of the latter mechanism. In either case, the hemorrhage is self-limited and usually minimal. There have been no reports of hemorrhage affecting the outcome of PR in any way.

Infection

Endophthalmitis is rare (28,97). No cases have been reported in eyes that have had 5% to 10% povidone–iodine (Betadine) solution instilled at the beginning of the procedure, as described in chapter 8 (42).

Proliferative Vitreoretinopathy

The significant late complication associated with PR, as with other retinal detachment repair techniques, is PVR. It can lead to visual loss by causing persistent or recurrent retinal detachment. The development of advanced PVR necessitates reoperation with vitrectomy and SB to achieve long-lasting retinal reattachment. A prospective, randomized comparison of PR and SB for selected, primary retinal detachments showed comparable rates of postoperative PVR at 3% and 5%, respectively (97).

Miscellaneous

Increased floaters, subretinal pigment fallout, cataract, choroidal detachment, delayed resorption of SRF, macular pucker, and macular hole have all been reported with PR (2,15,16,97). None of these complications, however, are unique to the procedure. Furthermore, no evidence indicates that any of them occur with any greater frequency in PR compared with the other retinal detachment repair techniques.

REFERENCES

1. Aaberg TM, Pawlowski GJ, Machemer R, Norton EW. Exudative retinal detachments following scleral buckling with cryotherapy: a new concept for vitreous surgery. 3. Indications and results. *Am J Ophthalmol* 1972;74:245–251.
2. Algvere P, Hallnas K, Palmqvist BM. Success and complications of pneumatic retinopexy. *Am J Ophthalmol* 1988;106:400–404.
3. Arribas NP, Olk RJ, Schertzer M, et al. Preoperative antibiotic soaking of silicone sponges: does it make a difference? *Ophthalmology* 1984;91:1684–1689.
4. Bacon AS, Davison CR, Patel BC, Frazer DG, Ficker LA, Dart JK. Infective endophthalmitis following vitreoretinal surgery. *Eye* 1993;7:529–534.
5. Beekhuis H, Talsma M, Vreugdenhil W, Eggink F, Peperkamp E, Van Meurs J. Changes in refraction after retinal detachment surgery corrected by extended wear contact lenses for early visual rehabilitation. *Retina* 1993;13:120–124.
6. Bell FC, Pruett RC. Effects of cryotherapy on extraocular muscles. *Ophthalmic Surg* 1977;8:71.
7. Benson WE, Morse PH, Nantawan P. Late complications following cryotherapy of lattice degeneration. *Am J Ophthalmol* 1977;84:514–516.
8. Berler DK, Goldstein B. Scleral buckles and rotation of the ciliary body. *Arch Ophthalmol* 1979;97:1518–1521.
9. Binder S. Repair of retinal detachments with temporary balloon buckling. *Retina* 1986;6:210–214.
10. Brown GC. Macular hole following rhegmatogenous retinal detachment repair. *Arch Ophthalmol* 1988;106:765–766.
11. Burton TC. Irregular astigmatism following episcleral buckling procedure with the use of silicone rubber sponges. *Arch Ophthalmol* 1973;90:447–448.
12. Campochiaro PA. Pathogenic mechanisms in proliferative vitreoretinopathy. *Arch Ophthalmol* 1997;115:237–241.
13. Campochiaro PA, Kaden IH, Vidaurri-Leal J, Glaser BM. Cryotherapy enhances intravitreal dispersion of viable retinal pigment epithelial cells. *Arch Ophthalmol* 1985;103:434–436.
14. Chan CK, Olk RJ, Arribas NP, et al. Supplemental photocoagulation on the buckle for prevention of surgical revision after scleral buckling procedures. *Arch Ophthalmol* 1987;105:490–496.
15. Chan CK, Wessels IF. Delayed fluid absorption after pneumatic retinopexy. *Ophthalmology* 1989;96:1691–1700.
16. Chen JC, Robertson JE, Coonan P, et al. Results and complications of pneumatic retinopexy. *Ophthalmology* 1988;95:601–608.
17. Chignell AH. Choroidal detachment following retinal detachment without drainage of subretinal fluid. *Am J Ophthalmol* 1972;73:860–862.
18. Chignell AH, Fison LG, Davies EWG, et al. Failure in retinal detachment surgery. *Br J Ophthalmol* 1973;57:525–530.
19. Chignell AH, Talbot J. Absorption of subretinal fluid after nondrainage retinal detachment surgery. *Arch Ophthalmol* 1978;96:635–637.
20. Curtin VT, Norton EW, Gass JD. Photocoagulation: its use in the prevention of reoperation after scleral buckling operations. *Trans Am Acad Ophthalmol Otolaryngol* 1967;71:432–441.
21. de Bustros S, Rice TA, Michels RG, Thompson JT, Marcus S, Glaser BM. Vitrectomy for macular pucker: use after treatment of retinal tears or retinal detachment. *Arch Ophthalmol* 1988;106:758–760.
22. Delaney WV Jr. Retinal tear extension through the cryosurgical scar. *Br J Ophthalmol* 1971;55:205–9.
23. Deutsch J, Aggarwal RK, Eagling EM. Removal of scleral explant elements: a 10–year retrospective study. *Eye* 1992;6:570–3.
24. Diddie KR, Ernest JT. Uveal blood flow after 360 degrees constriction in rabbit. *Arch Ophthalmol* 1980;98:729–730.
25. Dobbie JG. Circulatory changes in the eye associated with retinal detachment and its repair. *Trans Am Ophthalmol Soc* 1980;78:503–566.
26. Doft BH, Lipkowitz J, Kowalski R, et al. An experimental model to assess factors associated with scleral buckle infection. *Retina* 1983;3:212.
27. Eagle RC, Yanoff M, Morse PH. Anterior segment necrosis following scleral buckling in hemoglobin SC disease. *Am J Ophthalmol* 1973;75:426–433.

28. Eckhardt C. Staphylococcus epidermidis endophthalmitis after pneumatic retinopexy. *Am J Ophthalmol* 1987;103:720–721.
29. Fison PN, Chignell AH. Diplopia after retinal detachment surgery. *Br J Ophthalmol* 1987;71:521–525.
30. Freeman WR, Lipson BK, Morgan CM, Liggett PE. New posteriorly located retinal breaks after pneumatic retinopexy. *Ophthalmology* 1988;95:14–18.
31. Green SN, Yarian DL, Masciulli L, Leff SR. Office repair of retinal detachment using a Lincoff temporary balloon buckle. *Ophthalmology* 1996;103:1804–1810.
32. Griffiths PG, Richardson J. Causes of proliferative retinopathy following pneumatic retinopexy. *Arch Ophthalmol* 1990;108:1515.
33. Grupposo SS. Visual acuity following surgery for retinal detachment. *Arch Ophthalmol* 1975;93:327–330.
34. Gundry MF, Davies EW. Recovery of visual acuity after retinal detachment surgery. *Am J Ophthalmol* 1974;77:310–314.
35. Hagler WS, Aturaliya U. Macular pucker after retinal detachment surgery. *Br J Ophthalmol* 1971;55:451–457.
36. Hahn YS, Lincoff A, Lincoff H, Kreissig I. Infection after sponge implantation for scleral buckling. *Am J Ophthalmol* 1979;87:180–185.
37. Harris MJ, Blumenkrantz MS, Wittpenn J, et al. Geometric alterations produced by encircling scleral buckles: biometric and clinical considerations. *Retina* 1987;7:14–19.
38. Hayreh SS, Baines JAB. Occlusion of the vortex veins: an experimental study. *Br J Ophthalmol* 1973;57:217–238.
39. Hayreh SS, W.E. S. Anterior segment ischemia following retinal detachment surgery. *Mod Probl Ophthalmol* 1979;20:148–153.
40. Hilton GF. Subretinal pigment migration: effects of cryosurgical retinal reattachment. *Arch Ophthalmol* 1974;91:445–450.
41. Hilton GF, Brinton DA. Pneumatic retinopexy and alternative techniques. In: Ryan SJ, Glaser BM, eds. *Retina*, 2nd ed. St Louis: CV Mosby, 1994:2093–2112.
42. Hilton GF, Tornambe PE. Pneumatic retinopexy: an analysis of intraoperative and postoperative complications. The Retinal Detachment Study Group. *Retina* 1991;11:285–294.
43. Hilton GF, Wallyn RH. The removal of scleral buckles. *Arch Ophthalmol* 1978;96:2061–2063.
44. Hitchings RA, Levy IS, Chignell AH. Acute infection after retinal detachment surgery. *Br J Ophthalmol* 1974;58:588–590.
45. Kanski JJ, Elkington AR, Davies MS. Diplopia after retinal detachment surgery. *Am J Ophthalmol* 1973;76:38–40.
46. Kerrison JB, Marsh M, Stark WJ, Haller JA. Phacoemulsification after retinal detachment surgery. *Ophthalmology* 1996;103:216–219.
47. Kinoshita M, Tanihara H, Negi A, et al. Vector analysis of corneal astigmatism after scleral buckling surgery. *Ophthalmologica* 1994;208:250–253.
48. Landers MB, Robinson D, Olsen, et al. Slit-lamp fluid–gas exchange and other office procedures following vitreoretinal surgery. *Arch Ophthalmol* 1985;103:967–972.
49. Larsen JS, Syrdalen P. Ultrasonographic study on changes in axial eye dimensions after encircling procedure in retinal detachment surgery. *Acta Ophthalmol* 1979;57:337.
50. Lean JS, Chignell AH. Infection following retinal detachment surgery. *Br J Ophthalmol* 1977;61:593–594.
51. Lerner BC, Lakhanpal V, Schocket SS. Transient myopia and accommodative paresis following retinal cryotherapy and panretinal photocoagulation. *Am J Ophthalmol* 1984;97:704–708.
52. Lincoff H, Kreissig I, Goldbaum M. Reasons for failure in non-drainage operations. *Mod Probl Ophthalmol* 1974;12:20.
53. Lincoff H, Nadel A, P OC. The changing character of the infected scleral implant. *Arch Ophthalmol* 1970;84:421–423.
54. Lindsey PS, Pierce LH, Welch RB. Removal of scleral buckling elements: causes and complications. *Arch Ophthalmol* 1983;101:570–573.
55. Lobes LA, Bourgon P. Pupillary abnormalities induced by argon laser photocoagulation. *Ophthalmology* 1985;92:234–236.
56. Lobes LA Jr, Burton TC. The incidence of macular pucker after retinal detachment surgery. *Am J Ophthalmol* 1978;85:72–77.
57. Lobes LA Jr, Grand MG. Incidence of cystoid macular edema following scleral buckling procedure. *Arch Ophthalmol* 1980;98:1230–1232.
58. McAllister IL, Meyers SM, Zegarra H, Gutman FA, Zakov ZN, Beck GJ. Comparison of pneumatic retinopexy with alternative surgical techniques. *Ophthalmology* 1988;95:877–883.
59. McDonald HR, Abrams GW, Irvine AR, et al. The management of subretinal gas following attempted pneumatic retinal reattachment. *Ophthalmology* 1987;94:319–326.
60. Meredith TA, Reeser FH, Topping TM, Aaberg TM. Cystoid macular edema after retinal detachment surgery. *Ophthalmology* 1980;87:1090–1095.
61. Mets MB, Wendell ME, Gieser RG. Ocular deviation after retinal detachment surgery. *Am J Ophthalmol* 1985;99:667–672.
62. Miyake K, Miyake Y, Maekubo K, Asakura M, Manabe R. Incidence of cystoid macular edema after retinal detachment surgery and the use of topical indomethacin. *Am J Ophthalmol* 1983;95:451–456.

63. Munoz M, Rosenbaum AL. Long-term strabismus complications following retinal detachment surgery. *J Pediatr Ophthalmol Strabismus* 1987;24:309–314.
64. Newsome DA, Einaugler RB. Tonic pupil following retinal detachment surgery. *Arch Ophthalmol* 1971;86:233–234.
65. Norton EWD. Retinal detachments in aphakia. *Trans Am Ophthalmol Soc* 1963;61:770.
66. O'Connor PR, 1973. Absorption of subretinal fluid after external scleral buckling without drainage. *Am J Ophthalmol* 1973;76:30–34.
67. Ogasawara H, Feke GT, Yoshida A, Milbocker MT, Weiter JJ, McMeel JW. Retinal blood flow alterations associated with scleral buckling and encircling procedures. *Br J Ophthalmol* 1992;76:275–279.
68. Ophthalmology AAO. The repair of rhegmatogenous retinal detachments. *Ophthalmology* 1996;103:1313–1324.
69. Packer AJ, Maggiano JM, Aaberg TM, Meredith TA, Reeser FH, Kingham JD. Serous choroidal detachment after retinal detachment surgery. *Arch Ophthalmol* 1983;101:1221–1224.
70. Peduzzi M, Campos EC, Guerrieri F. Disturbances of ocular motility after retinal detachment surgery. *Doc Ophthalmol* 1984;58:115–118.
71. Perez RN, Phelps CD, Burton TC. Angle-closure glaucoma following scleral buckling operations. *Trans Am Acad Ophthalmol Otolaryngol* 1976;81:247–252.
72. Petitto VB, Buckley EG. Use of botulinum toxin in strabismus after retinal detachment surgery. *Ophthalmology* 1991;98:509–512 [discussion 512–513].
73. Phelps CD, Burton TC. Glaucoma and retinal detachment. *Arch Ophthalmol* 1977;95:418–422.
74. Poliner LS, Grand MG, Schoch LH, et al. New retinal detachment after pneumatic retinopexy. *Ophthalmology* 1987;94:315–318.
75. Poliner LS, Olk RJ, Grand MG, et al. Surgical management of premacular fibroplasia. *Arch Ophthalmol* 1988;106:761–764.
76. Portney GL, Campbell LH, Casebeer JC. Acquired heterotropia following surgery for retinal detachment. *Am J Ophthalmol* 1972;73:985–990.
77. Rachal WF, Burton TC. Changing concepts of failures after retinal detachment surgery. *Arch Ophthalmol* 1979;97:480–483.
78. Regillo CD, Sergott RC, Brown GC. Successful scleral buckling procedures decrease central retinal artery blood flow velocity. *Ophthalmology* 1993;100:1044–1049.
79. Robertson DM. Delayed absorption of subretinal fluid after scleral buckling procedures. *Am J Ophthalmol* 1979;87:57–64.
80. Rubin ML. The induction of refractive errors by retinal detachment surgery. *Trans Am Ophthalmol Soc* 1975;73:452.
81. Russo CE, Ruiz RS. Silicone sponge rejection. *Arch Ophthalmol* 1971;85:647.
82. Ryan SJ, Goldberg MF. Anterior segment ischemia following scleral buckling in sickle cell hemoglobinopathy. *Am J Ophthalmol* 1971;72:35–50.
83. Sabates NR, Sabates FN, Sabates R, Lee KY, Ziemianski MC. Macular changes after retinal detachment surgery. *Am J Ophthalmol* 1989;108:22–29.
84. Sarin LK, McDonald PR. Changes in the posterior pole following successful reattachment of the retina. *Trans Am Acad Ophthalmol Otolaryngol* 1970;74:75–79.
85. Schwartz PL, Pruett RC. Factors influencing retinal redetachment after removal of buckling elements. *Arch Ophthalmol* 1977;95:804–807.
86. Scott JD. Lens changes and retinal detachment. *Trans Ophthalmol Soc U K* 1979;99:241.
87. Seelenfreund MH, Silverstone BZ, Hirsch I, Arnon N, Sternberg I, Ivry M. Recurrent tears following successful retinal detachment surgery. *Ann Ophthalmol* 1986;18:319–323.
88. Sewell JJ, Knobloch WH, Eifrig DE. Extraocular muscle imbalance after surgical treatment for retinal detachment. *Am J Ophthalmol* 1974;78:321–323.
89. Smiddy WE, Flynn HW Jr, Nicholson DH, et al. Results and complications in treated retinal breaks. *Am J Ophthalmol* 1991;112:623–631.
90. Smiddy WE, Loupe D, Michels RG, Enger C, Glaser BM, deBustros S. Extraocular muscle imbalance after scleral buckling surgery. *Ophthalmology* 1989;96:1485–1489.
91. Smiddy WE, Loupe DN, Michels RG, et al. Refractive changes after scleral buckling surgery. *Arch Ophthalmol* 1989;107:1469–1471.
92. Smiddy WE, Michels RG, Stark WJ, Maumenee AE. Cataract extraction after retinal detachment surgery. *Ophthalmology* 1988;95:3–7.
93. Smiddy WE, Miller D, Flynn HW Jr. Scleral buckle removal following retinal reattachment surgery: clinical and microbiologic aspects. *Ophthalmic Surg* 1993;24:440–445.
94. Sudarsky RD, Yannuzzi LA. Cryomarcation line and pigment migration after retinal cryosurgery. *Arch Ophthalmol* 1970;83:395–401.
95. Tanenbaum HC, Schepens CL, Elzeneiny I, et al. Macular pucker following retinal detachment surgery. *Arch Ophthalmol* 1970;83:286–293.
96. Topilow HW, Ackerman AL. Massive exudative retinal and choroidal detachments following scleral buckling surgery. *Ophthalmology* 1983;90:143–147.
97. Tornambe PE, Hilton GF. Pneumatic retinopexy: a multicenter randomized controlled clinical trial comparing

pneumatic retinopexy with scleral buckling. The Retinal Detachment Study Group. *Ophthalmology* 1989;96:772–783.
98. Tornambe PE, Hilton GF. The steamroller maneuver and proliferative vitreoretinopathy [Letter]. *Arch Ophthalmol* 1992;110:15.
99. Tornambe PE, Hilton GF, Brinton DA, et al. Pneumatic retinopexy. A two-year follow-up study of the multicenter clinical trial comparing pneumatic retinopexy with scleral buckling. *Ophthalmology* 1991;98:1115–1123.
100. Tornambe PE, Hilton GF, Kelly NF, Salzano TC, Wells JW, Wendel RT. Expanded indications for pneumatic retinopexy. *Ophthalmology* 1988;95:597–600.
101. Uemura A, Ideta H, Nagasaki H, Morita H, Ito K. Macular pucker after retinal detachment surgery. *Ophthalmic Surg* 1992;23:116–119.
102. Ulrich RA, Burton TC. Infections following scleral buckling procedures. *Arch Ophthalmol* 1974;92:213–215.
103. Virdi PS, Hayreh SS. Anterior segment ischemia after recession of various recti: an experimental study. *Ophthalmology* 1987;94:1258–1271.
104. Wilson DJ, Green WR. Histopathologic study of the effect of retinal detachment surgery on 49 eyes obtained post mortem. *Am J Ophthalmol* 1987;103:167–179.
105. Wiznia RA. Removal of solid silicone rubber exoplants after retinal detachment surgery. *Am J Ophthalmol* 1983;95:495–497.
106. Wolff SM. Strabismus after retinal detachment surgery. *Trans Am Ophthalmol Soc* 1983;81:182.
107. Wright KW. The fat adherence syndrome and strabismus after retina surgery. *Ophthalmology* 1986;93:411–415.
108. Yeo JH, Vidaurri-Leal J, Glaser BM. Extension of retinal detachments as a complication of pneumatic retinopexy. *Arch Ophthalmol* 1986;104:1161–1163.
109. Yoshida A, Feke GT, Green GJ, et al. Retinal circulatory changes after scleral buckling procedures. *Am J Ophthalmol* 1983;95:182–188.
110. Yoshizumi MO, Friberg T. Erosion of implants in retinal detachment surgery. *Ann Ophthalmol* 1983;15:430–434.

12

Prophylactic Therapy

Autopsy and clinical studies have shown that 5% to 13% of the population has at least one retinal break, but most of these persons never develop retinal detachment (5,6,20,24,46). This chapter analyzes the evidence for and against prophylactic therapy for each type of retinal break (Table 12-1).

SYMPTOMATIC[1] TEARS IN PATIENTS WITH NO HISTORY OF RETINAL DISEASE

Flap (Horseshoe) Tears

Symptomatic flap tears are, by far, the most dangerous type of retinal break because 25% to 90% of them lead to retinal detachment (13,14,39). Prophylactic treatment of these tears reduces the incidence of retinal detachment to 0% to 19% (12,37,38,41,43). Such treatment therefore seems justified.

Operculated Tears

Fresh[2] operculated tears are less likely to cause detachment than are fresh flap tears because the traction on the retina is released when the operculum is pulled free. Two small studies have shown that one out of six patients with untreated fresh operculated tears will develop a retinal detachment (13,14). In evaluating operculated tears for therapy, one must examine carefully the vitreoretinal relationship in the region of the tear. If the vitreous is adherent to the edge of the retinal break, the break should be considered the equivalent of a flap tear and should be treated. Fresh operculated tears should also be treated if they are large, superiorly located, or associated with vitreous hemorrhage (Fig. 12-1).

TABLE 12-1. *General indications for prophylactic therapy*

	Fellow eye	Pseudophakic eye	Symptomatic	Asymptomatic
Flap tear	Treat	Sometimes treat	Treat	Rarely treat
Operculated tear	Treat	Sometimes treat	Sometimes treat	—
Round hole	Sometimes treat	—	—	—
Lattice degeneration (with/without holes)	Sometimes treat	—	—	—

[1] A symptomatic tear is a tear caused by posterior vitreous detachment in the eye of a patient complaining of light flashes (photopsias) or floaters (entopsias). An atrophic round hole in lattice degeneration in a patient with floaters should not be considered symptomatic, because it is unrelated to the posterior vitreous detachment.

[2] A fresh tear is either a symptomatic tear or a tear found in a location where no tear was seen on prior ophthalmic examination.

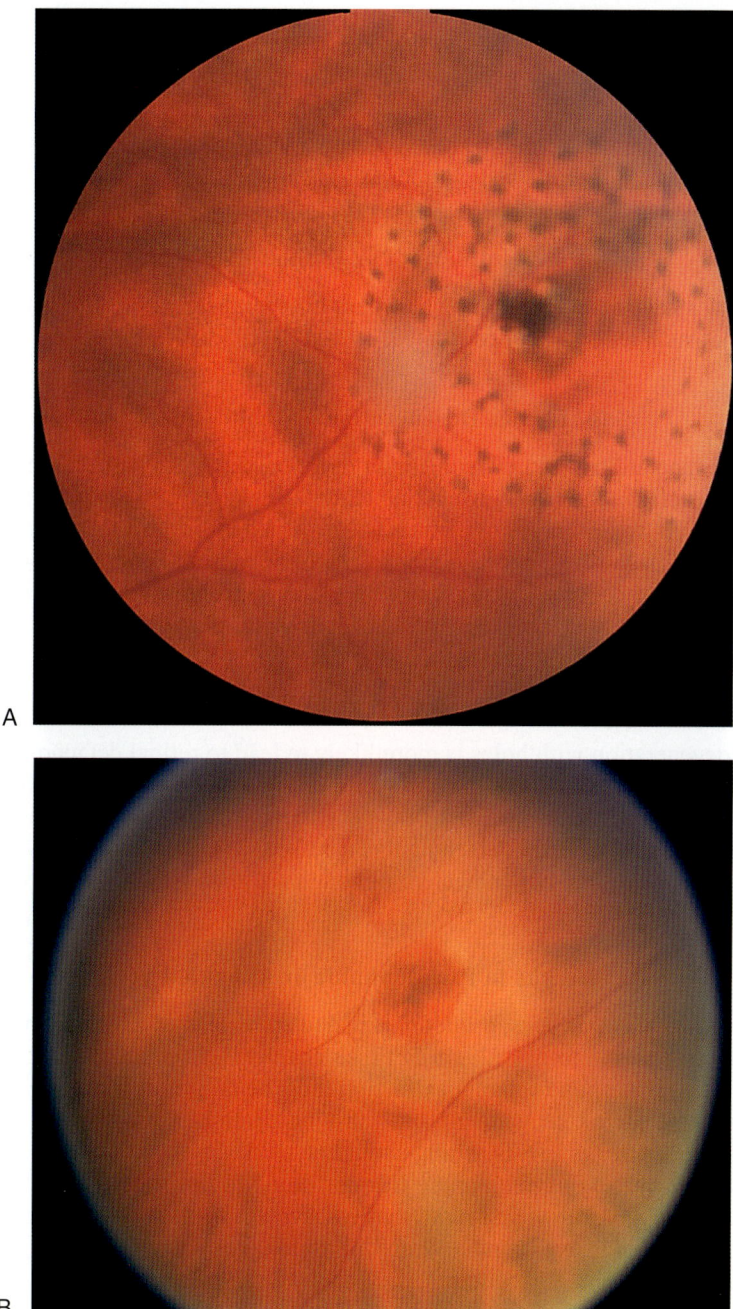

FIGURE 12-1. A: Operculated tear surrounded by argon laser burns. **B:** Operculated tear treated with a single spot of cryotherapy.

ASYMPTOMATIC BREAKS IN PATIENTS WITH NO HISTORY OF RETINAL DISEASE

Flap Tears

Eyes with asymptomatic flap tears have a low incidence of subsequent retinal detachment. Such tears can be followed without treatment (8,9,27,39).

Round Holes, With or Without Operculum

These holes have been found to be harmless in several series (8,9,27,39). No evidence suggests that such tears should be treated.

Lattice Degeneration Without Holes

Lattice degeneration is a known precursor of retinal detachment, because vitreous traction on its posterior edge may cause a flap tear (see chapter 3, Predisposing Conditions). This condition is found in approximately 41% of patients who undergo retinal detachment surgery (1). However, because it is known to be present in about 6% of the population (24), apparently only a few persons with lattice degeneration develop retinal detachment. No treatment is indicated for lattice degeneration without holes.

Lattice Degeneration With Holes

Lattice degeneration with holes is more likely to lead to retinal detachment than is lattice degeneration without holes because fluid may gain access to the subretinal space. Nevertheless, the risk is not great. Of the 66 patients with this entity followed by Byer (4), none developed a retinal detachment. Therefore, prophylactic therapy of lattice degeneration with holes is not indicated, although patients should be reexamined at 6-month intervals.

Breaks in Pseudophakic or Aphakic Eyes

Compared with phakic eyes, pseudophakic and aphakic eyes have a higher risk of retinal detachment, at 1% to 5% (29,40,52) (see chapter 3, Predisposing Conditions). Patients who have undergone cataract extraction must be aware of symptoms that could indicate a retinal tear or detachment and must be examined promptly and carefully if symptoms occur. Breaks in this setting should be treated.

The value of treating asymptomatic tears or round holes in pseudophakic or aphakic eyes, however, is not known. Several studies have shown that asymptomatic tears and round holes in aphakic eyes can be safely followed without treatment (28,39). However, if they are large or posteriorly located, they may warrant treatment.

BREAKS IN FELLOW EYES

Phakic Fellow Eyes

Approximately 10% of patients who develop retinal detachment in one eye later develop retinal detachment in the other, or fellow, eye (15,25,35). Davis and colleagues compiled the classic study on the natural history of "fellow" eyes (15). In their series, 7 of 42 fellow eyes with flap tears and 0 of 26 with operculated tears developed retinal detachment. They also found that 9 of 38 fellow eyes with lattice degeneration, 11 of 68 with focal pigmented spots, and 4 of 51 with vitreoretinal tags with traction had subsequent retinal detachment in the second eye. Hyams and associates followed 32 fellow eyes that developed fresh tears while under observation (27); 10 of these had retinal detachment soon after the advent of the fresh tear. In another study (35), 19% of 966 fellow eyes had retinal breaks, and 20% of these had subsequent retinal detachment. Clearly, patients who have had a retinal detachment in one eye are at high risk of detachment in the second eye.

Prophylactic therapy has proven beneficial in the treatment of fellow eye vitreoretinal abnormalities, particularly retinal tears (37,41). In Israel, after the introduction of prophylactic therapy, the incidence of retinal detachment in fellow eyes decreased from 11% to 3% (35,49). Routinely treating lattice degeneration (with or without holes) in fellow phakic eyes, however, has more recently been questioned. Although Folk and colleagues demonstrated a significant reduction in both new breaks and retinal detachments in eyes that received prophylactic treatment (18), the risk of detachment was low in both treated and untreated groups (1.8% and 5.1%, respectively). From the standpoint of the cost-to-benefit ratio, treatment of lattice in all fellow eyes may not be justified.

Pseudophakic or Aphakic Fellow Eyes With Breaks

The incidence of retinal detachment in pseudophakic and aphakic fellow eyes is two to three times that of phakic fellow eyes (2,10,15). In this high-risk group, prophylactic treatment of all retinal breaks, and possibly also lattice degeneration and vitreoretinal tags, is beneficial (2,34).

Fellow Eyes of Patients With Giant Tear

In a large study by Freeman (22), 59.8% of patients with a giant tear (defined as a tear that is 90 degrees or larger) in one eye subsequently developed retinal breaks or detachments in the other eye. Fellow eyes at high risk were those that had high myopia and extensive lattice degeneration. Even in fellow eyes that had normal-appearing fundi or just white with pressure, the rate of break formation was 24%. Needless to say, fellow eyes of patients with giant retinal tears need to be followed closely, regardless of how benign the fellow eye may appear to be on initial examination.

Treatment of the peripheral retina for 360 degrees, whether or not any vitreoretinal abnormalities are present, has been advocated for fellow eyes to prevent retinal detachment. Scatter laser photocoagulation from the equator to the ora can be easily applied with the laser indirect ophthalmoscope and is better tolerated than cryotherapy to the same area for 360 degrees (44). For fellow eyes with other risk factors as described earlier, prophylactic scleral buckling (SB) has been advocated (22).

BREAKS IN MYOPIC EYES

Because extremely myopic eyes have a relatively high risk of retinal detachment, some surgeons treat all breaks found, even asymptomatic round holes (see chapter 3, Predisposing Conditions). Data from Israel have shown that, even in myopes, asymptomatic breaks are unlikely to cause a subsequent detachment (28). Because many patients with myopic eyes with asymptomatic breaks never develop a retinal detachment, they need not be treated.

BREAKS IN DEGENERATIVE RETINOSCHISIS

On routine autopsy examination of eyes with no history of ocular disease, nearly 1% had degenerative (senile) retinoschisis with outer wall holes (21). Hirose and colleagues followed a large number of patients with degenerative retinoschisis to determine the natural history of the condition (26). Retinal detachment did not develop in any of the 25 eyes with outer wall holes or in any of the 6 eyes with both inner and outer wall holes. They also observed an additional 245 cases of retinoschisis without holes. Nine developed outer wall holes during the period of observation; retinal detachment occurred subsequently in 3 of them. Byer followed 14 patients with localized, asymptomatic retinoschisis–retinal detachments (7). None progressed to symptomatic detachment.

Because of the low incidence of retinal detachment and because retinal detachments caused by retinoschisis progress slowly, most outer wall holes should not be treated. Byer suggests that the sole indication for treatment should be progression of full-thickness detachment (7). However, treatment also may be considered for large, multiple, or posteriorly located holes or for holes found in the fellow eye of a patient who has had a retinoschisis–retinal detachment in the other eye (26).

SUBCLINICAL RETINAL DETACHMENT

Retinal detachment is referred to as "subclinical" if subretinal fluid (SRF) extends at least one disc diameter from the retinal break, but no more than two disc diameters posterior to the equator (Fig. 12-2) (14). Because 30% of such detachments progress (14), treatment is indicated. Surgical repair with SB, pneumatic retinopexy (PR), or temporary balloon buckling is generally necessary.

However, if little or no vitreous traction is present, cryotherapy or photocoagulation combined with bed rest may promote settling of the retina and sealing of the break. Treatment should be applied adjacent to the break, but also to a 3- to 4-mm band of attached retina surrounding the subclinical detachment (see Fig. 12-2). In this way, the

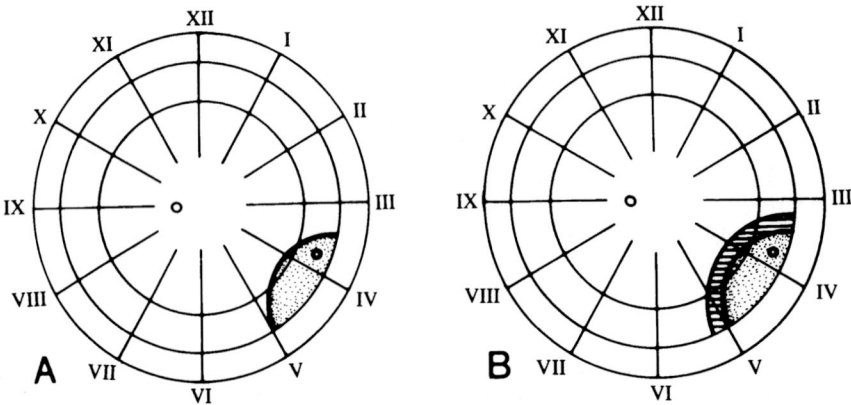

FIGURE 12-2. A: Subclinical retinal detachment. **B:** Walling-off technique used in selected cases (see text). The treatment *(dark band)* must extend 3 to 4 mm into attached retina and to the ora serrata.

detachment may be successfully walled off even if the retina does not settle (see also chapter 9, Alternative Techniques). It is of critical importance that such treatment extend to the ora serrata to prevent anterior leakage of SRF. This technique for containing a subclinical detachment may also be tried in the treatment of other types of detachment for patients who refuse or cannot undergo SB or other retinal reattachment procedures. Roseman and colleagues used this treatment in 228 eyes (45), 95% of which did not progress. Twelve of the 13 that progressed were successfully attached with SB.

RETINAL BREAKS WITH BRIDGING VESSELS

Generally, when vitreous traction tears the retina, it also tears the retinal vessels crossing the break. In some cases, however, an untorn vessel may cross over or "bridge" the break. The continued vitreous traction on this vessel can cause recurrent vitreous hemorrhage (42). It can also pull on the posterior edge of the retinal break (Fig. 12-3). This additional traction may prevent successful treatment of a flap tear by photocoagulation or cryotherapy alone. Therefore, any patient who has been treated with either of these modalities should be examined at intervals of 2 to 3 days until a firm adhesion develops. Some authors believe that tears with bridging vessels are sufficiently dangerous that all should be treated with SB procedures (51). Other investigators have found that hemorrhages are likely to recur no matter what the treatment until the vessel ruptures (16,42).

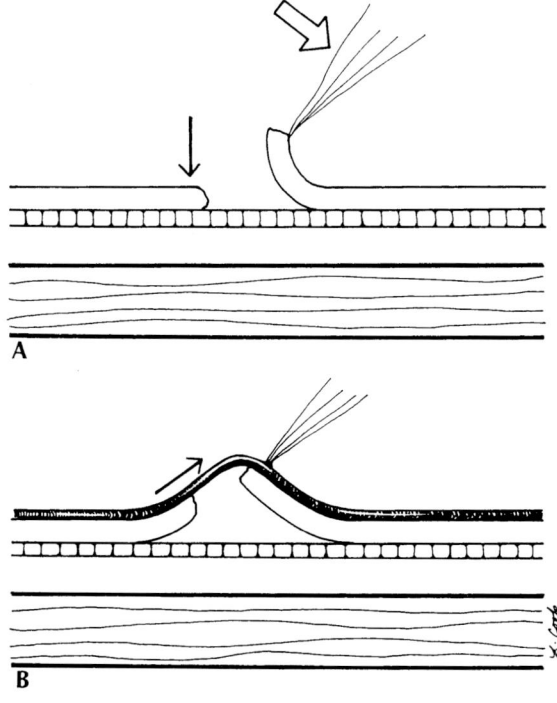

FIGURE 12-3. A: Bridging vessels: a flap tear with no bridging vessel. Vitreous traction (*open arrow*) on the flap is not transmitted to the posterior margin of the tear (*arrow*). **B:** When a vessel bridges a flap tear, vitreous traction is transmitted to the posterior margin. Cryotherapy may not suffice to close the break.

TREATMENT TECHNIQUE

Cryotherapy and laser photocoagulation are the modalities currently used in the prophylactic treatment of retinal breaks. Clinically, they are probably of equal efficacy, although animal studies show faster chorioretinal adhesion with laser photocoagulation (19,33,53). Complications of treatment with these techniques are comparably low (see later). With the advent of the laser indirect ophthalmoscope delivery system, most breaks are readily approachable with laser photocoagulation. Because patients usually have less ocular discomfort during and immediately after treatment with laser photocoagulation compared with cryotherapy, the former is more commonly used to treat breaks. However, cryotherapy is still sometimes preferred over photocoagulation for extremely anterior breaks, especially if the media are not entirely clear, such as from cataract or vitreous hemorrhage.

No matter which is chosen, the cardinal rule of treatment is to surround the break adequately. The most common cause of subsequent retinal detachment is inadequate treatment anterior to flap tears (Fig. 12-4) (3,17,43). Continued vitreous traction can extend

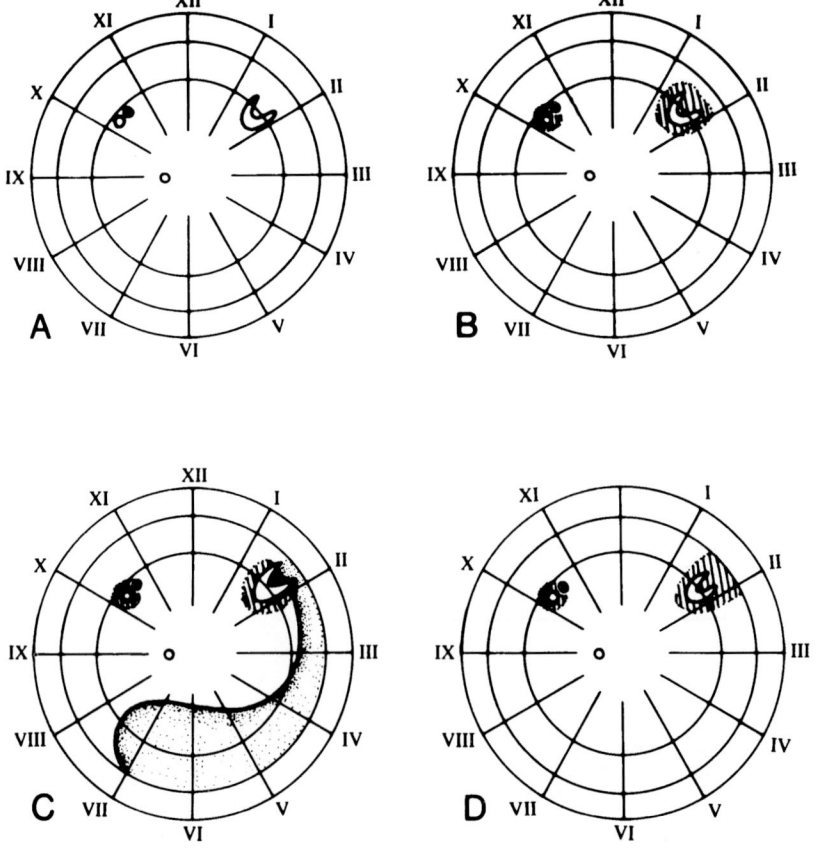

FIGURE 12-4. Proper treatment of retinal tears. **A:** Preoperative drawing: flap tear at the 1:30 position; operculated tear at the 10:30 position. **B:** Adequate treatment of the operculated tear and inadequate treatment of the flap tear. Its treatment should extend to the ora serrata. **C:** Increased vitreous traction has extended the flap tear through the cryotherapy scar. Anterior leakage causes a retinal detachment. **D:** Properly treated tears. Treatment of the flap tear extends to the ora serrata.

the flap anteriorly, allowing leakage of SRF and giving rise to a detachment. For breaks associated with lattice degeneration, both the tear and the adjacent patch of lattice should be completely surrounded.

Laser Photocoagulation

The technique consists of applying two or three rows of relatively large, nearly contiguous, moderate-intensity spots completely around the retinal tear (Fig. 12-5). For flap tears, treatment should extend to the ora serrata. Laser is delivered with either the slit-lamp biomicroscope and a mirrored fundus contact lens or the indirect ophthalmoscope and a handheld condensing lens. Indirect ophthalmoscope delivery systems are more versatile; with scleral depression, treatment to the ora can be performed routinely. No anesthesia is needed except for topical drops (proparacaine 0.5%) if a contact lens is used or if scleral depression directly on the globe is needed.

The usual laser parameters are as follows: green wavelength, 0.1- to 0.2-second duration, 200- to 500-µm spot size, and 200-mW power to start. Any visible light laser (or even diode laser infrared) wavelength can be used; argon green is most readily available and, if the media are clear, is most commonly used. For the same visible end point, diode infrared laser tends to be more painful. Heavier and larger spots provide better chorioretinal adhesion (30,31), but care must be taken not to produce too heavy a burn because this can cause retinal holes and breaks through Bruch's membrane with secondary choriovitreous anastomoses. The average spot size produced by the laser indirect ophthalmoscope is about 300 µm.

No significant pain or redness is present after laser treatment of a retinal tear. No postoperative drops are needed. Patients sometimes experience light flashes for the first few days after treatment, but they should not expect to have increased floaters or any loss of peripheral vision.

Cryotherapy

Cryotherapy is applied transconjunctivally using the indirect ophthalmoscope to visualize the effects on the retina. As with laser photocoagulation, the break must be completely surrounded. Applications are placed in a contiguous, slightly overlapping fashion, avoiding freezing of bare retinal pigment epithelium (RPE). In general, a 2-mm rim around operculated breaks and round holes suffices. As mentioned previously, treatment of flap tears is extended to the ora serrata, lest continued vitreous traction extend them through cryotherapy scars, allowing anterior leakage of SRF (see Fig. 12-4) (3,43). The end point of each application is whitening of the retina; significant freezing of the overlying vitreous gel, evident by visible crystal formation, should be avoided.

Some form of local anesthesia is needed with cryotherapy. With limited treatments, topical anesthesia alone is often adequate. Proparacaine 0.5% solution is instilled in the eye, and then a cotton pledget soaked in the same solution (or cocaine 10%) is placed for a few minutes in the quadrant in which the breaks are located. If this is not adequate anesthesia or if more extensive treatments are needed, lidocaine 1% solution is injected subconjunctivally. Retrobulbar anesthesia is rarely necessary. (Its complications are discussed in chapter 7, Scleral Buckling Procedure.)

Eyes after cryotherapy often have varying degrees of achiness, injection, and chemosis. Unless extensive cryotherapy is performed, signs and symptoms are usually mild and go away within a few days. Oral acetaminophen may be needed the first night after treat-

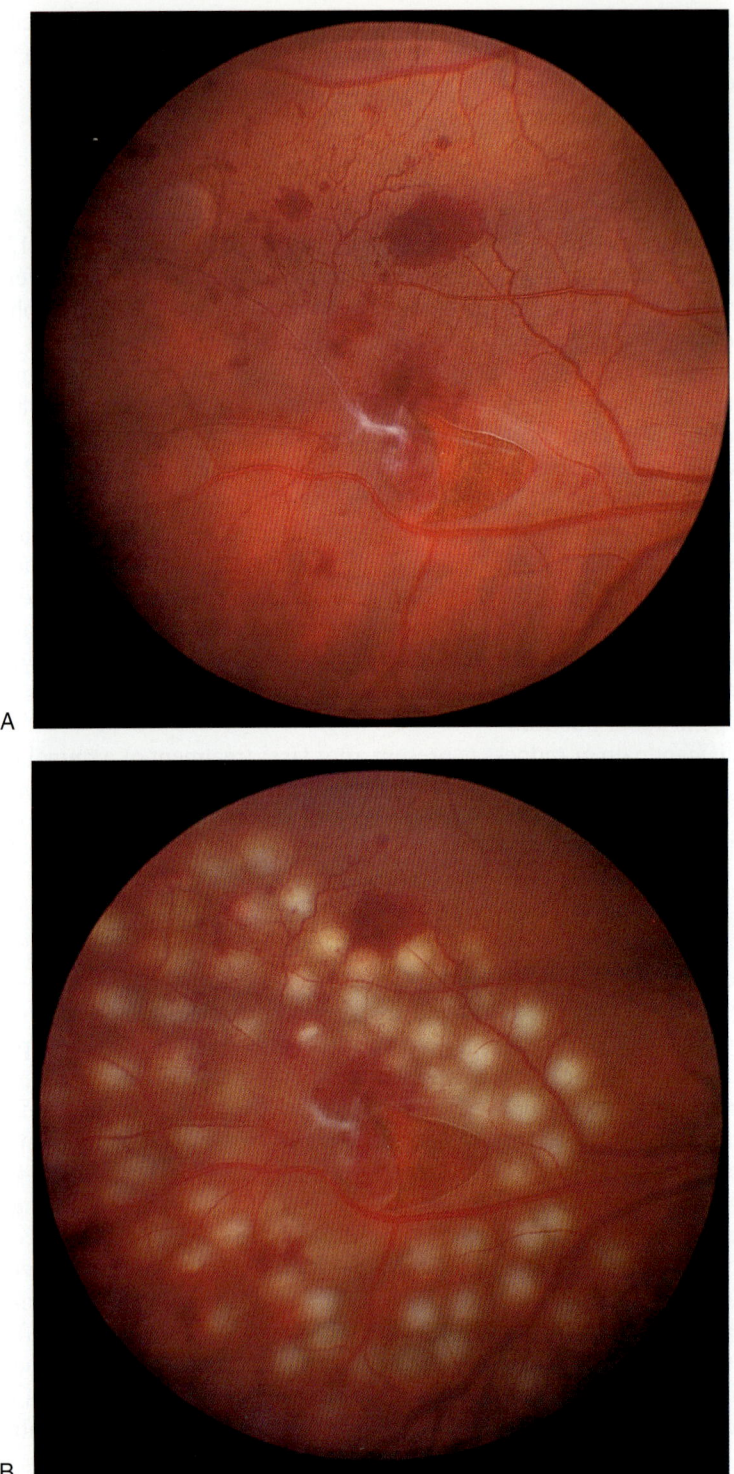

FIGURE 12-5. A: Posteriorly located flap tear before treatment. **B:** Same flap tear after photocoagulation. More treatment has been given anteriorly than posteriorly so the tear will still be contained if traction extends it.

ment. A mild topical corticosteroid drop such as fluorometholone 0.1% instilled four times daily may be used for several days.

TREATMENT FOLLOW-UP

All patients who receive prophylactic therapy for a retinal break must be followed closely and urged to return immediately if they have any visual field loss. Because the treatment may actually initially weaken the normal adhesion between the retina and RPE, a recheck about 1 week after the initial treatment is recommended to make sure that the break or any associated SRF has not extended beyond the treated area.

Even if a patient has had successful treatment, routine follow-up examinations thereafter are still important. Up to 14% of eyes develop new breaks, with or without detachment, at some point after treatment of a retinal tear (23,32,48). Although most new breaks manifest within the first few months after treatment and are symptomatic, nearly one-quarter of them may occur many months later and occasionally may be asymptomatic (48). Furthermore, patients who develop a retinal break in one eye are at risk for developing breaks in the fellow eye at some point during follow-up, and therefore both eyes should be examined.

MACULAR PUCKER

Complications related directly to the treatment of retinal breaks are rare with either laser photocoagulation or cryotherapy. In eyes with retinal tears, macular epiretinal membranes have been reported to occur in up to 10% of cases treated with cryotherapy and up to 14% of cases treated with laser photocoagulation (47). Significant surface wrinkling or macular pucker with decreased vision, however, occurs much less frequently, probably on the order of 1% to 2% of treated eyes (12,32,36,43).

Because epiretinal membranes and pucker can occur spontaneously, especially in eyes with retinal tears, the causative role of the therapy is difficult to determine (43). It seems likely, however, that the therapy can cause pucker in some cases, especially when extensive treatment has been given (44). However, despite experimental data that suggest that pucker would be more common after cryotherapy (11), clinical data have yet to show a significant difference between the treatment modalities (47).

ROLE OF EDUCATION IN PREVENTING VISUAL LOSS

A patient who is familiar with the symptoms of a retinal tear or detachment is much more likely to report promptly after its onset. In doing so, the chances of preserving vision are maximized. Many more retinal tears are likely to be detected before going on to retinal detachment. Preventing retinal detachment obviously preserves vision. Furthermore, by avoiding a retinal reattachment procedure, patients' suffering and inconvenience are minimized, and health care dollars are likely to be saved.

Once retinal detachment has started, patients who delay in presenting for treatment are more likely to have macular detachment or significant proliferative vitreoretinopathy (PVR). Visual acuity is lost as a result of the former, and retinal reattachment is jeopardized by the latter. In a large series of phakic retinal detachments, the macula was found to be involved in 65% of eyes (1). In contrast, a study of detachments in fellow phakic eyes had a macular involving rate of only 25% (15). The difference between the two figures seems to be largely caused by the prior experience of the patients in the latter study with retinal detachment.

Three studies that compare retinal detachments in first eyes with those in fellow eyes prove that this foreknowledge contributes to higher rates of reattachment as well as better visual results. In a series of phakic retinal detachments by Davis and colleagues (15), successful retinal reattachment was achieved in 91% of eyes in patients without a prior history of retinal detachment and in 98% of eyes in patients with a history of retinal detachment in the fellow eye. Similar differences in outcomes were reported in a series published by Tani and colleagues (50). More dramatically, a report on aphakic retinal detachments by Benson and colleagues showed rates of reattachment to be 83% in first eyes and 96% in fellow eyes (2). This study also showed that the rate of retaining a visual acuity of 20/50 or better in the two groups was 45% and 72%, respectively.

In general, all patients who have risk factors for developing retinal detachment—high myopia, pseudophakia or aphakia, and lattice degeneration—should be taught the symptoms of a retinal tear and detachment and urged to report promptly if any symptoms are perceived. They, as well as patients who have already had a retinal detachment, should be trained to check their own peripheral fields at regular intervals.

REFERENCES

1. Ashrafzadeh MT, Schepens CL, Elzeneiny IH, et al. Aphakic and phakic retinal detachment. *Arch Ophthalmol* 1973;89:476.
2. Benson WE, Grand MG, Okun E. Aphakic retinal detachment. Management of the fellow eye. *Arch Ophthalmol* 1975;93:245–249.
3. Benson WE, Morse PH, Nantawan P. Late complications following cryotherapy of lattice degeneration. *Am J Ophthalmol* 1977;84:514–516.
4. Byer NE. Changes in and prognosis of lattice degeneration of the retina. *Trans Am Acad Ophthalmol Otolaryngol* 1974;78:114–125.
5. Byer NE. Clinical study of lattice degeneration of the retina. *Trans Am Acad Ophthalmol Otolaryngol* 1965;69:1064–1081.
6. Byer NE. Clinical study of retinal breaks. *Trans Am Acad Ophthalmol Otolaryngol* 1967;71:461–473.
7. Byer NE. Long-term natural history of senile retinoschisis with implications for management. *Ophthalmology* 1986;93:1127–1136.
8. Byer NE. The natural history of asymptomatic retinal breaks. *Ophthalmology* 1982;89:1033–1039.
9. Byer NE. Prognosis of asymptomatic retinal breaks. *Arch Ophthalmol* 1974;92:208–210.
10. Campbell CJ, Rittler MC. Cataract extraction in the retinal detachment prone patient. *Am J Ophthalmol* 1972;73:17.
11. Campochiaro PA, Kaden IH, Vidaurri-Leal J, Glaser BM. Cryotherapy enhances intravitreal dispersion of viable retinal pigment epithelial cells. *Arch Ophthalmol* 1985;103:434–436.
12. Chignell AH, Schilling J. Prophylaxis of retinal detachment. *Br J Ophthalmol* 1973;57:291–298.
13. Colyear BHJ, Piscel DK. Clinical tears in the retina without detachment. *Am J Ophthalmol* 1956;41:773.
14. Davis MD. Natural history of retinal breaks without detachment. *Arch Ophthalmol* 1974;92:183–194.
15. Davis MD, Segal PP, MacCormack A. The natural course followed by the fellow eye in patients with rhegmatogenous retinal detachment. In: Pruett RC, Regan CDJ, eds. *Retinal Congress.* New York: Appleton-Century-Crofts, 1972:643–660.
16. deBustros S, Welch RB. The avulsed retinal vessel syndrome and its variants. *Ophthalmology* 1984;91:86–88.
17. Delaney WV Jr. Retinal tear extension through the cryosurgical scar. *Br J Ophthalmol* 1971;55:205–209.
18. Folk JC, Arrindell EL, Klugman MR. The fellow eye of patients with phakic lattice retinal detachment. *Ophthalmology* 1989;96:72–79.
19. Folk JC, Sneed SR, Folberg R, Coonan P, Pulido JS. Early retinal adhesion from laser photocoagulation. *Ophthalmology* 1989;96:1523–1525.
20. Foos RY. Posterior vitreous detachment. *Trans Am Acad Ophthalmol Otolaryngol* 1972;76:480–497.
21. Foos RY. Senile retinoschisis. *Trans Am Acad Ophthalmol Otolaryngol* 1970;74:33–51.
22. Freeman HM. Fellow eye of nontraumatic giant retinal breaks. In: Lewis H, Ryan SJ, eds. *Medical and Surgical Retina: Advances, Controversies, and Management.* St. Louis: Mosby–Year Book, 1994:222–225.
23. Goldberg RE, Boyer DS. Sequential retinal breaks following a spontaneous initial retinal break. *Ophthalmology* 1981;88:10–12.
24. Halpern JI. Routine screening of the retinal periphery. *Am J Ophthalmol* 1966;62:99.

25. Haut J, Massin M. Fréquence des décollements de rétine dans la population française: pourcente des décollements bilateraux. *Arch Ophthalmol* 1975;35:533.
26. Hirose T, Marcil G, Schepens CL, et al. Acquired retinoschisis, observations and treatment. In: Pruett RC, Regan CDJ, eds. *Retinal Congress*. New York: Appleton-Century-Crofts, 1972:489–504.
27. Hyams SW, Meir E, Ivry M, et al. Chorioretinal lesions predisposing to retinal detachment. *Am J Ophthalmol* 1974;78:429–437.
28. Hyams SW, Neumann E, Friedman Z. Myopia–aphakia. II. Vitreous and peripheral retina. *Br J Ophthalmol* 1975;59:483–485.
29. Javitt JC, Vitale S, Canner JK, Krakauer H, McBean AM, Sommer A. National outcomes of cataract extraction. I. Retinal detachment after inpatient surgery. *Ophthalmology* 1991;98:895–902.
30. Kain HL. A new model for examining chorioretinal adhesion experimentally. *Arch Ophthalmol* 1984;102:608–611.
31. Kain HL. Chorioretinal adhesion after argon laser photocoagulation. *Arch Ophthalmol* 1984;102:612–615.
32. Kanski JJ, Daniel R. Prophylaxis of retinal detachment. *Am J Ophthalmol* 1975;79:197–205.
33. Kita M, Negi A, Kawano S, Honda Y. Photothermal, cryogenic, and diathermic effects of retinal adhesive force in vivo. *Retina* 1991;11:441–444.
34. McCuen BWD, Azen SP, Stern W, et al. Vitrectomy with silicone oil or perfluoropropane gas in eyes with severe proliferative vitreoretinopathy: Silicone Study Report 3. *Retina* 1993;13:279–284.
35. Merin S, Feiler V, Hyams S, et al. The fate of the fellow eye in retinal detachment. *Am J Ophthalmol* 1971;71:477–481.
36. Mester U, Volker B, Kroll P, Berg P. Complications of prophylactic argon laser treatment of retinal breaks and degenerations in 2,000 eyes. *Ophthalmic Surg* 1988;19:482–484.
37. Morse PH, Scheie HG. Prophylactic cryoretinopexy of retinal breaks. *Arch Ophthalmol* 1974;92:204–207.
38. Nadel AJ, Gieser RG. The treatment of acute horseshoe tears by transconjunctival cryopexy. *Ann Ophthalmol* 1975;7:1568.
39. Neumann E, Hyams S. Conservative management of retinal breaks: a follow-up study of subsequent retinal detachment. *Br J Ophthalmol* 1972;56:482–486.
40. Ninn-Pedersen K, Bauer B. Cataract patients in a defined Swedish population, 1986 to 1990. V. Postoperative retinal detachments. *Arch Ophthalmol* 1996;114:382–386.
41. Pollak A, Oliver M. Argon laser photocoagulation of symptomatic flap tears and retinal breaks of fellow eyes. *Br J Ophthalmol* 1981;65:469–472.
42. Robertson DM, Curtin VT, Norton EW. Avulsed retinal vessels with retinal breaks; a cause of recurrent vitrous hemorrhage. *Arch Ophthalmol* 1971;85:669–672.
43. Robertson DM, Norton EWD. Long-term follow-up of treated retinal breaks. *Am J Ophthalmol* 1973;75:395–404.
44. Robertson DM, Priluck IA. 3600 prophylactic cryoretinopexy: a clinical and experimental study. *Arch Ophthalmol* 1979;97:2130–2134.
45. Roseman RL, Olk RJ, Arribas NP, et al. Limited retinal detachment: a retrospective analysis of treatment with transconjunctival retinocryopexy. *Ophthalmology* 1986;93:216–223.
46. Rutnin U, Schepens CL. Fundus appearance in normal eyes. IV. Retinal breaks and other findings. *Am J Ophthalmol* 1967;64:1063–1078.
47. Saran BR, Brucker AJ. Macular epiretinal membrane formation and treated retinal breaks. *Am J Ophthalmol* 1995;120:480–485.
48. Smiddy WE, Flynn HW, Jr., Nicholson DH, et al. Results and complications in treated retinal breaks. *Am J Ophthalmol* 1991;112:623–631.
49. Stein R, Feller-Ofry V, Romano A. The effect of treatment on the prevention of retinal detachment. In: Michaelson I, Berman E, eds. *Causes and Prevention of Blindness*. New York: Academic Press, 1972:409–410.
50. Tani P, Robertson DM, Langworthy A. Prognosis for central vision and anatomic reattachment in rhegmatogenous retinal detachment with macula detached. *Am J Ophthalmol* 1981;92:611–620.
51. Theodossiadis GP, Koutsandrea CN. Avulsed retinal vessels with and without retinal breaks: treatment and extended follow-up. *Trans Ophthalmol Soc U K* 1985;104:887.
52. Wilkes SR, Beard CM, Kurland LT, Robertson DM, O'Fallon WM. The incidence of retinal detachment in Rochester, Minnesota, 1970–1978. *Am J Ophthalmol* 1982;94:670–673.
53. Yoon YH, Marmor MF. Rapid enhancement of retinal adhesion by laser photocoagulation. *Ophthalmology* 1988;95:1385–1388.

Appendix

This appendix is intended to serve as a guide to the management of various types of retinal detachment and as a review of some of the principles of treatment.

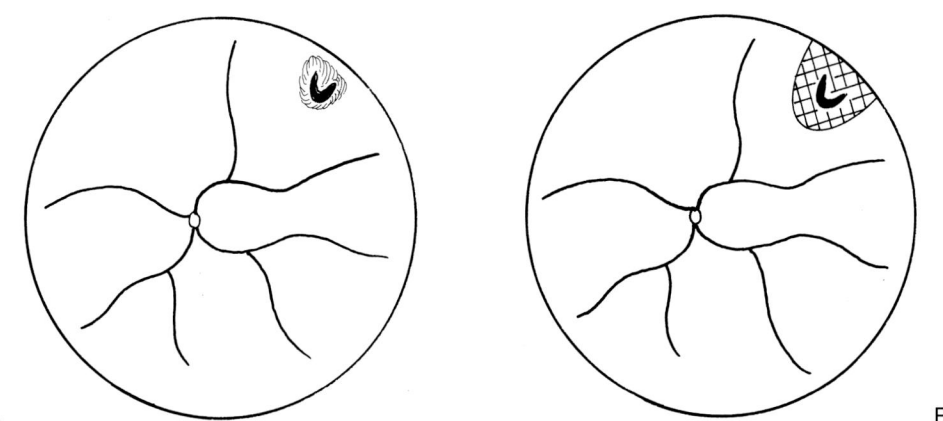

FIGURE A-1. *Case 1.* **A:** Flap tear with a small rim of subretinal fluid. **B**: Cryotherapy or laser photocoagulation without scleral buckling usually suffices to seal the break. After treatment, the patient must be examined at close intervals to ensure that a good chorioretinal scar develops and the subretinal fluid resolves. In some cases, the detachment may spread before a firm retinopexy adhesion forms.

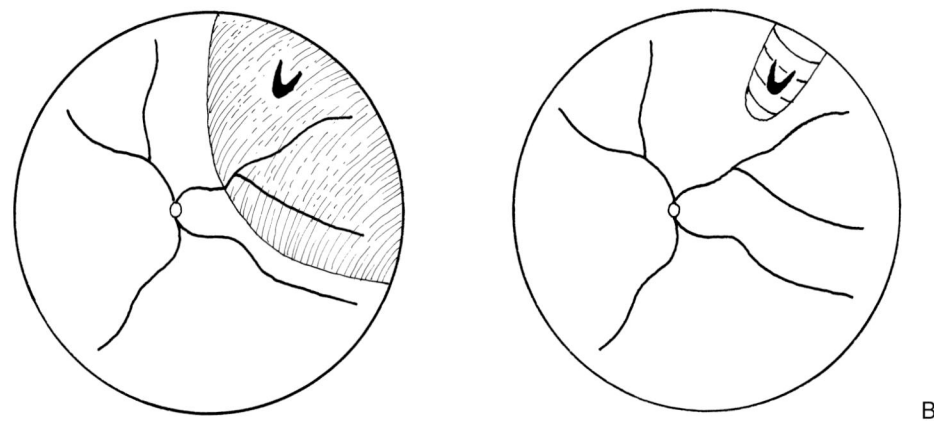

FIGURE A-2. *Case 2.* **A:** Flap tear with more extensive retinal detachment than was present in case 1. Treatment options include pneumatic retinopexy, temporary balloon buckling, and conventional scleral buckling. If pneumatic retinopexy is chosen, a steamroller maneuver should be considered to avoid detaching the macula. **B:** If scleral buckling is chosen, a radial sponge is the preferred technique; radial sponges cause less "fishmouthing" of flap tears than do circumferential elements.

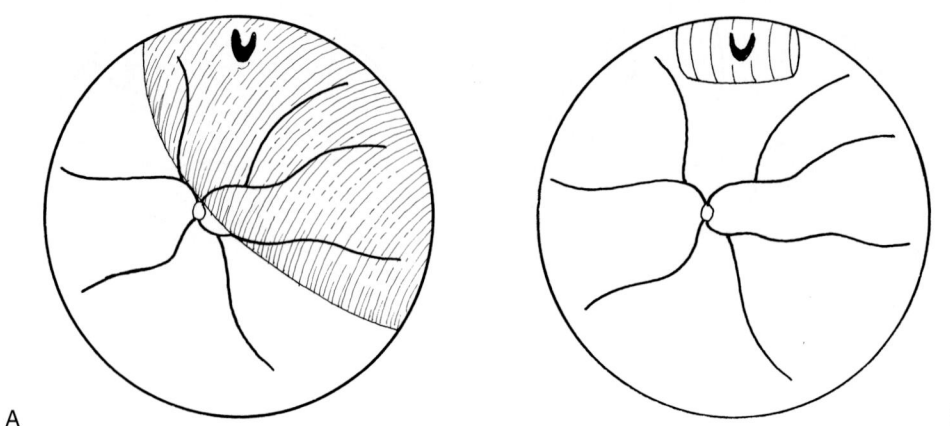

FIGURE A-3. *Case 3.* **A:** Retinal detachment caused by a flap tear under the superior rectus muscle. As with case 2, pneumatic retinopexy, temporary balloon buckling, and conventional scleral buckling are all options. **B:** If scleral buckling is chosen, a circumferential, rather than a radial, sponge is used to avoid placing excessive buckling material under the superior rectus muscle.

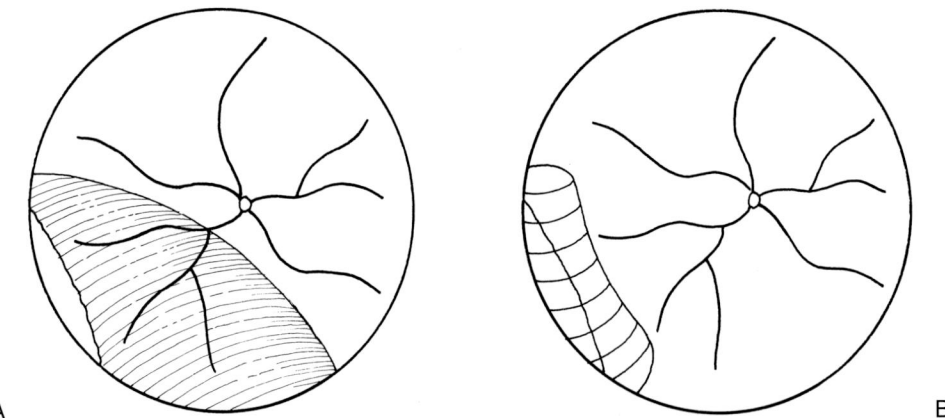

FIGURE A-4. *Case 4.* **A:** Retinal detachment caused by an inferotemporal dialysis. **B:** Scleral buckling with a circumferential sponge explant is the preferred approach.

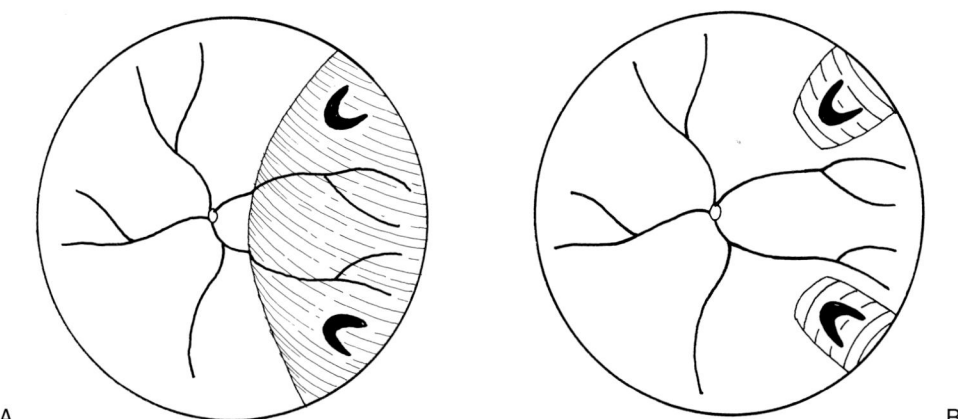

FIGURE A-5. *Case 5.* **A:** Retinal detachment caused by two, relatively large flap tears. **B:** This is best approached with scleral buckling using two radial sponges.

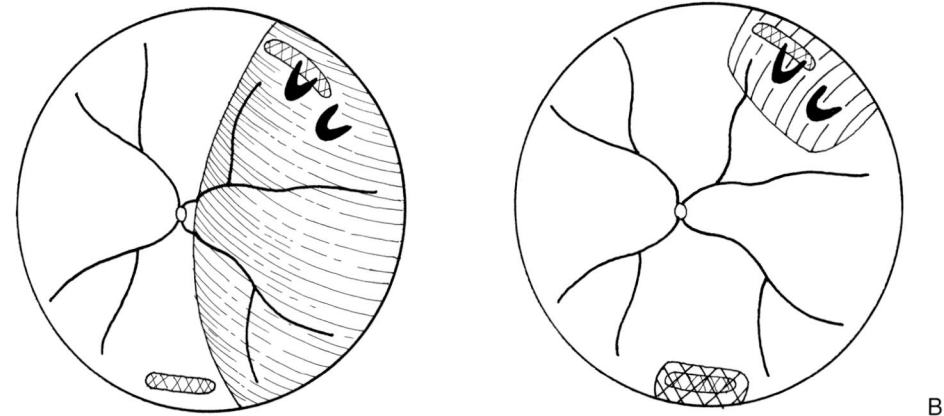

FIGURE A-6. *Case 6.* **A:** Retinal detachment caused by two flap tears. A small patch of lattice degeneration is present adjacent to the tears and another patch is seen inferiorly. **B:** Although this is approachable with pneumatic retinopexy or balloon buckling, we would opt for scleral buckling with a circumferential element to treat the detachment itself and cryotherapy or laser photocoagulation to treat the inferior lattice patch.

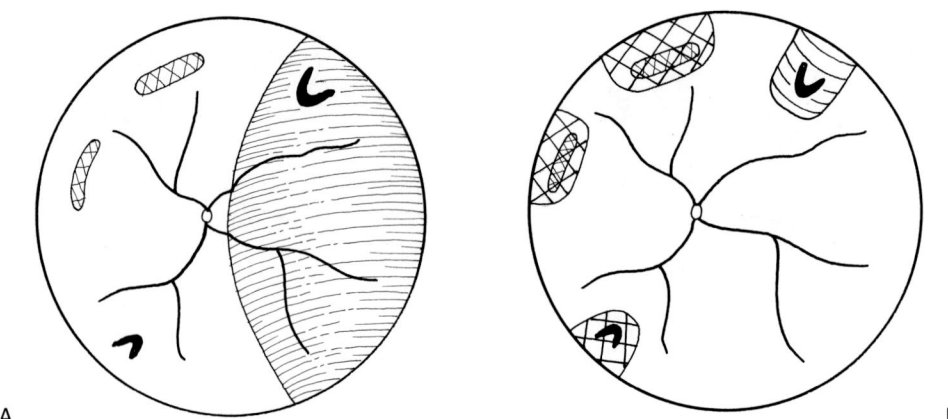

FIGURE A-7. *Case 7.* **A:** Retinal detachment caused by a superotemporal flap tear. Two large patches of lattice degeneration and a flap tear are present in attached retina. **B:** Compared with case 6, more extensive vitreoretinal disease occurs outside the detachment; scleral buckling should be performed. A radial sponge is best for the flap tear. The other abnormalities are treated with cryotherapy or laser photocoagulation.

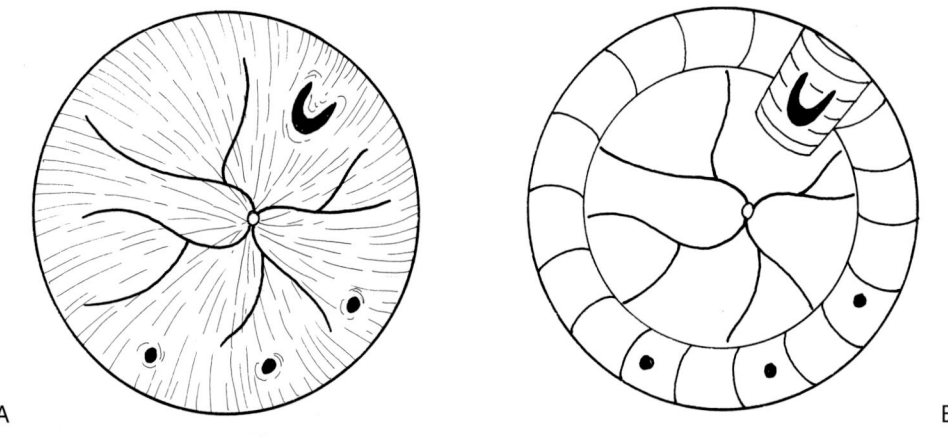

FIGURE A-8. *Case 8.* **A:** Total retinal detachment caused by a flap tear and three round holes. **B:** Scleral buckling repair consists of using a radial sponge to close the flap tear and an encircling band to support the round holes. Alternatively, the round holes can be closed with a segmental, circumferential element.

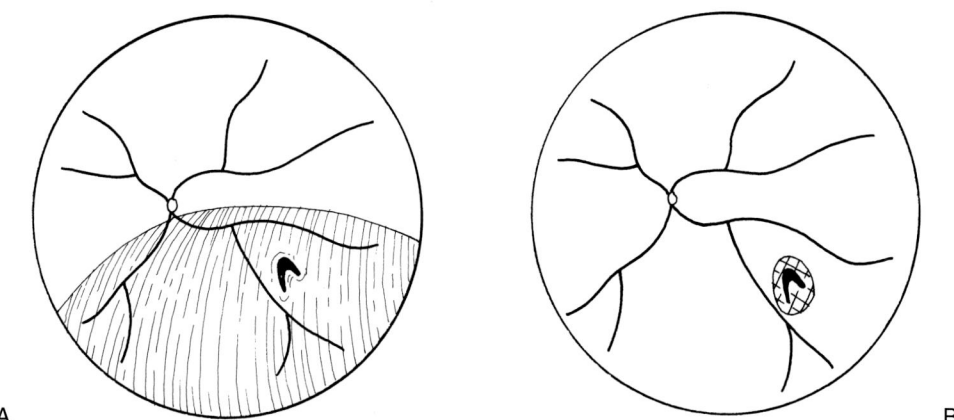

FIGURE A-9. *Case 9.* **A:** Retinal detachment caused by a posterior, inferior flap tear. Repair options include pneumatic retinopexy, temporary balloon buckling, and pars plana vitrectomy. **B**: For extremely posterior breaks, vitrectomy is the preferred approach. The subretinal fluid is drained internally through the break, and a complete fluid–gas exchange is performed for postoperative tamponade.

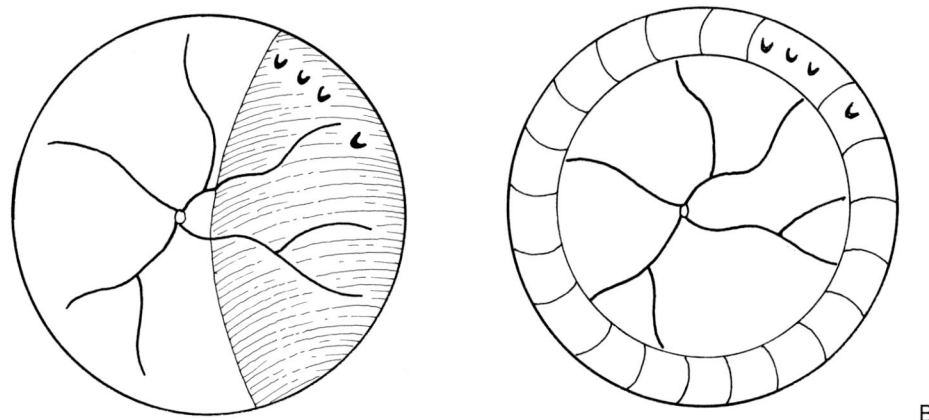

FIGURE A-10. *Case 10.* **A:** Pseudophakic retinal detachment caused by four small flap tears at the posterior vitreous base. **B:** The best approach is scleral buckling using an encircling band to close all the breaks and to support the entire vitreous base. Encircling allows one to close any small, undetected breaks and to counter any subsequent proliferative vitreoretinopathy, both of which are more common in pseudophakic or aphakic eyes compared with phakic eyes.

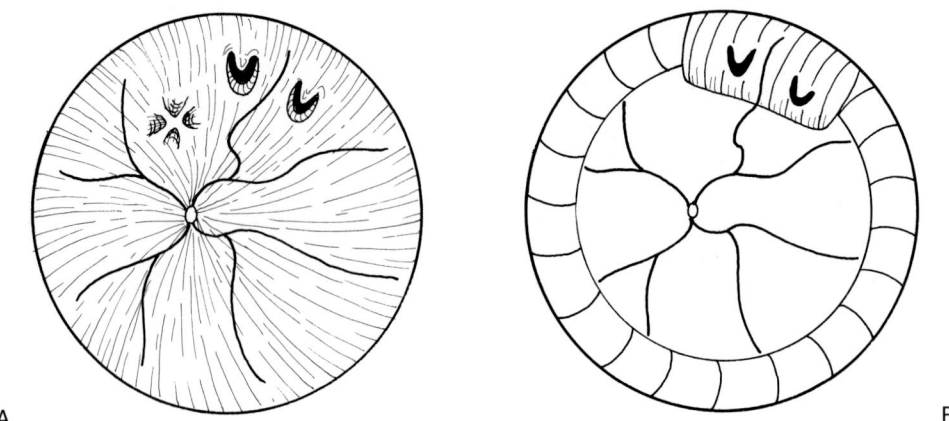

FIGURE A-11. *Case 11.* **A:** Retinal detachment caused by two flap tears. Early proliferative vitreoretinopathy is indicated by the posteriorly rolled edges of the tears and by the fixed fold superonasally. **B**: Many of these cases can be successfully managed with a scleral buckling procedure. The tears are closed by a circumferential explant, and, as in case 10, an encircling band is used to counter vitreous traction elsewhere.

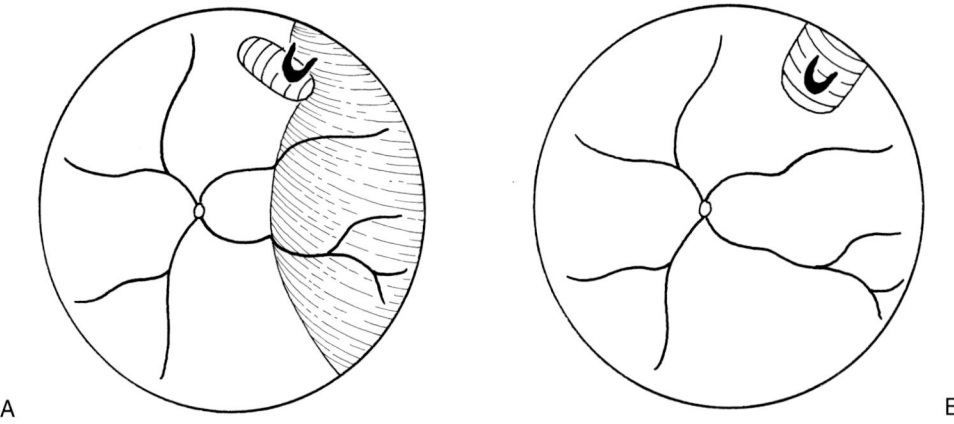

FIGURE A-12. *Case 12.* **A:** Failure to reattach the retina. The buckle does not support the anterior horns of the flap tear. Postoperative pneumatic retinopexy can often result in successful repair. **B**: Alternatively, one can revise the scleral buckling procedure by replacing the original element with a larger one.

APPENDIX

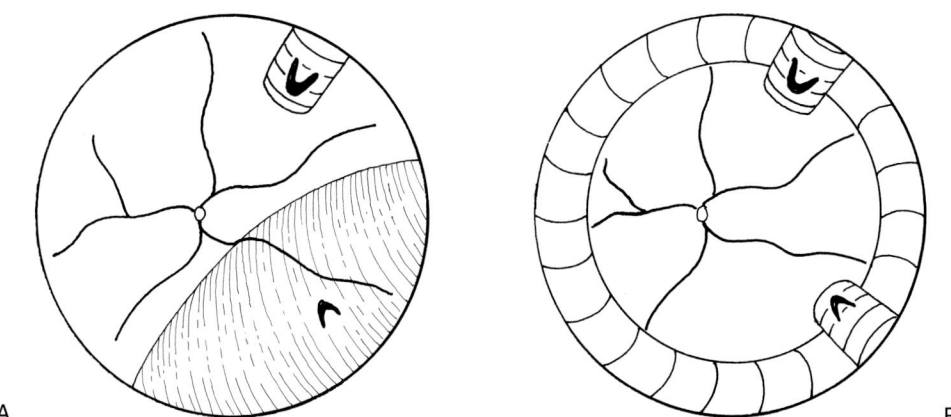

FIGURE A-13. *Case 13.* **A:** Redetachment of the retina caused by a new flap tear located inferiorly. A temporary balloon buckle could be used to close the new tear. **B**: However, because the new tear indicates increased vitreous traction, we would opt to treat the new tear with a radial sponge and use a band to encircle the eye as prophylaxis against future tears.

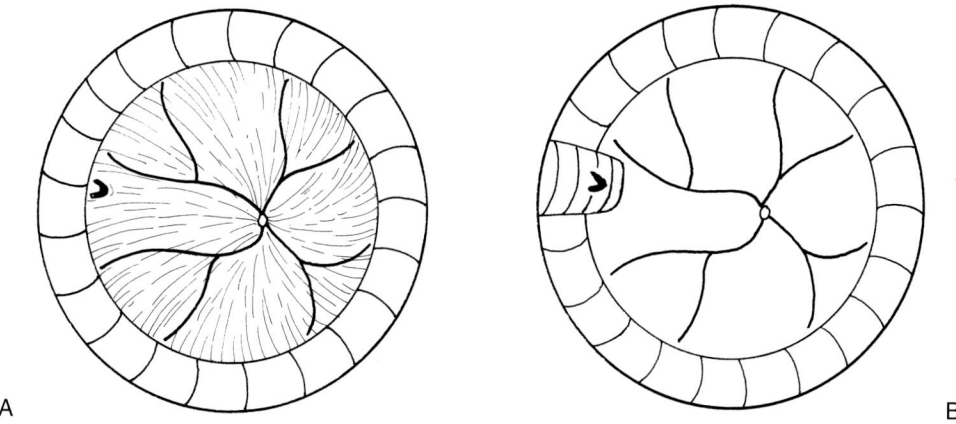

FIGURE A-14. *Case 14.* **A:** Redetachment of the retina caused by a new flap tear posterior to the original buckle. Pneumatic retinopexy is a good option in this setting. **B**: Alternatively, a radial sponge can be secured under the encircling band to close the break.

Subject Index

Page numbers followed by f refer to figures; page numbers followed by t refer to tables.

A

Acetaminophen
  after pneumatic retinopexy, 145
  cryotherapy, 201
Actin-containing sheaths, 11
Acute retinal necrosis syndrome, 38
Air tamponade, 53, 53f
Anesthesia
  pars plana vitrectomy, 155
  pneumatic retinopexy, 137
  scleral buckling procedure, 100
  temporary balloon buckling, 149
Anterior chamber
  nanophthalmos, 66
  paracentesis, 139–140
  pigment clumps in, 3–4
Anterior proliferative vitreoretinopathy, 25, 26f
Anterior segment ischemia, 177, 178f
Antibiotics
  after closure in scleral buckling, 128
  after pneumatic retinopexy, 145
  temporary balloon buckling, 151–152
Aphakic eye
  with breaks, 197
  examination for tiny flap tears, 96
  indication for encircling, 113t
  prophylactic treatment, 196
Apoptosis, 14
Atopic dermatitis, 41
Atrophic round hole, 7f, 8f, 9, 9f
  fundus examination, 84, 86f
Atrophy, anterior segment necrosis, 177, 178f
Autokines, 25
Avulsion of vitreous base, 33, 34f

B

Bed rest, 98
Binocular patching, 98
Biomicroscopy, 93
Blunt trauma, 33–35, 34f
Breaks, 4–10, 5–9f
  after pneumatic retinopexy, 188–189
  coloboma, 171
  Custodis operation, 54, 54f
  fundus drawing, 84f
  fundus examination, 84, 85f, 87f
  ignipuncture operation, 49f, 49–50
  Lindner operation, 52, 52f
  pneumatic retinopexy, 136, 136f

predisposing conditions, 29–44
  atopic dermatitis, 41
  cataract surgery, 31–32
  congenital choroidal coloboma, 39
  congenital optic disc abnormalities, 38–39
  congenital retinoschisis, 39, 40f
  Ehlers-Danlos syndrome, 41
  glaucoma, 33
  Goldmann-Favre syndrome, 41
  hereditary hyaloideoretinopathies, 38, 39f
  infections, 38
  lattice degeneration, 29–31, 30–31f
  Marfan syndrome and homocystinuria, 41
  myopia, 31
  proliferative retinopathies, 35–38, 36f
  trauma, 33–35, 34f
proliferative vitreoretinopathy, 24f
prophylactic therapy, 194t, 194–205
  asymptomatic breaks with no history of retinal disease, 196
  breaks in degenerative retinoschisis, 198
  breaks in fellow eyes, 196–197
  breaks in myopic eyes, 197
  breaks with bridging vessels, 199, 199f
  follow-up, 203
  macular pucker, 203
  role of education in preventing visual loss, 203–204
  subclinical retinal detachment, 198f, 198–199
  symptomatic tears with no history of retinal disease, 194–196, 195f
  treatment technique, 200f, 200–203, 202f
reopening
  after pneumatic retinopexy, 186–187
  after scleral buckling, 186–187
retinitis-related, 170
Šafář operation, 51, 51f
scleral buckling procedure, 100–134
  anesthesia, 100
  circumferential explants, 112f, 113
  closure, 127f, 127–130, 128f, 129–130f
  drainage of subretinal fluid, 116t, 116–122, 117t, 117–121f
  encircling, 113t, 113–115, 114f, 115f
  explant materials, 108, 109f
  incision, 101–104, 102–103f
  intraoperative problems, 123–127, 124f, 125f, 126f
  intravitreal injections, 122–123, 123f

Breaks, scleral buckling procedure *(contd.)*
    localization, 104f, 104–106, 105f, 106f
    preoperative preparation, 101
    principles, 100, 101f
    radial explants, 111–112
    retinopexy, 106–108, 107f
    routine postoperative management, 129
    surgical results, 131
    suture technique, 108–111, 109f, 110f, 111f
    without thermal adhesion, 115–116
  scleral depression, 87–90, 88–89f, 90f
  temporary balloon buckling, 149–154, 150f, 151f, 153t
  Weve operation, 51
Bridging vessels, retinal breaks with, 199, 199f
Bruch's membrane, 65
Buckle infection, 175–176, 176f
Bullous retinal detachment
  exudative, 65
  finding retinal breaks, 97
  localization technique, 105f, 105–106

C

Canthus, direct scleral depression, 90–91, 92f
Carcinoma, choroid, 61, 62f
Case studies, 207–213f
Cataract
  after scleral buckling, 186
  after vitrectomy, 157
  Goldmann-Favre syndrome, 41
  hereditary hyaloideoretinopathies, 38
  predisposition for retinal detachment after surgery, 31–32
  temporary balloon buckling, 153
Chemosis, infected scleral buckle, 176, 176f
Child
  juvenile retinoschisis, 39, 40f, 70, 171
  proliferative diseases, 171–172
Choriocapillaris, 106
Chorioretinal scar, 50, 50f, 84f
Chorioretinopathy, 65
Choroid
  bleeding after subretinal fluid drainage, 117, 118f
  carcinoma, 61, 62f
  coloboma, 39
  drainage by Graefe knife, 49, 49f
  fundus drawing, 84f
  melanoma, 61, 61f
  perforation during scleral buckling, 110
  Šafář operation, 51, 51f
  uveal effusion syndrome, 65–66
Choroidal detachment
  after scleral buckling, 177–178
  differential diagnosis, 71–73, 71–72f
  penetrating injuries, 168
  proliferative vitreoretinopathy risk, 26
Choroidopathy
  inadequate absorption of subretinal fluid after scleral buckling, 181
  senile, 116
Choroidotomy, 120–121f
Ciliary body
  abnormality after scleral buckling, 177
  uveal effusion syndrome, 65–66
Ciliochoroidal effusion, 71–73, 71–72f

Circumferential explant, 112f, 113
  closure, 127f, 127–128
  early proliferative vitreoretinopathy, 212f
  with encircling band, 115
  flap tear and round holes, 210f
  inferotemporal dialysis, 208f
  staphyloma, 125, 125f
Closure in scleral buckling procedure, 127f, 127–130, 128f, 129–130f
Cobblestones, 84f
Collagen
  Ehlers-Danlos syndrome, 41
  vitreous cavity, 1
Coloboma, 39, 171
Congenital cataract extraction, 32
Congenital conditions
  choroidal coloboma, 39
  juvenile retinoschisis, 70
  optic disc abnormalities, 38–39
  retinoschisis, 39, 40f
Conjunctiva
  pars plana vitrectomy, 155
  peritomy, 101, 102f, 103f
Cornea
  opacification during scleral buckling, 124
  stromal edema, 177
  temporary balloon buckling, 151
Corticosteroids
  after closure in scleral buckling, 128
  after pneumatic retinopexy, 145
Crescentic tear, 7f
Cryotherapy
  flap tear with small rim of subretinal fluid, 207f
  lattice degeneration, 209f
  Lincoff operation, 54
  macular pucker after, 203
  pigment fallout during, 178–179, 179f
  pneumatic retinopexy, 137–138, 138f
  prophylactic, 200–203
  scleral buckling, 106–108, 107f
  superotemporal flap tear, 210f
  temporary balloon buckling, 153
Custodis-Schepens-Lincoff era (1947–1971), 53f, 53–55, 54f, 55f
  instruments for examination, 53
  intravitreal air injection, 53, 53f
  scleral buckling explants, 53–54, 54f
  scleral buckling implants, 54–55, 55f
Cyanoacrylate glue
  coloboma, 171
  staphyloma, 125
Cyclopentolate, 101
Cycloplegia, 98
Cystoid configuration, 70
Cystoid degeneration
  fundus drawing, 84f
  retinoschisis, 68
Cystoid macular edema
  after scleral buckling, 185–186
  macular hole *versus,* 159
Cystoid spaces, 14, 18f
Cystoid spoking pattern, 39, 40f
Cytokines, 25
Cytomegalovirus
  retinal detachment, 38

retinitis, 170

D

Degeneration
  cystoid
    fundus drawing, 84f
    retinoschisis, 68
  lattice, 7f, 9f
    fellow eye, 197
    fundus drawing, 84f
    Goldmann-Favre syndrome, 41
    hereditary hyaloideoretinopathies, 38
    indication for encircling, 113t
    indication for prophylactic therapy, 194t
    localization technique, 104–105, 105f
    predisposition for retinal detachment, 29–31, 30–31f
    repair options, 209f
    superotemporal flap tear, 210f
    without holes, 196
  macular
    pneumatic retinopexy-induced, 144, 145f
    temporary balloon buckling, 153
  retinal detachment
    chronic, 16f
    early, 14
Degenerative retinoschisis, 9, 67, 68f, 171, 198
Dehydration spot, localization in scleral buckling, 104
Demarcation line, 14–17, 19f
  fundus drawing, 84f
  hole between line and ora serrata, 96, 96f
Dermatitis, atopic, 41
Diabetic retinopathy
  macula, 169
  surgical treatment, 169–170, 170f
  traction retinal detachment, 67f
Diagnosis and management, historical background, 45–59
  attempts at treatment, 47–48
  Custodis-Schepens-Lincoff era (1947–1971), 53f, 53–55, 54f, 55f
  Gonin era (1919–1947), 48–52, 49f, 50f, 51f, 52f
  incorrect theories of etiology, 45–46, 46f, 47f, 48f
  Machemer era (contemporary), 55–57
Dialysis, 10, 10f
  circumferential explant, 113
  fundus drawing, 84f
  inferotemporal, 208f
  localization technique, 104–105, 105f
Diathermy
  external subretinal fluid drainage, 120f
  scleral buckling localization, 104, 104f
Differential diagnosis, 60–73
  choroidal detachment, 71–73, 71–72f
  exudative retinal detachment, 60–66, 61f, 62f
  long-standing retinal detachment, 67–70
  retinoschisis, 68f, 69f, 68–70, 69f, 70f
  rhegmatogenous retinal detachment, 60
  traction retinal detachment, 66–67, 67f
Diplopia, 183
Disinsertion, 10, 10f, 84f
Distension, theory of, 45–46, 46f
Drainage in scleral buckling procedure, 116–122
  complications, 117f, 117t, 117–118, 118f
  indications, 116t, 116–117
  technique, 118–122, 119f, 120f, 121f

E

Early retinal detachment, 14–16, 15–16f
Edema
  cystoid macular
    after scleral buckling, 185–186
    macular hole *versus*, 159
  excessive scleral depression, 124
  intraretinal, 14, 15f
  retinal recovery after reattachment, 20f, 20–21
Ehlers-Danlos syndrome, 41
Encircling
  closure, 127, 128f
  early proliferative vitreoretinopathy, 212f
  flap tear and round holes, 210f
  penetrating injuries, 169
  persistent extraocular muscle imbalance, 183
  proliferative vitreoretinopathy, 166
  pseudophakic retinal detachment, 211f
  redetachment of retina, 213f
  scleral buckling procedure, 113t, 113–115, 114f, 115f
  staphyloma, 125
Endophthalmitis
  after cataract surgery, 38
  scleral buckling-induced, 176
Epipapillary glial tissue tear, 2, 3
Erosive vitreoretinopathy, 38
Etiology, incorrect theories, 45–46, 46f, 47f, 48f
Explant
  circumferential, 112f, 113
    closure, 127f, 127–128
    early proliferative vitreoretinopathy, 212f
    with encircling band, 115
    flap tear and round holes, 210f
    inferotemporal dialysis, 208f
    staphyloma, 125, 125f
  closure, 127, 127f, 128
  coverage by Tenon's capsule, 128
  extrusion or intrusion after scleral buckling, 184, 184f
  infected, 176, 176f
  materials, 108, 109f
  persistent extraocular muscle imbalance, 183
  radial, 111–112, 112f
    closure, 128
    under encircling band, 114
    extrusion, 184, 184f
    flap tear and round holes, 210f
    redetachment of retina, 213f
    superotemporal flap tear, 210f
    staphyloma, 125, 125f
External laser choroidotomy, 122
Extracapsular cataract extraction, 32
Extrusion of explant after scleral buckling, 184, 184f
Exudate
  fundus drawing, 84f
  over scleral buckle, 176, 176f
Exudation, theory of, 46, 47f, 48f
Exudative retinal detachment
  after scleral buckling, 180
  differential diagnosis, 60–66
    idiopathic central serous chorioretinopathy, 65

Exudative retinal detachment, differential diagnosis *(contd.)*
    inflammatory diseases, 61–63, 63f–64f
    nanophthalmos, 66
    neoplasms, 61, 62f
    posterior scleritis, 63–65, 65f
    uveal effusion syndrome, 65–66, 66f

F
Familial exudative vitreoretinopathy, 171
Fellow eye, breaks, 196–197
Fibronectin, 25
Fibrovascular proliferation, 35, 35f
    pediatric, 171–172
    penetrating injuries, 168, 168f
Fishmouth phenomenon, 126f, 126–127
Fixed fold
    early proliferative vitreoretinopathy, 212f
    fundus drawing, 84f
Flap tear, 4–9, 5f, 7f
    blunt trauma, 34
    detachment after extracapsular cataract extraction, 32
    double, 209f
    with extensive retinal detachment, 207f
    fundus drawing, 84f
    incorrectly buckled, 181, 182f
    localization technique, 104–105, 105f
    observation, 196
    photocoagulation, 202f
    posterior, inferior, 211f
    prophylactic treatment, 194
    reopening of original break, 186–187
    scleral depression, 87, 89f
    with small rim of subretinal fluid, 207f
    under superior rectus muscle, 208f
    superotemporal, 210f
Floaters
    differential diagnosis, 60
    posterior vitreous detachment, 2, 4
Fluorescein angiography
    Harada's disease, 61
    idiopathic central chorioretinopathy, 65
    temporal retinal detachment with thin macula, 160f
Fluorometholone, 203
Focal retinal atrophy, 8f, 9
Folds
    early proliferative vitreoretinopathy, 212f
    fundus drawing, 84f
    rhegmatogenous retinal detachment, 60
    traction retinal detachment, 67
Fovea
    cystoid macula, 40
    juvenile retinoschisis, 70
Fundus drawing, 82–87, 84f, 85–87f
Fundus examination, 75–97
    biomicroscopy, 93
    finding retinal breaks, 93–97, 94–96f, 97f
    indirect ophthalmoscopy, 75–92
        fundus drawing, 82–87, 84f, 85–87f
        principles and advantages, 75–76, 76f, 77f
        scleral depression, 87–92, 88–89f, 90f, 91f, 92f
        technique, 77–82, 79–81f, 82f, 83f

G
Gas injection in pneumatic retinopexy, 55–56, 135–148
    anesthesia, 137
    intraoperative problems, 142–145, 144f, 145f
    paracentesis, 139–140
    patient selection, 136f, 136–137, 137t
    retinopexy, 137–139, 138f
    routine postoperative management, 145–146
    surgical results, 146–147
    techniques, 137–142, 138f, 140t, 141f, 142f
General anesthesia
    pneumatic retinopexy, 137
    scleral buckling, 100
Giant retinal tear
    fellow eye, 197
    surgical treatment, 163f, 163–165, 164f
Glaucoma
    drainage of subretinal fluid, 116
    hereditary hyaloideoretinopathies, 38
    pneumatic retinopexy, 136–137
    predisposition for retinal detachment, 33
    scleral depression, 90
Globe
    complications of local anesthesia, 100
    cryotherapy in scleral buckling, 107
    gas injection for repressurization, 123f
    immobilization during scleral buckling, 109
    perforation during scleral buckling, 125
Glycosaminoglycans, 11
Goldmann-Favre syndrome, 41
Goldmann three-mirror lens, 53, 93
Gonin era (1919–1947), 48–52, 49f, 50f, 51f, 52f
    Guist operation, 50, 50f
    ignipuncture operation, 49f, 49–50
    Larsson operation, 50, 51f
    Lindner operation, 52, 52f
    rhegmatogenous theory, 48–49
    Šafář operation, 51, 51f
    Weve operation, 51
Guist operation, 50, 50f

H
Hand lens
    biomicroscopy, 93
    proper use, 77, 78f
Harada's disease, 61
Hemangioma, choroidal, 61
Hemorrhage
    after pneumatic retinopexy, 189
    complication of subretinal fluid drainage, 117, 117t
    contraindication to pneumatic retinopexy, 136–137, 137t
    diabetic patient, 36
    extrusion or intrusion of buckling element, 184
    fundus drawing, 84f
    penetrating injuries, 168
    peripheral punctate intraretinal, 4
    during pneumatic retinopexy, 144
    posterior vitreous detachment, 2, 3
    proliferative vitreoretinopathy risk, 26
    retinal breaks with bridging vessels, 199, 199f
    rhegmatogenous retinal detachment, 60
    during scleral buckling, 123
    sickle cell retinopathy, 37
    temporary balloon buckling, 153
Hereditary hyaloideoretinopathies, 38, 39f

Herpes simplex virus retinitis, 170
High myopia
  drainage of subretinal fluid, 116
  Ehlers-Danlos syndrome, 41
  examination for breaks, 96
  hereditary hyaloideoretinopathies, 38
  inadequate absorption of subretinal fluid after scleral buckling, 181
  indication for encircling, 113t
  lattice degeneration, 29
  predisposition for retinal detachment, 31
  prophylactic therapy, 197
History of diagnosis and management, 45–59
  attempts at treatment, 47–48
  Custodis-Schepens-Lincoff era (1947–1971), 53f, 53–55, 54f, 55f
  Gonin era (1919–1947), 48–52, 49f, 50f, 51f, 52f
  incorrect theories of etiology, 45–46, 46f, 47f, 48f
  Machemer era (contemporary), 55–57
Holes
  congenital retinoschisis, 39, 40f
  localization technique, 104–105, 105f
  macular, 9–10
    after scleral buckling, 179
    blunt trauma, 34
    surgical treatment, 159–162, 160–161f
    temporary balloon buckling, 153
  retinoschisis-retinal detachment, 69–70, 70f
  round, 8f, 9, 9f, 10f
    fundus drawing, 84f
    indication for prophylactic therapy, 194t
    inferotemporal retinal detachment, 17f
    with or without operculum, 196
    repair options, 210f
    scleral depression, 87–90, 88–89f, 90f
Homocystinuria, 41
Horseshoe tear, 4–9, 5f, 7f, 194
Human immunodeficiency virus, 170
Hyalinized retinal blood vessels, 29, 30f
Hyaloideoretinopathies, hereditary, 38, 39f
Hyaluronic acid molecules, 1
Hydrostatic pressure, 11
Hyphema, traumatic, 34
Hypotony
  after subretinal fluid drainage, 122
  anterior segment necrosis, 177
  choroidal detachment, 71, 177
  inadvertent perforation of globe, 125
  theory of, 46, 47f

I

Idiopathic central serous chorioretinopathy, 65
Ignipuncture operation, 49f, 49–52, 50f, 51f, 52f
Illumination beam
  binocular indirect ophthalmoscope, 76f
  examiner position, 79f
  pupillary aperture, 83f
Implant
  Schepens operation, 55
  scleral buckling, 54–55, 55f
Incision
  conjunctival peritomy, 101, 103f
  external subretinal fluid drainage, 120
  pars plana vitrectomy, 155
  scleral buckling procedure, 101–104, 102–103f

Indirect ophthalmoscope, 104
Indirect ophthalmoscopy, 75–92
  fundus drawing, 82–87, 84f, 85–87f
  idiopathic central chorioretinopathy, 65
  pneumatic retinopexy, 137
  posterior scleritis, 63
  principles and advantages, 75–76, 76f, 77f
  scleral depression, 87–92, 88–89f, 90f, 91f, 92f
  technique, 77–82, 79–81f, 82f, 83f
Infection
  after pneumatic retinopexy, 189
  after scleral buckling, 175–176, 176f
  predisposition for retinal detachment, 38
  preoperative prevention, 98
  retinal breaks, 170
Inferior retinal detachment, 94f, 95f
Inferonasal periphery examination, 78, 80f
Inferotemporal dialysis, 208f
Inferotemporal periphery examination, 78–82, 81f
Inferotemporal sclerotomy, 155
Inflammation, proliferative vitreoretinopathy risk, 26
Inflammatory disease, 60, 61–63, 64f
Informed consent, 98
Instruments for examination
  Custodis-Schepens-Lincoff era (1947–1971), 45
  early period (1851–1918), 45
Interleukin, 25
Interphotoreceptor matrix, 11
Intracapsular cataract extraction, 31–32
Intraocular gas, 143
Intraocular pressure
  after pneumatic retinopexy, 187
  after scleral buckling, 175
  external subretinal fluid drainage, 120
  increase during scleral buckling, 126
  intravitreal injections, 123
  pneumatic retinopexy, 139–140
  rhegmatogenous retinal detachment, 20, 60
  scleral depression, 90
  temporary balloon buckling, 151
Intraoperative problems
  pneumatic retinopexy, 142–145, 144f, 145f
  scleral buckling procedure, 123–127, 124f, 125f, 126f
Intraretinal edema, 14, 15f, 20f, 20–21
Intraretinal hemorrhage, 84f
Intraretinal pigmentation, 84f
Intravitreal injection
  pneumatic retinopexy, 55–56, 135–148
    anesthesia, 137
    gas injection, 140t, 140–142, 141f, 142f
    intraoperative problems, 142–145, 144f, 145f
    paracentesis, 139–140
    patient selection, 136f, 136–137, 137t
    retinopexy, 137–139, 138f
    routine postoperative management, 145–146
    surgical results, 146–147
    techniques, 137–142, 138f, 140t, 141f, 142f
  scleral buckling procedure, 122–123, 123f
    fishmouth phenomenon, 126
    inadequate absorption of subretinal fluid, 181
Intrusion of explant, 184, 184f
Iris
  abnormality after scleral buckling, 177
  incarceration during pneumatic retinopexy, 144

Iris *(contd.)*
    retractors to augment pupillary dilation, 124, 124f
Ischemia, anterior segment, 177, 178f

J
Jansen's disease, 38
Juvenile retinoschisis, 39, 40f, 70, 171

L
Larsson operation, 50, 50f
Laser photocoagulation, 157
    inadequate absorption of subretinal fluid after scleral buckling, 181
    lattice degeneration, 209f
    pars plana vitrectomy, 154, 154f, 156
    pneumatic retinopexy, 138–139, 139f
    prophylactic, 200–203, 202f
    subretinal fluid drainage, 122
    superotemporal flap tear, 210f
    temporary balloon buckling, 149, 152
Laser retinopexy, 153
Lattice degeneration, 7f, 9f
    contraindication to pneumatic retinopexy, 136–137, 137t
    fellow eye, 197
    fundus drawing, 84f
    Goldmann-Favre syndrome, 41
    hereditary hyaloideoretinopathies, 38
    indication for encircling, 113t
    indication for prophylactic therapy, 194t
    localization technique, 104–105, 105f
    predisposition for retinal detachment, 29–31, 30–31f
    repair options, 209f
    superotemporal flap tear, 210f
    without holes, 196
Lenses
    biomicroscopy, 93
    indirect ophthalmoscope, 77, 78f
Lidocaine, 201
Limbal peritomy, 102, 102f, 103f
Lincoff operation, 54
Lindner operation, 52
Local anesthesia
    cryotherapy, 201
    pneumatic retinopexy, 137
    scleral buckling, 100
Localization
    scleral buckling procedure, 104f, 104–106, 105f, 106f
    temporary balloon buckling, 150
Long-standing retinal detachment
    differential diagnosis, 67–70
    fundus examination, 84, 86f
    pathophysiology, 14–17, 16f, 17f, 18–19f

M
Machemer era (contemporary), 55–57
    pars plana vitrectomy, 55
    perfluorocarbon liquids, 56
    pneumatic retinopexy, 55–56
    primary vitrectomy, 56
    silicone oil, 56
    temporary balloon device, 56–57
Macrocyst, 84, 86f

Macula
    complicated proliferative vitreoretinopathy detachments, 168
    delay in retinal detachment treatment, 203
    Harada's disease, 63f–64f
    proliferative diabetic retinopathy, 169
    timing of surgery, 98–99
Macular degeneration
    pneumatic retinopexy-induced, 144, 145f
    temporary balloon buckling, 153
Macular edema
    after scleral buckling, 185–186
    macular hole *versus,* 159
Macular hole, 9–10
    after scleral buckling, 179
    blunt trauma, 34
    surgical treatment, 159–162, 160–161f
    temporary balloon buckling, 153
Macular pucker
    after scleral buckling, 184–185, 185f
    prophylactic therapy, 203
    temporary balloon buckling, 153
Mainster and Volk wide-field contact lenses, 93
Malignant melanoma
    choroidal detachment *versus,* 73
    rhegmatogenous retinal detachment, 61, 62f
Marfan syndrome, 41
Medical evaluation, preoperative, 98
Melanoma
    choroidal, 61, 61f
    choroidal detachment *versus,* 73
Meridional fold, 84f
Meridional lattice degeneration, 29, 31f
Metastatic carcinoma of choroid, 61, 62f
Miotic-induced retinal detachment, 33
Morning glory syndrome, 38
Mucopurulent discharge
    extrusion or intrusion of buckling element, 184
    infected scleral buckle, 176, 176f
Multiple trephination, 50, 50f
Mydriasis
    preoperative management, 98
    before scleral buckling, 101
Myopia
    drainage of subretinal fluid, 116
    Ehlers-Danlos syndrome, 41
    examination for breaks, 96
    hereditary hyaloideoretinopathies, 38
    inadequate absorption of subretinal fluid after scleral buckling, 181
    indication for encircling, 113t
    lattice degeneration, 29
    predisposition for retinal detachment, 31
    prophylactic therapy, 197

N
Nanophthalmos, 66
Nasal periphery, scleral depression, 92f
Necrosis
    acute retinal necrosis syndrome, 38
    anterior segment, 177, 178f
    scleral, 176
Neoplasm, exudative retinal detachment, 60, 61, 62f
Night blindness, 41
Nitrous oxide, 123

Nonrhegmatogenous traction retinal detachment, 36
Nonsteroidal antiinflammatory drugs, 145
Nuclear sclerosis, 157

O

Observation beam
   binocular indirect ophthalmoscope, 76f
   examiner position, 79f
   pupillary aperture, 83f
Ocular contusion, 33
Oncotic pressure, 11
Open-angle glaucoma, 33
Open-sky vitrectomy, 55
Operculated retinal tear, 8f
   fundus drawing, 84f
   prophylactic treatment, 194, 195f
Operculum, 9
Ophthalmoscope
   electrically illuminated binocular indirect, 53
   invention of, 45
   Schepens, 75
Ophthalmoscopy
   paracentesis, 142, 142f
   posterior vitreous detachment, 4
Optic atrophy, 38
Optic disc congenital abnormality, 38–39
Optic nerve, complications of local anesthesia, 100
Ora serrata
   hole between demarcation line and, 96, 96f
   scleral depression, 91f

P

Pain
   extrusion or intrusion of buckling element, 184
   scleral depression, 90
Papillitis, 61
Paracentesis
   pneumatic retinopexy, 139–140
   temporary balloon buckling, 151
Parallax, 105–106, 106f
Pars plana
   blunt trauma, 33
   choroidal detachment, 71, 72f
   fundus drawing, 84f
   gas under, 143
Pars plana vitrectomy, 55
   advanced proliferative vitreoretinopathy, 165, 166f
   macular hole, 162, 162f
   posterior, inferior flap tear, 211f
   without scleral buckling, 154f, 154–157
Pathophysiology, 14–28
   early retinal detachment, 14–16, 15–16f
   intraocular pressure, 20
   long-standing retinal detachment, 14–17, 16f, 17f, 18–19f
   proliferative vitreoretinopathy, 21f, 21–26, 22–24f, 25t
   retinal recovery after reattachment, 20f, 20–21
   subretinal fluid, 17–20
Patient positioning
   gas injection, 142, 142f, 143
   pars plana vitrectomy, 156
Patient selection in pneumatic retinopexy, 136f, 136–137, 137t
Pediatric proliferative diseases, 171–172

Penetrating diathermy, 51
Penetrating injuries
   surgical treatment, 168–169
   traction retinal detachment, 66–67
Perfluorocarbon liquids, 56
   giant retinal tear, 163, 164f
   pars plana vitrectomy, 155–156
   penetrating injuries, 169
   proliferative vitreoretinopathy, 166–167
Perfluorophenanthrene, 163
Perfluoropropane
   giant retinal tear, 163
   macular hole, 159
   pars plana vitrectomy, 156
   pneumatic retinopexy, 140t, 140–141
   proliferative vitreoretinopathy, 167
Perforation
   choroid
      during scleral buckling, 110
      during subretinal fluid drainage, 121f
   globe, during scleral buckling, 125
   retina, during subretinal fluid drainage, 117, 117t
Peribulbar block
   pars plana vitrectomy, 155
   pneumatic retinopexy, 137
   retinal artery occlusion after, 123
   scleral buckling, 100
Peripheral cystoid degeneration, 84f
Peripheral punctate intraretinal hemorrhage, 4
Peritomy, 101
Phakic eye
   after vitrectomy, 157
   fellow eye, 196–197
Phenylephrine, 101
Photocoagulation, 157
   lattice degeneration, 209f
   pars plana vitrectomy, 154, 154f, 156
   pneumatic retinopexy, 138–139, 139f
   prophylactic, 200–203
   scleral buckling procedure, 108
   subretinal fluid drainage, 122
   superotemporal flap tear, 210f
   temporary balloon buckling, 149, 152
Photopsia, 2
Pierre Robin malformation, 38
Pigment clumps in anterior chamber, 3–4
Pigment fallout after scleral buckling, 178–179, 179f
Pigmentary dispersion syndrome, 33
Pigmented lattice degeneration, 29, 30f
Platelet-derived growth factor, 25
Pneumatic retinopexy, 55–56, 135–148
   anesthesia, 137
   failure to reattach, 212f
   flap tear under superior rectus muscle, 208f
   flap tear with extensive retinal detachment, 207f
   gas injection, 140t, 140–142, 141f, 142f
   intraoperative problems, 142–145, 144f, 145f
   macular hole after, 179
   paracentesis, 139–140
   patient selection, 136f, 136–137, 137t
   posterior, inferior flap tear, 211f
   postoperative complications, 187–190
   redetachment of retina, 213f
   retinopexy, 137–139, 138f
   routine postoperative management, 145–146

Pneumatic retinopexy *(contd.)*
  surgical results, 146–147
  techniques, 137–139, 138f
  temporary balloon buckling *versus,* 152
Pneumocausis, 56
Posterior, inferior flap tear, 211f
Posterior scleritis, 63–65, 65f
Posterior segment, penetrating injuries, 35
Posterior vitreous detachment, 1–4, 2f, 3f
  diabetes, 35–36
  lattice degeneration, 29
  scleral depression, 87–92, 88–89f, 90f, 91f, 92f
  with vitreoretinal adhesion, 5f
Postoperative complications, 175–193
  pneumatic retinopexy, 187–190
  scleral buckling, 175–187
    anterior segment ischemia, 177, 178f
    cataract, 186
    choroidal detachment, 177–178
    ciliary body and iris abnormalities, 177
    cystoid macular edema, 185–186
    decreased or displaced scleral buckle, 187
    elevated intraocular pressure, 175
    extrusion or intrusion, 184, 184f
    exudative retinal detachment, 180
    infection, 175–176, 176f
    initial retinal reattachment failure, 180–182, 182f
    macular hole, 179
    macular pucker, 184–185, 185f
    new retinal tears, 186
    pigment fallout, 178–179, 179f
    proliferative vitreoretinopathy, 187
    refractive error, 182–183
    removal of scleral buckle, 187
    reopening of original break, 186–187
    slow absorption of subretinal fluid, 179–180, 180f
    strabismus, 183
Postoperative management
  pars plana vitrectomy, 156
  pneumatic retinopexy, 145–146
  scleral buckling procedure, 129
Predisposing conditions, 29–44
  atopic dermatitis, 41
  cataract surgery, 31–32
  congenital choroidal coloboma, 39
  congenital optic disc abnormalities, 38–39
  congenital retinoschisis, 39, 40f
  Ehlers-Danlos syndrome, 41
  glaucoma, 33
  Goldmann-Favre syndrome, 41
  hereditary hyaloideoretinopathies, 38, 39f
  infections, 38
  lattice degeneration, 29–31, 30–31f
  Marfan syndrome and homocystinuria, 41
  myopia, 31
  proliferative retinopathies, 35–38, 36f
  trauma, 33–35, 34f
Preoperative management, 98–99
  drawing of retinal tear, 200, 200f
  scleral buckling procedure, 101
  temporary balloon buckling, 150
Primary retinal detachment, 1–13
  incidence and epidemiology, 11–12
  mechanisms of retinal attachment, 10–11
  posterior vitreous detachment, 1–4, 2f, 3f
  retinal breaks, 4–10, 5–9f
Primary vitrectomy, 56, 154f, 154–157
Proliferative diabetic retinopathy
  surgical treatment, 169–170, 170f
  traction retinal detachment, 67f
Proliferative retinopathy, 35–38, 36f
Proliferative vitreoretinopathy
  after pneumatic retinopexy, 189
  after scleral buckling, 187
  complicated cases, 165f, 165–168, 166f, 167f
  contraindication to pneumatic retinopexy, 136–137, 137t
  delay in retinal detachment treatment, 203
  encircling, 166
  failure of scleral buckling, 182
  giant retinal tear, 163, 165
  indication for encircling, 113, 113t, 114f
  pars plana vitrectomy, 55, 165, 166f
  pathophysiology, 21f, 21–26, 22–24f, 25t
  perfluorocarbon liquids, 166–167
  repair options, 212f
  scleral buckling complications, 187
  surgical treatment, 165f, 165–168, 166f, 167f
  temporary balloon buckling, 153
  traction retinal detachment, 66–67
Proparacaine, 201
Prophylactic therapy, 194t, 194–205
  asymptomatic breaks with no history of retinal disease, 196
  breaks in degenerative retinoschisis, 198
  breaks in fellow eyes, 196–197
  breaks in myopic eyes, 197
  breaks with bridging vessels, 199, 199f
  follow-up, 203
  giant retinal tear, 165
  macular pucker, 203
  role of education in preventing visual loss, 203–204
  subclinical retinal detachment, 198f, 198–199
  symptomatic tears with no history of retinal disease, 194–196, 195f
  treatment technique, 200f, 200–203, 202f
Proteins in interphotoreceptor matrix, 11
Pseudodemarcation line, 179
Pseudomonas, scleral necrosis, 176
Pseudophakic eye
  with breaks, 197
  indication for encircling, 113t
  indication for prophylactic therapy, 194t
  prophylactic treatment, 196
Pseudophakic retinal detachment
  repair options, 211f
  risk after extracapsular cataract extraction, 32
Pupil
  complications during scleral buckling, 124, 124f
  examination, 82, 83f
  preoperative dilatation, 98
PVD; *see* Posterior vitreous detachment
PVR; *see* Proliferative vitreoretinopathy

R

Radial explant, 111–112, 112f
  closure, 128

under encircling band, 114
extrusion, 184, 184f
flap tear and round holes, 210f
redetachment of retina, 213f
superotemporal flap tear, 210f
Radial lattice degeneration, 29, 31f
Reattachment
  case studies, 207–213f
  complicated cases, 159–167
    coloboma, 171
    giant retinal tear, 163f, 163–165, 164f
    macular holes, 159–162, 160–161f
    pediatric proliferative diseases, 171–172
    penetrating injuries, 168–169
    proliferative diabetic retinopathy, 169–170, 170f
    proliferative vitreoretinopathy, 165f, 165–168, 166f, 167f
    retinitis-related, 170
    retinoschisis-related, 171
  congenital cataract surgery, 32
  failure, 212f
  historical background, 45–59
    Custodis-Schepens-Lincoff era (1947–1971), 53f, 53–55, 54f, 55f
    early attempts at treatment, 47–48
    Gonin era (1919–1947), 48–52, 49f, 50f, 51f, 52f
    incorrect theories of etiology, 45–46, 46f, 47f, 48f
    Machemer era (contemporary), 55–57
  ignipuncture operation, 49f, 49–50
  laser photocoagulation, 157
  pneumatic retinopexy, 135–148
    anesthesia, 137
    gas injection, 140t, 140–142, 141f, 142f
    intraoperative problems, 142–145, 144f, 145f
    paracentesis, 139–140
    patient selection, 136f, 136–137, 137t
    retinopexy, 137–139, 138f
    routine postoperative management, 145–146
    surgical results, 146–147
  postoperative complications, 175–193
    pneumatic retinopexy, 187–190
    scleral buckling, 175–187
  primary vitrectomy without scleral buckling, 154f, 154–157
  repair options, 213f
  retinal recovery, 20f, 20–21
  scleral buckling procedure, 100–134
    anesthesia, 100
    circumferential explants, 112f, 113
    closure, 127f, 127–130, 128f, 129–130f
    drainage of subretinal fluid, 116t, 116–122, 117t, 117–121f
    encircling, 113t, 113–115, 114f, 115f
    explant materials, 108, 109f
    incision, 101–104, 102–103f
    intraoperative problems, 123–127, 124f, 125f, 126f
    intravitreal injections, 122–123, 123f
    localization, 104f, 104–106, 105f, 106f
    preoperative preparation, 101
    principles, 100, 101f
    radial explants, 111–112
    retinopexy, 106–108, 107f
    routine postoperative management, 129
    surgical results, 131–132
    suture technique, 108–111, 109f, 110f, 111f
    without thermal adhesion, 115–116
  temporary balloon buckling, 149–154, 150f, 151f, 153t
  traumatic retinal break, 35
Rectus muscle, scleral buckling, 110
Redetachment
  finding retinal breaks, 96f, 97, 97f
  new retinal tears, 186
  reopening of original break, 186–187
Refractive error after scleral buckling, 182–183
Relaxing retinotomy, 166, 167f
Repair procedures; *see* Reattachment
Retina
  appearance when frozen, 107
  attachment mechanisms, 10–11
  complications during subretinal fluid drainage, 117, 117t, 118f
  examination scanning technique, 85f
  failure to reattach, 212f
  recovery after reattachment, 20f, 20–21
  redetachment, 213f
Retinal artery
  fundus drawing, 84f
  occlusion after retrobulbar or peribulbar anesthesia, 123
  temporary balloon buckling, 151
Retinal blood vessels
  breaks with, 199, 199f
  hyalinized, 29, 30f
  scleral buckling, 118, 119f
Retinal break; *see* Breaks
Retinal detachment
  differential diagnosis, 60–73
    choroidal detachment, 71–73, 71–72f
    exudative retinal detachment, 60–66, 61f, 62f, 63f
    long-standing retinal detachment, 67–70
    retinoschisis, 68f, 69f, 68–70, 69f, 70f
    rhegmatogenous retinal detachment, 60
    traction retinal detachment, 66–67, 67f
  history of diagnosis and management, 45–59
    attempts at treatment, 47–48
    Custodis-Schepens-Lincoff era (1947–1971), 53f, 53–55, 54f, 55f
    Gonin era (1919–1947), 48–52, 49f, 50f, 51f, 52f
    incorrect theories of etiology, 45–46, 46f, 47f, 48f
    Machemer era (contemporary), 55–57
  laser photocoagulation, 157
  pathophysiology, 14–28
    early, 14–16, 15–16f
    intraocular pressure, 20
    long-standing, 14–17, 16f, 17f, 18–19f
    proliferative vitreoretinopathy, 21f, 21–26, 22–24f, 25t
    retinal recovery after reattachment, 20f, 20–21
    subretinal fluid, 17–20
  pneumatic retinopexy, 135–148
    anesthesia, 137
    gas injection, 140t, 140–142, 141f, 142f
    intraoperative problems, 142–145, 144f, 145f

Retinal detachment, pneumatic retinopexy *(contd.)*
    paracentesis, 139–140
    patient selection, 136f, 136–137, 137t
    retinopexy, 137–139, 138f
    routine postoperative management, 145–146
    surgical results, 146–147
  predisposing conditions, 29–44
    atopic dermatitis, 41
    cataract surgery, 31–32
    congenital choroidal coloboma, 39
    congenital optic disc abnormalities, 38–39
    congenital retinoschisis, 39, 40f
    Ehlers-Danlos syndrome, 41
    glaucoma, 33
    Goldmann-Favre syndrome, 41
    hereditary hyaloideoretinopathies, 38, 39f
    infections, 38
    lattice degeneration, 29–31, 30–31f
    Marfan syndrome and homocystinuria, 41
    myopia, 31
    proliferative retinopathies, 35–38, 36f
    trauma, 33–35, 34f
  primary, 1–13
    incidence and epidemiology, 11–12
    mechanisms of retinal attachment, 10–11
    posterior vitreous detachment, 1–4, 2f, 3f
    retinal breaks, 4–10, 5–9f
  primary vitrectomy without scleral buckling, 154f, 154–157
  prophylactic therapy, 194t, 194–205
    asymptomatic breaks with no history of retinal disease, 196
    breaks in degenerative retinoschisis, 198
    breaks in fellow eyes, 196–197
    breaks in myopic eyes, 197
    breaks with bridging vessels, 199, 199f
    follow-up, 203
    macular pucker, 203
    role of education in preventing visual loss, 203–204
    subclinical retinal detachment, 198f, 198–199
    symptomatic tears with no history of retinal disease, 194–196, 195f
    treatment technique, 200f, 200–203, 202f
  scleral buckling procedure, 100–134
    anesthesia, 100
    circumferential explants, 112f, 113
    closure, 127f, 127–130, 128f, 129–130f
    drainage of subretinal fluid, 116t, 116–122, 117t, 117–121f
    encircling, 113t, 113–115, 114f, 115f
    explant materials, 108, 109f
    incision, 101–104, 102–103f
    intraoperative problems, 123–127, 124f, 125f, 126f
    intravitreal injections, 122–123, 123f
    localization, 104f, 104–106, 105f, 106f
    preoperative preparation, 101
    principles, 100, 101f
    radial explants, 111–112
    retinopexy, 106–108, 107f
    routine postoperative management, 129
    surgical results, 131–132
    suture technique, 108–111, 109f, 110f, 111f
    without thermal adhesion, 115–116
  subclinical, 198f, 198–199
  surgery of complicated cases, 159–167
    coloboma, 171
    giant retinal tear, 163f, 163–165, 164f
    macular holes, 159–162, 160–161f
    pediatric proliferative diseases, 171–172
    penetrating injuries, 168–169
    proliferative diabetic retinopathy, 169–170, 170f
    proliferative vitreoretinopathy, 165f, 165–168, 166f, 167f
    retinitis-related, 170
    retinoschisis-related, 171
  temporary balloon buckling, 149–154, 150f, 151f, 153t
Retinal dialysis, 10, 10f
  circumferential explant, 113
  fundus drawing, 84f
  inferotemporal, 208f
  localization technique, 104–105, 105f
Retinal hemorrhage, 84f
Retinal holes; *see* Holes
Retinal pigment epithelial cell pump, 11
Retinal pigment epithelial cell sheath, 10–11
Retinal pigment epithelium
  cryotherapy in scleral buckling, 106
  early retinal detachment, 14, 16f
  idiopathic central serous chorioretinopathy, 65
  osmotic forces, 11
  pigment clumps, 4
  pneumatic retinopexy, 138
  proliferative vitreoretinopathy, 25
  retinal detachment, 1
  retinoschisis-retinal detachment, 69–70
  scleral depression, 87, 88f
  traction retinal detachment, 66–67
Retinal tear; *see* Tears
Retinitis-related retinal detachment, 170
Retinopathy, 35–38, 36f
  predisposition for retinal detachment, 35–38, 36f
  of prematurity, 171
  sickle cell, 37
Retinopexy
  pneumatic, 55–56, 135–148
    anesthesia, 137
    failure to reattach, 212f
    flap tear under superior rectus muscle, 208f
    flap tear with extensive retinal detachment, 207f
    gas injection, 140t, 140–142, 141f, 142f
    intraoperative problems, 142–145, 144f, 145f
    macular hole after, 179
    paracentesis, 139–140
    patient selection, 136f, 136–137, 137t
    posterior, inferior flap tear, 211f
    postoperative complications, 187–190
    redetachment of retina, 213f
    retinopexy, 137–139, 138f
    routine postoperative management, 145–146
    surgical results, 146–147
    techniques, 137–139, 138f
    temporary balloon buckling *versus,* 152
  scleral buckling procedure, 106–108, 107f
  temporary balloon buckling, 153
Retinoschisis
  congenital, 39, 40f
  differential diagnosis, 68f, 69f, 68–70, 69f, 70f

Goldmann-Favre syndrome, 41
hereditary hyaloideoretinopathies, 38
juvenile, 70
prophylactic treatment, 198
surgical treatment, 171
Retinotomy, 166, 167f
Retrobulbar block
  pars plana vitrectomy, 155
  pneumatic retinopexy, 137
  retinal artery occlusion after, 123
  scleral buckling, 100
  temporary balloon buckling, 149
Retrobulbar hemorrhage
  complication of local anesthesia, 100
  during scleral buckling, 123
Rhegmatogenous retinal detachment, 1
  branch retinal vein occlusion, 36, 37f
  with choroidal detachment, 71–73, 73f
  coloboma, 171
  cystoid macular edema, 159
  differential diagnosis, 60
  intraocular pressure, 20
  intraretinal edema, 15f
  pneumatic retinopexy, 136
  retinitis-related, 170
  retinopathy of prematurity, 37
  retinoschisis *versus,* 69
  scleral buckling procedure, 100–134
    anesthesia, 100
    circumferential explants, 112f, 113
    closure, 127f, 127–130, 128f, 129–130f
    drainage of subretinal fluid, 116t, 116–122, 117t, 117–121f
    encircling, 113t, 113–115, 114f, 115f
    explant materials, 108, 109f
    incision, 101–104, 102–103f
    intraoperative problems, 123–127, 124f, 125f, 126f
    intravitreal injections, 122–123, 123f
    localization, 104f, 104–106, 105f, 106f
    preoperative preparation, 101
    principles, 100, 101f
    radial explants, 111–112
    retinopexy, 106–108, 107f
    routine postoperative management, 131
    surgical results, 131–132
    suture technique, 108–111, 109f, 110f, 111f
    without thermal adhesion, 115–116
  subretinal fluid, 17–20
Rhegmatogenous theory, 48–49
Rosengren operation, 53, 53f
Round hole, 8f, 9, 9f, 10f
  fundus drawing, 84f
  indication for prophylactic therapy, 194t
  inferotemporal retinal detachment, 17f
  with or without operculum, 196
  repair options, 210f
RRD; *see* Rhegmatogenous retinal detachment

S
Šafář operation, 51
Schepens binocular indirect ophthalmoscope, 75
Schepens operation, 54–55, 55f
Sclera
  Custodis operation, 54, 54f

  drainage by Graefe knife, 49, 49f
  Guist operation, 50, 50f
  Lindner operation, 52, 52f
  nanophthalmos, 66
  Šafář operation, 51, 51f
  Schepens operation, 55
Scleral buckling, 100–134
  after failed pneumatic retinopexy, 146
  anesthesia, 100
  closure, 127f, 127–130, 128f, 129–130f
  double flap tears, 209f
  drainage of subretinal fluid, 116–122
    complications, 117f, 117t, 117–118, 118f
    indications, 116t, 116–117
    technique, 118–122, 119f, 120f, 121f
  early proliferative vitreoretinopathy, 212f
  encircling, 113t, 113–115, 114f, 115f
  explants
    circumferential, 112f, 113
    historical background, 53–54, 54f
    materials, 108, 109f
    radial, 111–112
  flap tear and round holes, 210f
  flap tear under superior rectus muscle, 208f
  flap tear with extensive retinal detachment, 207f
  implants, 54–55, 55f
  incision, 101–104, 102–103f
  inferotemporal dialysis, 208f
  intraoperative problems, 123–127, 124f, 125f, 126f
  intravitreal injections, 122–123, 123f
  localization, 104f, 104–106, 105f, 106f
  pediatric proliferative diseases, 171
  penetrating injuries, 169
  postoperative complications, 175–187
    anterior segment ischemia, 177, 178f
    cataract, 186
    choroidal detachment, 177–178
    ciliary body and iris abnormalities, 177
    cystoid macular edema, 185–186
    decreased or displaced scleral buckle, 187
    elevated intraocular pressure, 175
    extrusion or intrusion, 184, 184f
    exudative retinal detachment, 180
    infection, 175–176, 176f
    initial retinal reattachment failure, 180–182, 182f
    macular hole, 179
    macular pucker, 184–185, 185f
    new retinal tears, 186
    pigment fallout, 178–179, 179f
    proliferative vitreoretinopathy, 187
    refractive error, 182–183
    removal of scleral buckle, 187
    reopening of original break, 186–187
    slow absorption of subretinal fluid, 179–180, 180f
    strabismus, 183
  preoperative preparation, 101
  principles, 100, 101f
  proliferative vitreoretinopathy, 24f
  pseudophakic retinal detachment, 211f
  retinopexy, 106–108, 107f
  revision, 212f
  routine postoperative management, 131
  sickle cell retinopathy, 37

Scleral buckling *(contd.)*
  superotemporal flap tear, 210f
  surgical results, 131–132
  suture technique, 108–111, 109f, 110f, 111f
  temporary balloon buckling *versus,* 152
  without thermal adhesion, 115–116
Scleral depression, 87–92, 88–89f, 90f, 91f, 92f
  posterior vitreous detachment, 4
Scleral necrosis, 176
Scleral resection, 52
Scleritis, 63–65, 65f
Sclerosis, 157
Sclerotomy, 120
Senile choroidopathy, 116
Senile retinoschisis, 9, 67, 68f, 171
  fundus drawing, 84f
  prophylactic therapy, 198
Shapland and Paufique operation, 52, 52f
Sickle cell retinopathy, 37
Silicone explant, 108, 109f, 111, 112f
Silicone oil, 56, 166
Simultaneous multiple puncture, 51
Slit lamp, 45
Spatula needle, 110, 111f
Staphylococcus, buckle infection, 175
Staphyloma
  macular hole, 162, 162f
  scleral buckling, 125, 125f
Steamroller maneuver, 144, 145f
Stickler's syndrome, 38, 39f
Strabismus, after scleral buckling, 183
Stretch tear, 34
Striate keratopathy, 177
Sub-Tenon's space, temporary balloon buckling, 150, 151
Subclinical retinal detachment, 198f, 198–199
Subconjunctival anesthesia
  pneumatic retinopexy, 137
  temporary balloon buckling, 149
Subconjunctival gas, 145
Subconjunctival hemorrhage, 184
Subretinal fluid, 17–20
  congenital optic disc abnormalities, 38
  drainage by Graefe knife, 49, 49f
  drainage in pars plana vitrectomy, 154f, 155
  drainage in scleral buckling procedure, 116–122
    complications, 117f, 117t, 117–118, 118f
    before cryotherapy, 108
    indications, 116t, 116–117
    technique, 118–122, 119f, 120f, 121f
  exudative retinal detachment, 60–61, 61f, 180
  finding retinal breaks, 84–96f, 93–97, 97f
  Guist operation, 50, 50f
  inadequate absorption after scleral buckling, 181
  Larsson operation, 50, 50f
  primary vitrectomy, 56
  rhegmatogenous retinal detachment, 60
  Šafář operation, 51, 51f
  Schepens operation, 55
  shifting after pneumatic retinopexy, 189
  slow absorption after scleral buckling, 179–180, 180f
  uveal effusion syndrome, 65–66, 66f
Subretinal gas, 142–143
  after pneumatic retinopexy, 188

Subretinal hemorrhage
  after pneumatic retinopexy, 189
  complication of subretinal fluid drainage, 117, 117t
  fundus drawing, 84f
  during pneumatic retinopexy, 144
Sulfur hexafluoride, 55–56
  macular hole, 159
  pars plana vitrectomy, 156
  pneumatic retinopexy, 140t, 140–141
Superior retinal detachment, 93, 94f
Superonasal dialyses, 34
Superonasal periphery examination, 78, 80f
Superotemporal flap tear, 210f
Superotemporal periphery examination, 78–82, 81f
Suprachoroidal hemorrhage, 117, 117t
Supratrochlear block, 100
Surface diathermy, 50, 50f
Surgery
  case studies, 207–213f
  cataract
    endophthalmitis, 38
    predisposition for retinal detachment, 31–32
  complicated cases, 159–167
    coloboma, 171
    giant retinal tear, 163f, 163–165, 164f
    macular holes, 159–162, 160–161f
    pediatric proliferative diseases, 171–172
    penetrating injuries, 168–169
    proliferative diabetic retinopathy, 169–170, 170f
    proliferative vitreoretinopathy, 165f, 165–168, 166f, 167f
    retinitis-related, 170
    retinoschisis-related, 171
  contraindication to scleral depression, 91
  historical background, 45–59
    attempts at treatment, 47–48
    Custodis-Schepens-Lincoff era (1947–1971), 53f, 53–55, 54f, 55f
    Gonin era (1919–1947), 48–52, 49f, 50f, 51f, 52f
    incorrect theories of etiology, 45–46, 46f, 47f, 48f
    Machemer era (contemporary), 55–57
  laser photocoagulation, 157
  pars plana vitrectomy
    advanced proliferative vitreoretinopathy, 165, 166f
    macular hole, 162, 162f
    posterior, inferior flap tear, 211f
    without scleral buckling, 154f, 154–157
  pneumatic retinopexy, 135–148
    anesthesia, 137
    gas injection, 140t, 140–142, 141f, 142f
    intraoperative problems, 142–145, 144f, 145f
    paracentesis, 139–140
    patient selection, 136f, 136–137, 137t
    results, 146–147
    retinopexy, 137–139, 138f
    routine postoperative management, 145–146
  postoperative complications, 175–193
    pneumatic retinopexy, 187–190
    scleral buckling, 175–187
  preoperative management, 98–99
  scleral buckling procedure, 100–134

SUBJECT INDEX

anesthesia, 100
circumferential explants, 112f, 113
closure, 127f, 127–130, 128f, 129–130f
drainage of subretinal fluid, 116t, 116–122, 117t, 117–121f
encircling, 113t, 113–115, 114f, 115f
explant materials, 108, 109f
incision, 101–104, 102–103f
intraoperative problems, 123–127, 124f, 125f, 126f
intravitreal injections, 122–123, 123f
localization, 104f, 104–106, 105f, 106f
preoperative preparation, 101
principles, 100, 101f
radial explants, 111–112
retinopexy, 106–108, 107f
routine postoperative management, 131
surgical results, 131–132
suture technique, 108–111, 109f, 110f, 111f
without thermal adhesion, 115–116
temporary balloon buckling, 149–154, 150f, 151f, 153t
vitrectomy
  advanced proliferative vitreoretinopathy, 165, 166f
  congenital cataracts, 32
  diabetic patient, 36
  endophthalmitis vitrectomy study, 38
  macular hole, 162, 162f
  pars plana, 55
  penetrating injuries, 169
  posterior, inferior flap tear, 211f
  primary, 56, 154f, 154–157
  proliferative diabetic retinopathy, 169
  retinitis-related retinal detachment, 171
  sickle cell retinopathy, 37
  traction retinal detachment, 67
  without scleral buckling, 154f, 154–157
Suture
  circumferential explant, 113
  Custodis operation, 54, 54f
  increased intraocular pressure, 126
  posteriorly located breaks, 124
  radial explant, 111
  scleral buckling, 108–111, 109f, 110f, 111f
  staphyloma, 125, 125f
  subretinal fluid drainage, 122

T

Tears, 4–9, 5–8f
  after scleral buckling, 186
  flap, 4–9, 5f, 7f
    blunt trauma, 34
    detachment after extracapsular cataract extraction, 32
    double, 209f
    with extensive retinal detachment, 207f
    fundus drawing, 84f
    incorrectly buckled, 181, 182f
    localization technique, 104–105, 105f
    observation, 196
    photocoagulation, 202f
    posterior, inferior, 211f
    prophylactic treatment, 194
    reopening of original break, 186–187
    scleral depression, 87, 89f
    with small rim of subretinal fluid, 207f
    under superior rectus muscle, 208f
    superotemporal, 210f
  Guist operation, 50, 50f
  localization technique, 104–105, 105f
  operculated, 8f
    fundus drawing, 84f
    prophylactic treatment, 194, 195f
  penetrating injuries, 35
  perfluorocarbon liquids, 56
  posterior vitreous detachment, 2–3
  proliferative vitreoretinopathy risk, 26
  prophylactic therapy, 194t, 194–205
    asymptomatic breaks with no history of retinal disease, 196
    breaks in degenerative retinoschisis, 198
    breaks in fellow eyes, 196–197
    breaks in myopic eyes, 197
    breaks with bridging vessels, 199, 199f
    follow-up, 203
    macular pucker, 203
    role of education in preventing visual loss, 203–204
    subclinical retinal detachment, 198f, 198–199
    symptomatic tears with no history of retinal disease, 194–196, 195f
    treatment technique, 200f, 200–203, 202f
  redetachment, 186
  scleral buckling procedure, 100–134
    anesthesia, 100
    circumferential explants, 112f, 113
    closure, 127f, 127–130, 128f, 129–130f
    drainage of subretinal fluid, 116t, 116–122, 117t, 117–121f
    encircling, 113t, 113–115, 114f, 115f
    explant materials, 108, 109f
    incision, 101–104, 102–103f
    intraoperative problems, 123–127, 124f, 125f, 126f
    intravitreal injections, 122–123, 123f
    localization, 104f, 104–106, 105f, 106f
    preoperative preparation, 101
    principles, 100, 101f
    radial explants, 111–112
    retinopexy, 106–108, 107f
    routine postoperative management, 131
    surgical results, 131–132
    suture technique, 108–111, 109f, 110f, 111f
    without thermal adhesion, 115–116
Weve operation, 51
Temporal periphery
  examination, 82, 82f
  scleral depression, 92f
Temporary balloon buckling, 149–154, 151f
  device, 56–57, 150f
  flap tear under superior rectus muscle, 208f
  flap tear with extensive retinal detachment, 207f
  macular hole after, 179
  posterior, inferior flap tear, 211f
  surgical results, 152–154, 153t
  technique, 149–152
Tenon's capsule
  coverage of explant, 128
  pars plana vitrectomy, 155

Tenon's capsule *(contd.)*
  peritomy, 101, 102f
  temporary balloon buckling, 149
Theory
  distension, 45–46, 46f
  exudation, 46, 47f, 48f
  hypotony, 46, 47f
  rhegmatogenous, 48–49
Thermocautery operation, 49f, 49–50
Timing of surgery, 98–99
Tissue growth factor beta, 25
Tobacco dust phenomenon, 3f, 3–4
  rhegmatogenous retinal detachment, 60
  traumatic retinal breaks, 34
Traction retinal detachment
  diabetic patient, 36
  differential diagnosis, 66–67, 67f
Transcleral cryotherapy
  pneumatic retinopexy, 137–138, 138f
  temporary balloon buckling, 149
Transcleral diode laser probe, 108
Transillumination, 118–120, 120f
Trauma
  penetrating
    surgical treatment, 168–169
    traction retinal detachment, 66–67
  predisposition for retinal detachment, 33–35, 34f
  retinal detachment, 12
Tropicamide, 101

U

Ultrasonography
  choroidal detachment, 71, 73f
  posterior scleritis, 63–65, 65f
  posterior vitreous detachment, 4
Uveal effusion syndrome, 65–66, 66f
Uveitis, 61

V

Varicella zoster virus retinitis, 170
Visual loss
  Goldmann-Favre syndrome, 41
  role of education in prevention, 203–204
  temporary balloon buckling, 153
Vitrectomy
  congenital cataracts, 32
  diabetic patient, 36
  endophthalmitis vitrectomy study, 38
  pars plana, 55
    advanced proliferative vitreoretinopathy, 165, 166f
    macular hole, 162, 162f
    posterior, inferior flap tear, 211f
    without scleral buckling, 154f, 154–157
  penetrating injuries, 169
  primary, 56, 154f, 154–157
  proliferative diabetic retinopathy, 169
  retinitis-related retinal detachment, 171
  sickle cell retinopathy, 37
  traction retinal detachment, 67
Vitreoretinal adhesion, 5f
Vitreoretinal traction tuft, 6f
Vitreoretinopathy
  erosive, 38
  familial exudative, 171
  proliferative
    after pneumatic retinopexy, 189
    after scleral buckling, 187
    complicated cases, 165f, 165–168, 166f, 167f
    contraindication to pneumatic retinopexy, 136–137, 137t
    delay in retinal detachment treatment, 203
    encircling, 166
    failure of scleral buckling, 182
    giant retinal tear, 163, 165
    indication for encircling, 113, 113t, 114f
    pars plana vitrectomy, 55, 165, 166f
    pathophysiology, 21f, 21–26, 22–24f, 25t
    perfluorocarbon liquids, 166–167
    repair options, 212f
    scleral buckling complications, 187
    surgical treatment, 165f, 165–168, 166f, 167f
    temporary balloon buckling, 153
    traction retinal detachment, 66–67
Vitreous
  fundus drawing of opacity, 84f
  incarceration during pneumatic retinopexy, 144
  operculated tears, 194, 195f
  role in retinal attachment, 11
Vitreous base, 1, 2f
  anterior proliferative vitreoretinopathy, 25
  atopic dermatitis, 41
  avulsion, 33, 34f
  blunt trauma, 33
  giant retinal tears and proliferative vitreoretinopathy, 165
  pars plana vitrectomy, 155
Vitreous hemorrhage
  after pneumatic retinopexy, 189
  contraindication to pneumatic retinopexy, 136–137, 137t
  diabetic patient, 36
  penetrating injuries, 168
  during pneumatic retinopexy, 144
  posterior vitreous detachment, 2, 3
  proliferative vitreoretinopathy risk, 26
  retinal breaks with bridging vessels, 199, 199f
  sickle cell retinopathy, 37
  temporary balloon buckling, 153
Vitreous infusion suction cutter, 55
Vitreous traction
  failure of scleral buckling, 182
  proliferative diabetic retinopathy, 169
  reopening of original break, 186–187
  retinal breaks with bridging vessels, 199, 199f
Vogt-Koyanagi-Harada syndrome, 61
Volk aspheric lenses, 93
Vortex vein ampulla, 84f

W

Wagner's disease, 38
Walling-off technique in subclinical retinal detachment, 198f, 198–199
Watzke sleeve, 109f, 127, 128f
Weiss ring, 2, 3f
Weve operation, 51
Wide-field contact lenses, 93